Immunotoxicology

Proceedings of the First International Symposium
on Immunotoxicology held at the University of Surrey,
13-17 September 1982

Immunotoxicology

Edited by

G. Gordon Gibson

Ronald Hubbard

Dennis V. Parke

University of Surrey
Guildford
Surrey
England

1983

ACADEMIC PRESS
A Subsidiary of Harcourt Brace Jovanovich, Publishers
London   New York
Paris   San Diego   San Francisco   São Paulo
Sydney   Tokyo   Toronto

ACADEMIC PRESS INC. (LONDON) LTD.
24/28 Oval Road
London NW1

United States Edition published by
ACADEMIC PRESS INC.
111 Fifth Avenue
New York, New York 10003

British Library Cataloguing in Publication Data
Immunotoxicology.
 1. Drugs—Toxicology—Congresses
 I. Gibson, G.G.   II. Hubbard, R.   III. Parke, D.V.
 615.9   RA1238

 ISBN 0-12-282180-7

 LCCCN 83-70717

Printed in Great Britain by
Galliard (Printers) Limited, Great Yarmouth

CONTENTS

CONTRIBUTORS

M.J.P. ADOLFS Department of Pharmacology, Faculty of Medicine, Erasmus University of Rotterdam, PO Box 1738, 3000 DR Rotterdam, Netherlands

H.E. AMOS Medical Department, ICI plc, Pharmaceuticals Division, Macclesfield, Cheshire, England

J.G. BEKESI Department of Neoplastic Diseases, Mount Sinai School of Medicine, New York, New York 10029, USA

I.L. BONTA Department of Pharmacology, Faculty of Medicine, Erasmus University of Rotterdam, PO Box 1738, 3000 DR Rotterdam, Netherlands

W.D. BRIGHTON Allergy Advisory Services, 33 Bedhampton Hill, Havant, Hampshire, England

G.M.J. BROUWER National Institute of Public Health, PO Box 1, 3720 BA Bilthoven, Netherlands

E.V. BUEHLER Proctor and Gamble Company, Miami Valley Laboratories, PO Box 391, Southern 5, Cincinati, Ohio 45239, USA

F.M. CUNNINGHAM Department of Clinical Pharmacology, Cardio-thoracic Institute, Fulham Road, London SW3 6HP, England

M.L. CUZNER The Multiple Sclerosis Society Laboratory, Department of Neurochemistry, Institute of Neurology, London WC1N 2NS, England

G.E. DAVIES Central Toxicology Laboratory, ICI plc, Alderley Park, Macclesfield, Cheshire SK10 4TJ, England

M. DAVIS Dudley Road Hospital, Birmingham B18 7QH, England

J.H. DEAN Chemical Industry Institute of Toxicology Research Triangle Park, North Carolina 27709, USA

J.M. DEWDNEY Biosciences Research Centre, Beecham Pharmaceuticals, Great Burgh, Yew Tree Bottom Road, Epsom, Surrey, England

J.E. DOE Central Toxicology Laboratory, ICI plc, Alderley Park, Macclesfield, Cheshire SK10 4TJ, England

P. DRUET Hospital Broussais, 96 rue Didot, 75674 Paris Cedex 14, France

R.G. EDWARDS Beecham Pharmaceuticals, Research Division, Biosciences Research Centre, Yew Tree Bottom Road, Epsom, Surrey KT18 5XQ, England

G.R. ELLIOTT Department of Pharmacology, Faculty of Medicine, Erasmus University of Rotterdam, PO Box 1738, 3000 DR Rotterdam, Netherlands

M.W. ELVES Cell Biology Division, Glaxo Group Research Limited, Greenford Road, Greenford, Middlesex, England

S. FILIPPESCHI Laboratory of Tumour Chemotherapy and Immunology, Institute of Pharmaceutical Research, Mario Negri, Milan, Italy

A. FISCHBEIN Environmental Sciences Laboratory, Mount Sinai School of Medicine, New York, New York 10029, USA

B.M.J. FOXWELL Imperial Cancer Research Fund, PO Box 123, Lincoln's Inn Fields, London WC2A 3PX, England

D.E. GARDNER U.S. Environment Protection Agency, Health Effects Research Laboratory, Inhalation Toxicology Division, Toxicology Branch, Research Triangle Park, North Carolina 27711, USA

P.G.H. GELL Department of Pathology, University of Cambridge, Cambridge, England

G.G. GIBSON Department of Biochemistry, University of Surrey, Guildford, Surrey GU2 5XH, England

B.F.J. GOODWIN Environmental Safety Laboratory, Unilever Research, Colworth House, Sharnbrook, Bedford MK44 1LQ, England

E.C. GORDON-SMITH, Royal Postgraduate Medical School, Du Cane Road, London W12 OHS, England

J.A. GRAHAM   U.S. Environmental Protection Agency, Health
    Effects Research Laboratory, Inhalation Toxicology Division,
    Toxicology Branch, Research Triangle Park, North Carolina
    27711, USA

B. GUERIN   Labaratoire des Stallergenes, 160 quai de Polangis,
    94349 Joinulle Le Pont, France

J.W. HADDEN   Immunopharmacology Program, University of South
    Florida, Medical College, 12901 North 30th Street, Tampa,
    Florida 33612, USA

J.G. HALL   Institute of Cancer Research, Clifton Avenue,
    Sutton, Surrey, England

G. HARRIS   The Kennedy Institute of Rheumatology, Division of
    Experimental Pathology, Bute Gardens, London W6 7DW,
    England

B. HEWITT   Laboratoire des Stallergenes, 160 quai de Polangis,
    94349 Joinulle Le Pont, France

F. HIRSCH   Hopital Broussais, 96 rue Didot, 75674 Paris Cedex
    14, France

R. HUBBARD   Biochemistry Department, University of Surrey,
    Guildford, Surrey GU2 5XH, England

A.W. JOHNSON   Environmental Safety Laboratory, Unilever
    Research, Colworth House, Sharnbrook, Bedford MK44 1LQ,
    England

L.D. LAUER   National Institute of Environmental Health
    Sciences, Research Triangle Park, North Carolina 27709, USA

F.X.R. van LEEUWEN   National Institute of Public Health, PO
    Box 1, 3720 BA Bilthoven, Netherlands

W. LORENZ   Department of Theoretical Surgery, Centre of
    Operative Medicine 1, University of Marburg (Lahn),
    Federal Republic of Germany

M.I. LUSTER   Chemical Industry Institute of Toxicology
    Research, Triangle Park, North Carolina 27709, USA

K. MILLER   Immunotoxicology Department, The British Industrial
    Biological Research Association, Woodmansterne Road,
    Carshalton, Surrey, England

J. MORLEY Department of Clinical Pharmacology, Cardiothoracic
Institute, Fulham Road, London SW3 6HP, England

M.J. MURRAY National Institute of Environmental Health
Sciences, Research Triangle Park, North Carolina 27709, USA

S. NICKLIN Immunotoxicology Department, The British Industrial
Biological Research Association, Woodmansterne Road,
Carshalton, Surrey, England

C.P. PAGE Department of Clinical Pharmacology, Cardiothoracic
Institute, Fulham Road, London SW3 6HP, England

A.L. PARKE Department of Rheumatology, Hammersmith Hospital,
London, England

D.V. PARKE Department of Biochemistry, University of Surrey,
Guildford, Surrey GU2 5XH, England

D. PARKER Department of Pathology, Royal College of Surgeons
of England, Lincoln's Inn Fields, London WC2A 3PN, England

R. PASQUIER Hopital Broussais, 96 rue Didot, 75674 Paris
Cedex 14, France

L. PELLETIER Hopital Broussais, 96 rue Didot, 75674 Paris
Cedex 14, France

A.H. PENNICKS Working-Group Pathology-Toxicology, Faculty of
Veterinary Sciences, State University of Utrecht,
Netherlands

J. PEPYS Brompton Hospital, London, England

A.L. REEVES Wayne State University, Detroit, Michigan, USA

D.W. ROBERTS Unilever Research, Port Sunlight Laboratory,
Quarry Road East, Bebington, Wirral, Merseyside L63 3JW,
England

J.P. ROBOZ Department of Neoplastic Diseases, Mount Sinai
School of Medicine, New York, New York 10029, USA

C. SAPIN Hopital Broussais, 96 rue Didot, 75674 Paris Cedex
14, France

W. SEINEN Working-Group Pathology-Toxicology, Faculty of
Veterinary Sciences, State University of Utrecht, Netherlands

M.J.K. SELGRADE U.S. Environment Protection Agency, Health
Effects Research Laboratory, Inhalation Toxicology Division,
Toxicology Branch, Research Triangle Park, North Carolina
27711, USA

I.J. SELIKOFF Environmental Sciences Laboratory, Mount Sinai
School of Medicine, New York, New York 10029, USA

M. SIRONI Laboratory of Tumour Chemotherapy and Immunology,
Institute of Pharmaceutical Research, Mario Negri, Milan,
Italy

S. SOLOMON Department of Neoplastic Diseases, Mount Sinai
School of Medicine, New York, New York 10029, USA

F. SPREAFICO Laboratory of Tumour Chemotherapy and Immunology,
Institute of Pharmaceutical Research, Mario Negri, Milan,
Italy

D.R. STANWORTH Rheumatology and Allergy Research Unit,
University of Birmingham, Vincent Drive, Birmingham B15 2TJ,
England

J.L. TURK Department of Pathology, Royal College of Surgeons
of England, Lincoln's Inn Fields, London WC2A 3PN, England

A. VECCHI Laboratory of Tumour Chemotherapy and Immunology,
Institute of Pharmaceutical Research, Mario Negri, Milan,
Italy

J.G. VOS National Institute of Public Health, PO Box 1,
3720 BA Bilthoven, Netherlands

E.D. WACHSMUTH Research Department of Pharmaceuticals Division, CIBA-GEIGY Limited, 4002 Basel, Switzerland

Sj. WAGENAAR National Institute of Public Health, PO Box 1,
3720 BA Bilthoven, Netherlands

D.L.WILLIAMS Unilever Research, Port Sunlight Laboratory,
Quarry Road East, Bebington, Wirral, Merseyside L63 3JW,
England

PARTICIPANTS

M. ARLMAN-HOEKE Gesondheidsraad, Princes Margreit Plantsoen 20, PO Box 95379, 2520C7 Den Haag, Netherlands

D.F. ARNOLD Ciba-Geigy Pharmaceuticals Division, Stamford Lodge, Altrincham Road, Wilmslow, Cheshire, England

S.C. BAIRD Boehringer Ingelheim Ltd., Southern Industrial Estate, Bracknell, Berkshire, England

M. BATER Toxicology Department, Smith Kline and French Ltd., The Frythe, Welwyn, Hertfordshire, England

R.R. BALMBRA Procter and Gamble Ltd., Whitley Road, Longbenton, Newcastle Upon Tyne, England

D. BECKER INBIFO Institut fur biologische Forschung, Fuggerstrasse 3, 5000 Cologne 90, Federal Republic of Germany

M.F. BEESON Beecham Pharmaceuticals, Yew Tree Bottom Road, Epsom, Surrey, England

A. BERLIN Commission of European Communities, Health and Safety Directorate, Jean Monnet Building, Luxembourg

J. BONNET Centre De Recerche Anhar-Rolland, 4 rue de la Division Leclerc, 91380 Chilly Mazarin, France

P.A. BOTHAM Central Toxicology Laboratory, ICI plc, Alderley Park, Macclesfield, Cheshire SK10 4TJ, England

J.N. BREMMER Medical and Toxicology Division, Shell Centre, London SE1, England

J. BROCK Central Toxicology Laboratory, ICI plc, Alderley Park, Macclesfield, Cheshire SK10 4IJ, England

G.T. BROPHY Lilly Research Laboratories, PO Box 708, Greenfield, Indiana 46140, USA

J.H. BYRNE General Foods Europe, 14 ave de l'Astronomie,
   1030 Brussels, Belgium

M.J. BUTCHER Toxicology Laboratories Ltd., Bromyard Road,
   Ledbury, Herefordshire, England

L. CAPRINO Assoreni — Via Ercole Ramarini, 00015 Monterotondo,
   Rome, Italy

M. CARAZ Pasteur Institute, rue Pasteur, Lyon 69365, France

F.A. CHARLESWORTH Association of the British Pharmaceutical
   Industry, 12 Whitehall, London SW1, England

A.J. CLARKE Fisons plc, S and T Laboratory, Bakewell Road,
   Loughborough, Leicestershire, England

A. COCKBURN Beecham Pharmaceuticals, 4th Avenue, Harlow,
   Essex, England

R.W.R. CREVEL E.S.L. Unilever Research, Colworth House,
   Sharnbrook, Bedfordshire, England

W. GORDON CREWTHER SCIRO Division of Protein Chemistry,
   343 Royal Parade, Parkville, Victoria 3052, Australia

P. DELORT Searle R and D., Sophia Antipolis, 06561 Valbonne,
   Cedex, France

D.A. EICHLER Roche Products Ltd., PO Box 8, Welwyn Garden
   City, Hertfordshire, England

A.E.J. EVANS ICI plc, Organics Division, PO Box 42, Blackley,
   Manchester M9 3DA, England

J.M. FACCINI Robens Institute of Industrial and Environmental
   Health and Safety, University of Surrey, Guildford, Surrey
   GU2 5XH, England

R. FALCHETTI Serono Institute, Rome, Italy

S. FERRINI Rbm C.P. 226, 10015 Evrea, Turin, Italy

R.J. FIELDER Health and Safety Executive, Baynards House,
   1 Chepstow Place, London W2, England

J. PETER FINN Merck Sharp-Dohme-Chibret, Research Centre-
   Route de Marsat, 63203 RIOM Cedex, France

C.E. FISHER   Food Science Division, Ministry of Agriculture, Fisheries and Food, Horseferry Road, London SW1, England

D. FORBES   Central Toxicology Laboratory, ICI plc, Alderley Park, Macclesfield, Cheshire SK10 4TJ, England

R.A. FORD   RIFM, 375 Sylvan Avenue, Englewood Cliffs, New Jersey 07632, USA

J. FULLER   Adverse Reactions Unit, Glaxo Group Research Ltd., Ware, Hertfordshire, England

E.W. GILL   Pharmacology Department, South Parks Road, Oxford, England

H. GLEICHMANN   The Netherlands Cancer Institute, Plesmanlaan 121, 1066 CX Amsterdam, Netherlands

P. GREAVES   Centre de Recherche, Laboratoires Pfizer, PO Box 109, 37401 Amboise, Cedex, France

R.W. GREENHILL   Beecham Pharmaceuticals Research Division, Coldharbour Road, The Pinnacles, Harlow, Essex, England

G. HALLIWELL   Pfizer Central Research, Sandwich, Kent, England

D. HANNANT   Institute of Occupational Medicine, City Hospital, Greenbank Drive, Edinburgh, Scotland

S. HATTERSLEY   Department of Health and Social Security, Market Towers, 1 Nine Elms Lane, London SW8, England

R.F. HARLAND   Toxicology Department, Smith Kline and French Research Laboratory, The Frythe, Welwyn, Hertfordshire, England

C. HEWETT   Boehringer Ingelheim KG, Act. Exp. Pathologie u. Toxikologie, 6507 Ingelheim/Rhein, Federal Republic of Germany

P.M. HOLMES   Beecham Products Research Department, Randalls Road, Leatherhead, Surrey

J.J. HOSTYNEK   The Clorox Company, 7200 Johnson Drive, Pleasanton, California, USA

S.N. JENKINS   Fisons plc, Pharmaceutical Division, Bakewell Road, Loughborough, Leicestershire, England

M. JONSSON Kabivitrum, Stockholm, Sweden

J. KIPLING Biological Research Department, May and Baker Ltd.,
Dagenham, Essex, England

N.G. LINDQUIST, National Board of Health and Welfare, Department of Drugs, Division of Pharmacology and Toxicology,
PO Box 607, S-751 25 Uppsala, Sweden

E.-ARNOLD LOBBECKE Institut of Toxikology, Bayer AG, 56-
Wuppertal 1, Federal Republic of Germany

S. LEWIS Hoechst Pharmaceutical Research Laboratory, Walton
Manor, Milton Keynes, England

C.M. LUCZYNSKA Occupational Medical Laboratory, 403 Edgware
Road, London NW2, England

A.R. MACKENZIE, Cell Biology Division, Glaxo Group Research
Ltd., Greenford Road, Greenford, Middlesex, England

B. MACGIBBON Department of Health and Social Security,
Market Towers, 1 Nine Elms Lane, London SW8, England

C. MADSEN Institute of Toxicology, National Food Institute,
Morkhoj Bygade 19, DK 2860 Soborg, Denmark

I. MAINS Boots Company plc, Research, The Priory, Thurgarton,
Nottingham, England

A. MANLEY Safety of Medicines, ICI Pharmaceuticals, Mereside,
Alderley Park, Macclesfield, Cheshire, England

L. MELDGAARD, Strandgade 29, DK-1401, Copenhagen K, Denmark

J.L. MILLER Safety of Medicines Department, ICI Pharmaceuticals, Mereside, Alderley Park, Macclesfield, Cheshire,
England

A.M. MONRO Laboratoires Pfizer, BP 109, 37401 Amboise,
Cedex, France

B. MORRIS Biochemistry Department, University of Surrey,
Guildford, Surrey GU2 5XH, England

L.A. MOUSTAFA, World Health Organization/Irru, PO Box 12233-
NIEHS, M.D. A2-06, Research Triangle Park, North Carolina
27709, USA

Z. NIEWOLA Immunology Section, Central Toxicology Laboratory, ICI plc, Alderley Park, Macclesfield, Cheshire, England

H. OBENHAUS c/o Sandoz Forschungsinstitut, Brunnerstrasse 59, A-1235 Vienna, Austria

G.J.A. OLIVER Central Toxicology Laboratory, ICI plc, Alderley Park, Macclesfield, Cheshire, England

R. OERTINE Solco, Basle, Switzerland

F. OSIYEM Biochemistry Department, University of Ibadan, Ibadan, Nigeria

J.J. OSTYNEK Clorox Company, 7200 Johnson Drive, Pleasanton, California 94566, USA

F. POLLITT Toxicology Department, Smith Kline and French Research Ltd., The Frythe, Welwyn, Hertfordshire, England

T.W. POOLE Sandoz Products Ltd., Sandoz House, Feltham, Middlesex, England

F. POULSEN Danish National Institute of Occupational Health, Baunegardsvej 73, 2900 Hellerup, Denmark

G.H. PRINCE Apple Tree House, Highfield Road, West Byfleet, Surrey, England

A.H. PULSFORD Huntingdon Research Centre, Huntingdon, Cambridgeshire, England

J. RANCE Smith Kline and French Research Ltd., The Frythe, Welwyn, Hertfordshire, England

C. RHODES Central Toxicology Laboratory, ICI plc, Alderley Park, Macclesfield, Cheshire, England

H. RONNEBERGER Behringwerke AG, PO Box 1140, D 355 0 Marburg/ Lahn 1, Denmark

B. RYFFEL Sandoz Ltd., Preclinical Research, 4133 Prattein 4, Switzerland

M. SARGIACOMO Lab id Biologia Cellulare, 1st Sup. di Sanita, Viale Reg. Elene 299, Rome Italy

A.H.W.M. SCHUURS Organon SDG, PO Box 20, 5340 BH Oss, Netherlands

J.T.B. SHAW Chalk Hill, Kingsdown, Deal, Kent, England

D.N. SKILLETER MRC Toxicology Unit, Woodmansterne Road, Carshalton, Surrey, England

P.R. SIBLEY Department of Toxicology, Glaxo Group Research Ltd., Ware, Hertfordshire, England

R.G. SIMMONDS Lilly Research Centre Ltd., Earl Wood Manor, Windlesham, Surrey, England

P. SLANINA The National Food Administration, PO Box 622, S-751 26 Uppsala, Sweden

M. SHARRATT Group Occupational Health Centre, BP Research Centre, Chertsey Road, Sunbury, Middlesex, England

P.N. SKELTON-STROUD Ciba-Geigy Pharmaceuticals Division, Stamford Lodge, Altrincham Road, Wilmslow, Cheshire, England

M.D.B. STEPHENS Adverse Reactions Unit, Glaxo Group Research Ltd., Ware, Hertfordshire, England

T.G. TERRELL Syntex Research, R2-201, 3401 Hillview Avenue, Palo Alto, California 94304, USA

S. SULLMAN Smith Kline and French Research Ltd., The Frythe, Welwyn, Hertfordshire, England

P. TAUPIN Hazleton Laboratories Europe Ltd., Otley Road, Harrogate, North Yorkshire HG3 1PY, England

C.M. TOWLER Reg. Affairs Planning Division, Glaxo Group Research Ltd., Greenford Road, Greenford, Middlesex, England

P.M. TRENCHARD Welsh Regional Transfusion Centre, Rhydlafar, St Fagans, Cardiff, Wales

P.F. UPHILL Department of Cell Biology, Huntingdon Research Centre, Huntingdon, Cambridgeshire, England

R.R. VERCOE Ciba-Geigy Pharmaceutical Division, Horsham, Sussex, England

F. WAGNIART ERS 22, rue Garbier 92201, Neuilly s/Seine, France

J.M. WAL INRA CNRZ Lab. des Sciences de la Consommation,
    78350 Jouy den Josas, France

S. WALSH Immunology Section, Central Toxicology Laboratory,
    ICI plc, Alderley Park, Macclesfield, Cheshire SK10 3TJ,
    England

E. WEIDMANN Behringwerke AG, PO Box 1140, D-3550 Marburg/
    Lahn 1, Denmark

D.J. WHITE Beecham Pharmaceuticals Research Division,
    Coldharbour Road, The Pinnacles, Harlow, Essex, England

R.N. WOODWARD Health and Safety Executive, Baynards House,
    1-13 Chepstow Place, London W2, England

FOREWORD

Sir Francis Avery Jones C.B.E., M.D., F.R.C.P.,
D. Univ. (Surrey), Hon. M.D. (Melb), Hon. F.R.C.S. (England)

Consulting Gastroenterologist,
Central Middlesex Hospital, London,
and St. Marks Hospital, London, England

Immunotoxicology is a new aspect of the many facets of drug
and chemical toxicity and it is likely to prove particularly
important and difficult, needing all the international co-
operation that can be achieved. At the present time new drugs
are screened by animal testing for organ toxicity, teratology
and carcinogenicity, and are then subjected to prolonged
clinical trials before being finally released. It is disturb-
ing for the public, for the pharmaceutical industry and for
the medical profession, that drugs of great therapeutic value
can then, after one to three years of continued monitoring of
the drug, be shown to have significant and sometimes deadly
longer-term hazards. The latest of such problems relates to
the recently withdrawn anti-arthritic drug, benoxaprofen,
marketed in the U.K. as Opren since 1980. It had been heralded
as opening a new era in the treatment of arthritis and count-
less sufferers from continued incapacity and pain clamoured
for the new drug, and in no time over half a million people in
Britain were taking it. It had certain recognized side-effects
which were accepted as a reasonable price for the benefit
achieved but now, after two years, it seems that a number of
them are more serious, and sometimes fatal complications can
apparently be related to its use. A total of 61 deaths have
been reported but these are mainly concentrated in the older
age groups. We have of course, to maintain a sense of perspective and realize that new drugs, like new stars, are being
formed the whole time and it is only occasionally that we have
a super-nova explosion! When they do happen it is an occasion
to re-double all our efforts, toxicological testing, surveillance, fundamental scientific studies and international co-
operation. This book is concerned with examining a new concept

which has been emerging recently. Toxicology in man is no longer just a matter of chemical reactivity directly on organs but relates more and more to the effects of drugs on the body's own defence system — the immune system, and a considerable time interval may elapse before secondary and tertiary side-effects can appear. We are also learning that no amount of animal testing is a full safeguard against such effects which relate to the much more highly developed immunity systems in man. The pharmaceutical industry is learning the hard way the significance of Pope's epigram, "that the proper study of mankind is man".

It is particularly appropriate that an international symposium on immunotoxicology should be held at Surrey University. Professor Dennis Parke and his Department of Biochemistry, together with Professor J.W. Bridges, the Director of the Robens Institute of Industrial and Environmental Health and Safety, are pathfinders in the field of toxicology. Although the University may not appreciate it, one of their strengths is that they do not have a medical school! This means that their interests and great expertise across the medico-biological field can better be concentrated in depth on new problems of importance to health. The University provides immense backing to the National Health Service. Last year I undertook an exercise bringing together the contributions within the University to the National Health Service and was able to identify nine departments with forty fields of relevant research. The Department of Biochemistry, with its Divisions of Clinical Biochemistry, Nutrition and Food Science, and Toxicology and Pharmacology, naturally led the field but most interesting work is being done by others, including the Departments of Microbiology, Human Biology and Health, Engineering, Chemistry, and Physics. Of further relevance in the present context is the work of the Epidemiology and Health Care Research Unit, linking the Royal College of General Practitioners and the University's Department of Mathematics, facilitating drug surveillance in general practice.

The conference covered a wide spectrum, with sessions on basic immunology, hypersensitivity, models for predicting hypersensitivity, immunotoxicology, complex phenomena of immune tissue damage, therapeutic aspects, and regulatory aspects. The new and bold concept of immunotoxicology develops the idea of some drugs acting like delayed-action bombs with immediate therapeutic benefit but longer-term damage to the defence mechanisms of the body. This may account for the delayed side-effects now being reported after new drugs have passed earlier clinical trials and have been accepted for general use. Such are the pitfalls still facing the present day pharmaceutical firms after their vast

injections of development funds! The complex human immunity
mechanisms have a potential for being damaged that has not
been fully appreciated or explored. Paradoxically, some drugs
may be too successful because some degree of aggression should
be preserved, as otherwise immune defences could deteriorate
for lack of use. For example, although inhibition of gastric
acid formation by the effective H_2 receptor antagonists meant
that peptic ulcers healed quickly, they then broke down again
sooner than expected because the defences had been impaired
by disease. Furthermore, over-growth of lumenal bacteria
brings a new set of problems. The mechanisms of gastrointestinal defence are gradually being unravelled and it is
now known that prostaglandins play a major role so that, when
inhibited by anti-inflammatory drugs, gastrointestinal inflammation and ulceration may follow. The complexity of this
chemical sequence, for example, the various pathways of
arachidonate metabolism, will be unfolded in this book. Of
great interest to us is that certain chemicals, such as these
H_2-receptor antagonists, not only inhibit acid secretion but
also block receptor sites on lymphocytes and hence may weaken
natural defence mechanisms. It has, of course, been long
known that synthetic drugs can be associated with a hyper-
immune response which may be an individual idiosyncrasy, and
patient sensitivity to aspirin, penicillin and hydrazides
still needs further investigation; and sensitive individuals
have shown cross-reactivity between chemically-similar drugs,
indicating that a common pathway may be involved. It is now
well recognized that drugs and other chemicals can be metabolized in the body into reactive intermediates which may then
form covalent complexes with proteins in the circulating
blood and in the tissues, especially the liver, and that such
drug-protein complexes may then act as antigens. It is not
only drugs which may precipitate immune responses, but some
naturally occurring substances present in food may also be
absorbed from the gut to act as antigens, and food allergies
are now associated with certain diseases.

Medical progress depends largely on steady, painstaking
effort but every now and then a new concept emerges which
acts like a catalyst, greatly speeding up the activity.
Immunotoxicology is one such concept and is indeed a very new,
complex and exciting aspect of toxicology and of the greatest
value and importance for the human subject. A better understanding of the interaction of drugs and chemicals with the
normal immunological defence systems of the body, and how
drugs and chemicals can augment and inhibit immune processes,
will result in a higher degree of drug safety and could lead
to the discovery of new medicines for the treatment of
inflammatory injury, allergies, rheumatoid diseases and possibly malignancy.

INTRODUCTION

Although drugs are designed to prevent or ameliorate disease,
it is a well recognized fact that no drug is completely safe
and adverse side effects are a common feature of therapy.
These adverse side effects can be expressed in many ways and
may arise from either an exaggerated pharmacological response
or be unrelated to the therapeutic action of the drug. One
of the premises of the science of toxicology is that the
design and development of safer drugs can only proceed on a
rational basis if we can fully characterize the drug-induced
lesion and more importantly, understand the basic chemical,
biochemical and pathophysiological mechanisms that ultimately
lead to overt toxicity. A particular problem in toxicology
is how do we rationalize target organ toxicity for a particular
group of compounds? Why do certain drugs induce lesions in
one particular tissue and yet leave other organs relatively
unscathed?

An excellent example of specific target organ toxicity is
the susceptibility of the immune system to the deleterious
effects of drugs and environmental chemicals. This is clearly
an important area of public health as competent immune surveillance is a prerequisite for resistance to infection, and
immuno-compromised individuals subjected to microbiological
or chemical challenge would be in substantial jeopardy.
Damage to the immune system can be a very sensitive indicator
of toxicity since substances which are described as "immunotoxic" may be active in extremely minute doses. A close in-
spection of our knowledge of drug-induced immune dysfunction
reveals that much has to be learned concerning our understanding of immunotoxicology, and towards this end it was
clear that a forum for discussion was long overdue.

Accordingly, an International Organizing Committee was
assembled, resulting in the First International Symposium

on Immunotoxicology held at the University of Surrey, England
in late 1982. This publication represents the edited contributions to this Symposium. The prime objective of the Symposium, reflected in the contents of this publication, was to
bring leading clinicians, toxicologists, immunologists and
other basic scientists together in an informal and pleasant
environment to crystallize the nature of the problems, the
experimental approaches, and the future directions of immunotoxicology.

The Organizing Committee are grateful to the many eminent
scientists who contributed to the meeting with presentations
and discussions, and to the secretariat and graduate students
of the University of Surrey who gave unstintingly, in a variety
of roles, to ensure the success of the Symposium. In particular, the editors would like to thank Jan McCall, Richard
Makowski and Ann Hanson. The Organizing Committee are also
most grateful to our sponsors including Beechams, Boehringer
Ingelheim, Glaxo, ICI, May and Baker, Merrell, Pfizer, Roche,
Servier, Seward Laboratories, Smith, Kline and French and
Wellcome Research, whose financial assistance was indispensable.
Finally, the editors wish to record their thanks to the production and editorial staff of Academic Press, who gave us
every encouragement to realize this project.

G. Gordon Gibson
Ron Hubbard
Dennis V. Parke

University of Surrey

October 1983

IMMUNOTOXICOLOGY —
OUTLINE OF MAJOR PROBLEMS

H.E. Amos

Medical Department, I.C.I. PLC, Pharmaceuticals Division, Macclesfield, Cheshire, U.K.

The interest in immunotoxicology is undoubtedly on the increase. Immunologists, of course, have always been concerned with the mechanisms by which an immunological reaction can cause tissue damage but toxicologists have only recently appreciated that the immunological system may be a target organ for chemically-induced toxic damage which may be expressed as a health hazard.

Toxicology can be thought of as a discipline in which toxic products are used to induce specific biochemical or pathological lesions in order to study mechanisms of biological processes. This academic view of toxicology is distinct from the safety evaluation aspect which uses *in vivo* and *in vitro* models in an attempt to evaluate the risk to man of chemical exposure. Since risk is quantifiable, the toxicologist should be able to devise systems for its measurement and use such data to make judgements on the hazard to man of exposure to a toxic compound. The basic assumption inherent in this assertion is that methods exist for measuring risk, and in the field of immunotoxicity it is very much a debatable point.

Consider first, the problems involved in assessing the risk of a drug causing hypersensitivity tissue damage. It is an accepted principle among immunologists that there is a minimum molecular weight for a substance to activate the immunological system. But with low molecular weight compounds, termed haptens, combined with macromolecular carriers, a complete antigen is formed (hapten-carrier) which can then induce a hapten specific allergic state.

The first problem, therefore, is one of chemical linkage between hapten and carrier. Based on Landsteiner and Jacobs' observation on the sensitizing capacity of various halogen substitutions into benzene [1], it is generally held that

the linkage must be a covalent one. Although it is now possible to argue against a rigid requirement for covalent binding, any alternate linkage must maintain stability of the
hapten protein complex under adverse equilibrium conditions
for it to function as an antigen.

Since protein binding is an important restriction on the
therapeutic availability of a drug, compounds are designed to
limit the degree and strength of drug-protein interactions.
Yet many compounds of different structural and chemical reactivity have been implicated in hypersensitivity reactions.
The fact that phase I metabolism, by mixed function oxygenases
generates reactive products with increased protein-binding
capacity is often quoted as a mechanism for drug-antigen
formation. Undoubtedly it is an attractive theory but it does
not command much experimental support, apart from the β-lactam
antibiotic models and the incompletely worked-out examples of
halothane and practolol.

Halothane has been blamed as a causative agent in fulminat-
ing hepatic necrosis but only recently has a metabolite of
halothane been shown to be involved in a hypersensitivity
process. Davies and co-workers were able to demonstrate in
a rabbit model that a product of halothane oxidative metabolism reacted with hepatocytes in such a way that they subsequently stimulated an autoantibody [2].

It is not clear from this latter work, what role the autoantibody plays in the pathogenesis of hepatic necrosis;
Davies and co-workers speculate that antibody-hepatocyte
interaction may have an adjuvant effect for direct toxic
damage caused by a product of the reductive metabolic pathway; this, however, still needs to be proven. In the halothane example, no specific halothane-metabolite antibodies
have been demonstrated nor is it clear what is the antigenic
specificity of the autoantibody. But its association with
signs of liver cell damage does merit further work to determine toxicological significance of the particular metabolite.

The antigenicity of practolol differs from halothane in
that metabolite(s) specific antibodies have been claimed.
Using an *in vitro* mixed oxygenase system Amos and co-workers
generated a product which reacted specifically with antibodies
present in sera of patients being treated with the drug [3].
Subsequent experiments failed to demonstrate conclusively
that the product was primarily involved in the oculo-
mucocutaneous syndrome as it could be detected in most
patients under treatment with practolol [4]. The critical
challenge experiments were never completed due to the company
withdrawing the drug but those that were carried out were
sufficiently instructive to justify further work.

Thus halothane and practolol serve as examples to support

hard data derived from β-lactam antibiotic studies, for a metabolite role in hypersensitivity responses. Severe anaphylaxis induced by penicillin is directly attributable to the action of IgE antibodies for penicillin metabolic products. The complexity of penicillin degradation and metabolism has made it impossible in most instances to define precisely the ultimate metabolite antigen, but there is no doubt that some of the minor metabolites are responsible. Attempts have been made, based on an analysis of the antigenic profile of penicillin metabolites, to produce reagents for selective skin testing. These have been used in trials, but not found universal acceptance due to their poor predictive value; this is a direct consequence of penicillin-metabolite antigen heterogeneity.

Methods exist which can be used to monitor perturbations in immune responsiveness both *in vitro* and *in vivo*, but it is not yet established how the results can be used in safety assessment schemes. Reduction in immunological parameters, as recorded in such tests, cannot be assumed to equate with a state of immune suppression which will compromise the host. There are, of course, various models using bacterial or tumour cells which attempt to measure the host's ability to adapt to an "immunosuppressed state" but for safety evaluation use, the methodology still requires rigid standardization to establish reproducibility.

No doubt during this symposium much will be discussed on the effects of substances on the immune response, but as this is the first international meeting of this kind, we must be careful not to be too hasty in extrapolating interesting academic experiments into schemes for safety evaluation of chemicals. We are at the stage of defining problems and investigating procedures which might be useful in attempting to answer them.

REFERENCES

1. Landsteiner, K. and Jacobs, J. (1935). *J. Exp. Med.* **61**, 643-656.
2. Davies, M., Vergani, D., Miele-Vergani, G., Eddleston, A.L.W.F., Neuberger, J. and Williams, R. (1981). In "Drug Reaction and the Liver" (eds. M. Davis, J.M. Tredger and R. Williams), pp.237-244. Pitman Medical, Tunbridge Wells.
3. Amos, H.E., Lake, B.G. and Atkinson, H.A.C. (1977). *Clin. All.* **7**, 423-428.
4. Amos, H.E., Lake, B.G. and Artis, J. (1978). *Brit. Med. J.* **1**, 402-404.

FUNDAMENTALS OF IMMUNOLOGY AND IMMUNOGLOBULINS

R. Hubbard

Biochemistry Department,
University of Surrey, Guildford, Surrey GU2 5XH, UK

INTRODUCTION

This international symposium has brought together many experts
in various fields of immunology and toxicology and I consider
that it is my role to set the immunological scene for the
toxicologists. I have thus given myself the impossible task
of reviewing the whole field of immunology in but a few pages.

PRINCIPLES OF IMMUNOLOGY

The body has two principal defence mechanisms, humoral and
cell-mediated immunity. Humoral immunity involves the synthesis and secretion of soluble antibodies into the blood and
other body fluids. Cell-mediated immunity involves the production of "sensitized" lymphocytes which are the effectors
of cellular defence. These mechanisms are adaptive immunological phenomena (rather than innate) and are largely dependent on B- and T-lymphocytes respectively.

The underlying principles of immunological defence mechanisms are:

    (i) recognition of self and non-self,
   (ii) specificity,
  (iii) memory.

These principles can give rise to certain other immunological phenomena, for example, breakdown of recognition of
self, leading to autoimmune disease. Cross-reactivity of an
antibody with different antigens may occur because of identical antigenic determinants on different antigens or it may
occur because of the very similar chemical structure of different determinants. Memory and memory cells are, of course,
the basis of immunization and long-term immunity against
various pathogens.

IMMUNOTOXICOLOGY
ISBN 0-12-282180-7

In terms of immune response itself, memory ensures that the
secondary response to an immunogen quickly produces higher
levels of antibody as shown in Fig. 1.

The major antibody class of the primary immune response is
immunoglobulin M (IgM) whilst that in the secondary response
is immunoglobulin G (IgG). Specificity is also indicated
(see Fig. 1) since if antigen Y, instead of X, is injected at
28 days, then only a primary response to Y is produced.

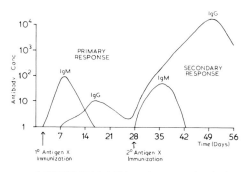

**Fig. 1 Studies of antibodies produced in primary and
secondary immune responses.** The major antibody class formed
in a primary immune response is IgM, while that in the secondary response is IgG. In the more rapid secondary response,
antibody levels are considerably higher and longer lasting
than in the primary response. Specificity is shown by the
primary response produced against antigen Y. (Antibody concentration units are arbitrary and are comparative only.)

Memory and specificity can also be illustrated in transplantation reactions. For example in Fig. 2 the first strain
B skin transplant (allograft) is rejected in 1 to 2 weeks,
but the second strain B skin transplant onto the same mouse
(strain A) is intensely rejected in 3-4 days. On the other
hand the skin transplant from strain C is rejected more
slowly in 1 to 2 weeks. The ability to "memorize" can be
transferred with the lymphocytes themselves but not in the
serum alone, and therefore is a cellular phenomenon. The
lymphocytes may be transferred to an immuno-incompetent syngeneic animal, months, or years later and will produce a
secondary response to a "memorized" antigen.

One of the major theories in immunology which has very
largely stood the test of time is the Clonal Selection theory

[1], proposed by Jerne (1955) and Burnet (1959) and elaborated by Mitchison (1967). The most important proposals of the Clonal Selection theory are shown in Table 1.

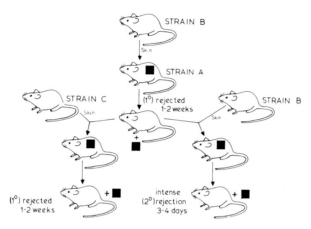

Fig. 2 Transplantation: specificity and memory. A skin transplant from strain B mouse to strain A mouse is rejected in 1 to 2 weeks, the equivalent of a primary response. If the same mouse receives a second skin transplant from strain B then the skin is intensely rejected in 3 to 4 days, the equivalent of a secondary response, indicating strain A has "memory" of the first skin transplant. However, if the same strain A mouse receives a strain C skin transplant instead of the second strain B skin transplant, it is more slowly rejected in the equivalent of a primary response. Thus transplantation experiments show both specificity and memory in respect of the transferred cells.

Table 1 *Clonal selection theory*

---

1. Specific receptors are present on lymphocytes,

2. All antibody structures are represented,

3. Clonal expansion of cells,

4. (a) Receptor specificity is identical to the specificity of the secreted antibody,

   (b) One cell is committed to one specificity prior to antigenic stimulation,

   (c) Progeny remain committed to this specificity.

THE CELLS OF THE IMMUNE RESPONSE

Stem cell differentiation in haemopoiesis produces the cells
of the immune response (see Table 2). All the white blood
cells are involved to some degree in immune function.

Table 2 *Haemopoiesis*

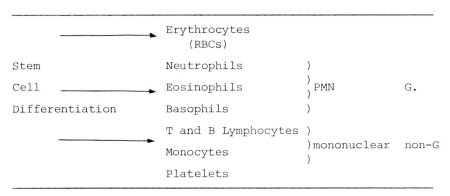

	Erythrocytes (RBCs)			
Stem	Neutrophils	)		
Cell	Eosinophils	) PMN	G.	
Differentiation	Basophils	)		
	T and B Lymphocytes	)		
	Monocytes	) mononuclear	non-G	
	Platelets			

PMN = Polymorphonuclear cells
G = Granules present in cells

Polymorphonuclear Cells

The neutrophils, basophils and eosinophils possess granules
which contain a battery of mediators and enzymes. The polymorphonuclear leukocytes constitute about 60 to 70% of the
total circulating leukocytes and are divided into the three
types based on their staining characteristics. The normal
range of total polymorphonuclear leukocytes (PMNs) is 4000-
8000 per mm^3 of blood, greater than 90% of these being neutrophils. The neutrophils are powerful phagocytic cells but
have a short half-life in the blood (about 6 to 8 h). The
complete neutrophil maturation process (in the bone marrow)
requires approximately 9 to 11 days and hence the estimated
neutrophil turnover rate is about 126 billion cells per day
in a normal 70 kg man [2]. Neutrophils and basophils possess
Fc and C3b receptors on their surface.

Mast Cells

These are mononuclear, long-lived cells which exist in the
connective tissue although their exact origin is not known.
They possess granules which can be released extracellularly,
and which contain histamine, heparin, mucopolysaccharides,
prostaglandins, platelet activating factor (PAF), slow reacting substance of anaphylaxis (SRS-A), and a variety of enzymes but no myeloperoxidase. Mast cells are capable of

phagocytosis and possess receptors for IgE, IgG and C3a* and
C5a* (anaphylatoxins). Mast cells are, of course, intimately
involved in allergic reactions, the mechanisms of which will
be discussed by Dennis Stanworth (see p. 71).

Monocytes and Macrophages

The blood monocytes develop into macrophages in the tissues
e.g. alveolar and peritoneal macrophages, Kupffer cells in the
liver, and osteoclasts of the bone marrow. They are large,
very active phagocytic cells (20 to 40 μm) having a kidney
shaped nucleus, and a long life span (approximately three
months). They are capable of ingesting bacteria, viruses,
protozoa, antigen-antibody complexes and inorganic materials
such as silica, charcoal and asbestos. Macrophages respond
to chemotaxis and possess Fc and C3b receptors on their cell
surface.

B- and T-lymphocytes

Resting B- and T-lymphocytes have a very large nucleus and
appear morphologically identical. They represent some 20 to
40% of human peripheral blood leukocytes (3,000 lymphocytes
per mm^3). Generally the majority of lymphocytes have a life
span of around 100 to 200 days but for some human small
lymphocytes, it may be as long as several years [2]. In the
peripheral blood, the lymphocyte composition is approximately
70 to 80% T and 15 to 20% B, whilst the remaining lymphocytes
are difficult to classify. In lymphoid tissue the ratio of
T- and B-lymphocytes is quite variable e.g. thoracic duct
(85% T), lymph nodes (80% T), and spleen (35% T).

The B- and T-lymphocytes mature and become immunocompetent
in the primary lymphoid tissue, the T-cells in the thymus and
the B-cells in the bone marrow or gut-associated lymphoid
tissue (G.A.L.T.). The lymphocytes become distributed in the
secondary lymphoid tissue and await appropriate antigenic
stimulation (see Fig. 3).

The B-lymphocytes are stimulated to differentiate into
plasma cells which have extensive endoplasmic reticulum,
enabling each cell to secrete a large amount of a single antibody directed against one particular determinant on the antigen. Plasma cells are mainly in the spleen, lymph nodes and
bone marrow and are not found extensively in the blood.

---

* C3 = complement component number 3.
  C3a and C5a are molecular fragments released during the
  complement cascade sequence (see p. 18)

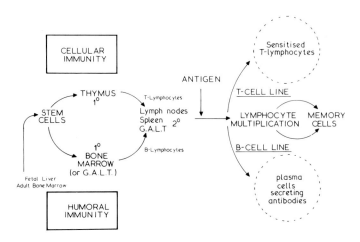

Fig. 3 Humoral and cellular immunity. Cellular immunity is
dependent on T-lymphocytes, so called because they differentiate and become immunocompetent in the thymus, which is described as primary (1°) lymphoid tissue. Humoral immunity is
dependent on antibodies secreted by plasma cells, which are
produced after antigenic stimulation of B-lymphocytes.
B-lymphocytes (so called originally because they are derived
from the Bursa of Fabricius in birds), become immunocompetent
in the bone marrow or possibly the gut-associated lymphoid
tissue (G.A.L.T.) (1° lymphoid tissue) in humans. The immunocompetent B- and T-lymphocytes become distributed in the
lymphoid system of the body (secondary (2°) lymphoid tissue)
and await stimulation by their appropriate antigen. This
triggers further differentiation and multiplication, producing
sensitized T-lymphocytes, plasma cells, and "memory" cells for
both T- and B-cell lineage.

Plasma cells develop in only 2 to 3 days from stimulated
B-cells and die within a few days. The T-lymphocytes differentiate in a more complex manner and a number of T-cell subpopulations are produced (see Table 3).
   These subpopulations include the regulatory T-suppressor
and T-helper cells which act to turn off or on both humoral
and cell-mediated immune responses. Human Ts and Th cells
differ in respect of their surface markers, the Ts cells
having Fc receptor for γ chains and Th, Fc receptors for
μ chains. Human T-cells can be differentiated from B-cells
in that they spontaneously form rosettes with sheep erythrocytes. Cytotoxic T-cells can kill either foreign cells or
virally-invaded self cells, by direct cell-cell contact.
The Tc cells operate with exquisite specificity and are able

Table 3 *T-cell subpopulations*

Subpopulation			Function
Th	T-helper	T_H	B-cell differentiation in the humoral response
		T_D	Delayed hypersensitivity, release soluble factors (lymphokines)
		T_A	Stimulation of killer Tc precursor cell differentiation
Ts	T-suppressor		Suppression of humoral and cell-mediated responses
Tc	T-cytotoxic		Specific lysis of antigen-bearing target cells

to precisely recognize major histocompatibility complex (MHC) antigens. Syngeneic cells which have been modified by a virus, hapten or possibly tumour transformation can be lysed by cytotoxic T-cells. Certain types of effector T-cells secrete a whole host of "lymphokines" which are soluble mediators of immune function, one of the main effects being to activate macrophages.

The cell surface receptors of B-lymphocytes are well-known to be membrane-bound antibody molecules which, after antigenic stimulation and conversion to plasma cells, can be secreted as free molecules with identical specificity. On the other hand the T-cell surface receptor has long been an area of controversy and several models have been proposed over the years. Current investigations indicate that the T-cell receptors are based upon the presence of a V_H fragment of an antibody molecule, combined with an I-region associated antigenic structure [3].

Natural Killer Cells

Natural killer (NK) cells are of unknown lineage but may be related to killer (K) cells and to T-cells, but they are not thymus dependent. NK cells are found in normal and T-cell deficient mice and can kill a variety of target cells [4,5]. NK cells are thought to play a significant role in immune surveillance. T-cells were ruled out for this role when it was found that nude mice, having no T-cells, had a very low

incidence of tumours. Nude mice however do have a high NK
activity. The natural cytotoxicity of NK cells appears to
require no prior sensitization and occurs by direct cell-cell
contact. Cytotoxicity is directed against virally-modified
cells and it is believed against certain tumour cells, particularly those of the lymphatic system. There is evidence that
certain interferons and interleukins* are involved in the
stimulation of NK system activity [5,6].

Killer Cells

Killer (K) cells are another cell type of unknown lineage
having lytic activity. The K population is quite heterogeneous (40% having the T-cell marker). The cytotoxic reaction mediated by K cells is an antibody dependent phenomenon
and is therefore often referred to as ADCC (antibody dependent cellular cytotoxicity). No activation is required for
this, unless activation is needed in order to express the Fc
receptors.

K cells express Fc receptors for IgG antibodies and these
mediate the cytotoxic process which appears to be identical
to that of cytotoxic T-cells.

Phagocytic Cells

The main phagocytic cells, the macrophages and neutrophils
are intimately involved in body defence and are considerably
aided in this respect by antibody and complement. Immunoglobulin G for example can "fix" complement (CH2 domain) and
can bind to macrophages (CH3 domain). Once the complement
cascade is underway, certain components e.g., C3a, C5a, and
C5b67 are produced which are chemotactic for phagocytes and
are also anaphylatoxic.

The generation of the immune response is dependent upon the
co-operation of many of the above cells [2]. In particular

---

* Interleukins were defined at the Second International
Workshop in Lymphokines as soluble factors produced by and
acting on leukocytes. Interleukin-1 (IL1) is a macrophage
derived factor which enhances lymphocyte proliferation.
Interleukin-2 (IL2) is a T-cell product (Th) and is a T-cell
growth factor (TCGF) which enhances the proliferation of
cytotoxic T-cells. There are two factors known as inter-
leukin-3 (IL3), one a product of antigen-activated T helper
cells, which acts as a differentiation and growth factor for
T-helper cells [7] while the other is defined as a T-cell
product that is required by macrophages to produce IL-1 [8].

the regulatory T-cells, the suppressors and helpers are
inevitably involved and there are a vast array of immune
molecular messengers such as the leukotrienes, prostaglandins
and interleukins [2]. The major histocompatibility complex
(MHC) is the driving force behind the immune response and acts
as controller of T-cell subpopulation activity. The MHC thus
controls the immune response, T-B co-operation, transplantation
reactions, and complement activity. It is not surprising then
to find the various mouse T-cell subpopulations possessing
specialized receptors for Ia, K, D and J molecules.

IMMUNITY TO INFECTION

General immunity and defence is often divided into innate and
adaptive mechanisms (see Table 4).

Table 4 *Innate and adaptive immune mechanisms*

Innate	Adaptive
No increase in efficiency on repeated exposure	Improves with repeated exposure
Lysozyme	Expansion of committed antigen-specific B and T lymphocytes through clonal expansion
Complement (Alternative pathway)	
Interferons	Antibody (activates complement and phagocytes when bound)
Phagocytic cells	
Natural killer cells	

The innate mechanisms include non-specific agents and cell
functions. Innate humoral mechanisms include lysozyme
(which splits muramic acid in bacterial cell walls), the
multi-enzyme complement system (leading to phagocytosis or
lysis), and interferons (anti-viral activity). Innate
cellular activity includes "non-specific" phagocytosis and
natural killer cytotoxicity. The adaptive mechanisms are
based on sensitized lymphocytes and "memory" cells and of
course the exquisite specificity of antibodies.

ANTIBODIES

Antibodies are universal "adaptor" molecules which can bind
to virtually any antigen and by so doing can enhance its
phagocytosis. Once bound to antigen, IgG and IgM can

activate complement and thus the phagocytes are chemotactically
"called" to that locality.

Remarkably, the vertebrate animal is able to produce some 10^7
maybe 10^8 different antibody specificities. This creates a
considerable problem in terms of explaining the genetics of
this process, often called G.O.D. or Generation of Diversity
[9-11].

There are five main classes of antibody, the basic unit
structure being a four-chain polypeptide of about 1300 amino
acids with two identical heavy chains and two identical light
chains [12,13]. (See Table 5).

Table 5 *Classes of antibody*

WHO designation	IgG	IgM	IgA	IgD	IgE
Heavy chain	γ	μ	α	δ	ε
Light chain	k or λ	k or λ	k or λ	k or λ	k or λ
Chain structure	$\gamma_2 k_2$	$(\mu_2 k_2)_5 J^*$	$(\alpha_2 k_2)_2 JS$	$\delta_2 k_2$	$\varepsilon_2 k_2$
	$\gamma_2 \lambda_2$	$(\mu_2 \lambda_2)_5 J$	$(\alpha_2 \lambda_2)_2 JS$	$\delta_2 \lambda_2$	$\varepsilon_2 \lambda_2$

* J chain: M.W. 15,000 present in polymeric antibodies and
produced in the plasma cell. Rich in cysteine.

A more detailed structure (see Fig. 4) reveals that the
heavy and light chains have constant and variable regions of
amino acid sequence** (when antibody sequences are compared)
and there is a flexible hinge region rich in proline.
Enzymic degradation can produce the familiar fragments
(i) Fc, "fragment crystallizable", (ii) Fab, "fragment antigen binding" (monovalent) and (iii) F(ab')$_2$, the divalent
antigen-binding fragment.

** Comparison of amino acid sequences in different antibodies
shows certain positions and areas are more variable than
others [14]. Variability has been defined as:

$$\text{Variability} = \frac{\text{number of different amino acids at a given position}}{\text{frequency of the most common amino acid at that position}}$$

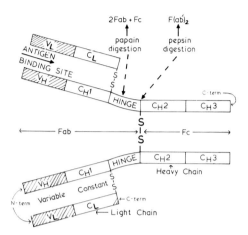

Fig. 4 IgG antibody structure. Immunoglobulin G consists of
two identical heavy (H) chains and two identical light (L)
polypeptide chains linked by disulphide bonds. The antigen-
binding sites are located at the variable (V) regions of amino
acid sequence shown as the shaded areas. The structure was
elucidated by enzymic digestion using pepsin and papain, which
gave the characteristic antibody fragments shown. Papain
digestion of IgG produces three fragments (2 Fab + Fc) whilst
pepsin produces a larger divalent antigen-binding fragment
designated F(ab')$_2$. The disulphide bridges between the chains
may be reduced and stabilized by alkylation, and then the
light and heavy chains can be isolated, separated and
characterized. H = heavy chain; L = light chain; C = constant
region, V = variable region, in respect of amino acid sequence
studies. Numbers on chains refer to the globular domains in
the structure. Fab = Fragment antigen-binding, monovalent;
F(ab')$_2$ = Fragment antigen-binding, divalent; Fc = Fragment
crystallizable; C-term, N-term, amino acid terminal end.

Within the V regions there are several hypervariable (HV)
regions of amino acid sequence and it is five such HV regions
which are folded to form the antigen binding site [14-16].
The 3-dimensional structure consists of globular constant and
variable homologous domains, each of which is independent and
consists of two β-pleated sheets held together by S-S bonds.
The class of antibody confers certain physiological properties on that antibody and hence on that particular antibody

Table 6 *Properties of human immunoglobulins*

IgG	IgM	IgA	IgD	IgE
monomer	pentamer	dimer monomer polymers	monomer	monomer
major serum Ig	mainly confined to blood and effective against blood borne infections	body secretions	low serum concentration	very low serum concentration
2° immune response	1° immune response			
defence against bacteria, viruses and toxins		secretory piece in dimer	unknown function	fixes to mast cell surface
fixes complement	excellent complement fixation	does not fix complement	present on surface of certain lymphocytes	responsible for immediate hypersensitivity
binds to macrophages				
crosses the placenta				raised levels in parasitic infection

specificity. A B-cell can change its antibody class without changing antibody specificity thus providing a particular specificity with a variety of biological capabilities. The proposed molecular mechanisms of the immunoglobulin class switch are most fascinating [17]. The important physiological properties of the human immunoglobulin classes are shown in Table 6.

Secretory IgA is a dimer and is present in virtually all body secretions. It possesses a glycoprotein chain known as secretory piece* which aids secretion of the molecule and may protect it against proteases. IgA can remove antigens via immune complex formation, transport to the liver, and excretion through the bile and this aspect will be expanded by Joe Hall (see p. 317). The function of IgD is unknown but its role may be more related to a receptor than to a conventional antibody [18,19]. IgD and monomeric IgM can be simultaneously expressed on differentiating B-lymphocytes and indeed on some mature B-cells. In fact IgD is thought to be synthesized and expressed at some stage of differentiation of all B-lymphocytes [2]. IgE is an antibody we shall hear much more about because it binds to mast cell and basophil cell surfaces and is involved in immediate hypersensitivity.

COMPLEMENT

Complement is an enzymic cascade system of plasma proteins which is intimately involved in inflammation, phagocytosis and lysis. There are two pathways of complement activation, one via antibody, the Classical, and one direct pathway via for example microbial polysaccharide, the Alternative [20], (see Fig. 5).

The important consequences of complement activation are the production of C3a, C5a and C5b67 which are anaphylatoxic and chemotactic for polymorphonuclear cells. The fragment C3b is able to bind to foreign cells or bacteria whilst the phagocytes can thus adhere to them using their C3b receptors. If phagocytosis does not occur, the invading cell will finally be lysed by C8, C9 components. However, C3 activation is vital and is the central event which is required.

RECENT ADVANCES

Probably the most important discovery of recent years is that of monoclonal antibodies by Milstein and Köhler [21-23]. One

---

* Secretory piece S: M.W. 60,000 produced in epithelial cells and attached during secretion.

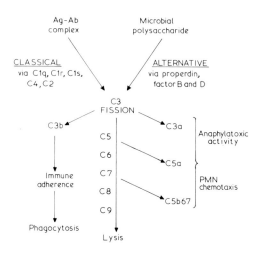

Fig. 5 Complement. Complement is a series of plasma proteins which play a vital role in inflammation and defence against infection. There are nine numbered basic components although the first component C1 actually consists of three proteins C1q, C1r, C1s which is involved in the "Classical" pathway of complement activation by C1q binding to the Fc region of an antibody. The other pathway to complement activation is the "alternative" pathway which is independent of antibody and is initiated by microbial polysaccharides, e.g. endotoxin. The central event in complement activation is the cleavage of complement component three (C3) and this leads to the production of physiologically active fragments, C3a and C3b as shown. C3b is able to coat the surface of invading bacteria and eventually lead to phagocytosis by the phagocytes (which possess C3b receptors). C3a and other fragments produced (C5a, C5b67), cause inflammation (anaphylatoxic) and are also chemotactic for polymorphonuclear cells which rapidly arrive in the locality due to the chemical gradient produced. They meet the C3b coated bacteria and phagocytose them. If this process does not occur then the complement cascade continues on the bacterial cell surface until complement components C8 and C9 bind and these "punch" a functional hole in the bacterial cell which leads to its rapid death by lysis.

application of these reagents will be discussed later in the symposium by Brian Foxwell (see p. 359).

Conventional antibodies are actually mixtures of antibodies and have several disadvantages notably unwanted cross-reactions and they can never be reproduced exactly (see Table 7).

Table 7 *Disadvantages of conventional antisera*

---

1. Heterogeneous mixture of antibodies.

2. Cross reactions may not be genuine.

3. Can never be reproduced exactly.

4. Need a pure immunogen and/or

5. Require purification for specificity.

Monoclonal antibodies, however, are pure antibodies, having a high specificity for their antigenic determinant.

The basic principle in making monoclonal antibodies is the fusion of an antigen-primed antibody-secreting lymphocyte with a suitable cancer cell line (see Fig. 6).

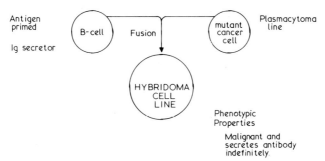

Fig. 6 Basic principle of monoclonals. Hybridoma cells secreting a single antibody of one specificity are the result of the fusion of an antigen-primed immunoglobulin-secreting B-cell with a suitable plasmacytoma line. The cell fusion is carried out in 50% polyethylene glycol M.W. 1500 → 4000 at 37°C, but its precise mechanism is unknown. Culture super-natants are screened for the required specific antibody to isolate the desired hybridomas. The excess unfused B-cells die after 3 to 4 days, whilst the excess plasmacytoma cells could survive indefinitely in culture. They are thus killed selectively using hypoxanthine, aminopterin, thymidine ('HAT') medium which prevents nucleic acid biosynthesis in cells lacking hypoxanthine guanine phosphoribosyl transferase (HGPRT) or thymidine kinase (TK) enzymes.

This produces hybridoma cells which have the properties of both its parents, i.e. the ability to secrete a single antibody of one specificity, and to grow and proliferate indefinitely in an appropriate medium. The cloned hybridomas may be grown *in vitro* or *in vivo* to produce an unlimited supply of the pure identical antibody.

It is hoped that this short overview of immunology will provide adequate background for this symposium.

REFERENCES

1. Sigal, N.H. and Klinman, N.R. (1978). *Adv. in Immunol.* **26**, 255-337.
2. Bier, O.G., Dias da Silva, W., Gotze, D. and Mota, I. (1981). "Fundamentals of Immunology" Springer-Verlag, New York.
3. Marchalonis, J.J. (1982). *Immunology Today* **3**, 10-17.
4. Kiesslinger, R., Klein, E. and Wigzell, H. (1975). *Eur. J. Immunol.* **5**, 112-117.
5. Herberman, R.B. (Ed.) (1980). Natural Cell-mediated Immunity Against Tumors, Academic Press, New York.
6. Henney, C.S., Kuribayashi, K., Kern, D.E. and Gillis, S. (1981). *Nature (London)* **291**, 335-338.
7. Ihle, J.N., Pepersack, L. and Rebar, L. (1981). *J. Immunol.* **126**, 2184.
8. Wagner, H., Hardt, C., Rollinghoff, M., Pfizenmaier, K. and Solbach, W. (1981). *Immunobiol.* **159**, 183.
9. Gough, N. (1981). *Trends in Biological Sciences*, August, 203-205 and November, 300-302.
10. Givol, D. (1981). *Nature* **292**, 426-430.
11. Gearhart, P.J. (1982). *Immunology Today* **3**, 107-112.
12. Porter, R.R. (1967). *Scientific American* **217**, 81-90.
13. Edelman, G.M. (1970). *Scientific American* **223**, 34-42.
14. Capra, J.D. and Edmundson, A.B. (1977). *Scientific American* **236**, 50-59.
15. Arnzel, L.M. and Poljak, R.J. (1979). *Ann. Rev. Biochem.* **48**, 961-997.
16. Marquart, M. and Deisenhofer, J. (1982). *Immunology Today* **3**, 160-166.
17. Honjo, T. (1982). *Immunology Today* **3**, 214-217.
18. Jefferis, R. (1981). *Trends in Biological Sciences*, April, 111-113.
19. Calvert, J.E. and Jefferis, R. (1981). *Trends in Biological Sciences*, May, 125-127.
20. Porter, R.R. and Reid, K.B.M. (1981). *Ann. Rev. Biochem.* **50**, 433-464.
21. Köhler, G. and Milstein, C. (1975). *Nature* **256**, 495-497.
22. Köhler, G. and Milstein, C. (1976). *Eur. J. Immunol.* **6**, 511-519.
23. Milstein, C. (1980). *Scientific American* **243**, 56-64.

THE CELL-MEDIATED IMMUNE RESPONSE AND ITS MODULATION

P.G.H. Gell

Department of Pathology,
University of Cambridge, Cambridge, UK

I want to consider the cell-mediated immune response, the so-called delayed response from a pragmatic, indeed teleologic point of view — what is it for? Therapists and toxicologists find it apparently just a nuisance, thwarting their well-meant attempts to pump ever more complicated organic ring systems into our tissues. At one time delayed hypersensitivity (DH) was considered to play an essential part in what was called immune surveillance. The concept of immune surveillance was first presented by Lewis Thomas in about 1957, primarily as a possible means of getting rid of deleterious somatic mutants, in particular, cancerous cells. This line of thought was strengthened when the circulation of T-cells was demonstrated; clearly the T-cells could readily penetrate nooks and crannies of the body and sample for the presence of any foreign, that is mutated, cell. This very attractive hypothesis, however, has been steadily eroded by the development of further knowledge of immunosuppression, gained from thymus-less nude mice, and immunosuppressed or naturally T-cell-deficient human beings.

The development of non-lymphoid tumours after clinical immunosuppression has come to be less and less of a problem as régimes become better controlled: yet this is exactly the situation where one would expect immune surveillance to be compromised, that is where responses to small differences of homograft antigens have been eliminated. So although now the case for immune surveillance by T-cells, as a major and frequently used defence against spontaneous tumours, is not as strong as it was, it is still necessary to analyse how the organism becomes aware of small antigenic differences, in small doses, such as occur in somatic mutation. A blueprint for effective immune responsiveness of this type would entail,

IMMUNOTOXICOLOGY
ISBN 0-12-282180-7

firstly, that the response is rapid and, secondly, that very
small amounts of antigen, even those produced by a single cell
or a single clone of cells, should be recognizable. Two T-cell
functions which are candidates for this are the killer cell
system and delayed hypersensitivity. But can any killer cell
be sufficiently sensitive to such very low doses of antigen,
and does DH in fact protect by producing an effectively cytotoxic cell of any sort? I do not want to talk here about
killer cells, but rather to consider how the DH-cell, assuming
that it exists at all, may be involved in this quick response
mechanism. There seems little doubt that there is a pre-
existing population of epitope-specific DH cells which can be
clonally multiplied *in vitro*. This is demonstrated by the
well-known techniques by which DH type reactivity can be
generated *in vitro* as for instance against sheep red blood
cells (SRBC) [1] and against viruses [2]. There is no reason
to suppose that in a normal animal a single T-cell or a small
clone of cells could not reach and respond to a single rogue
mutant cell by the local release of lymphokines, which would
then presumably lead to activation of the macrophage system
and a potential destruction of the aberrant clone. Such a
system would be liable to be far more rapid and sensitive
than anything depending on say, the production of antibody or
antibody-dependent cellular cytotoxicity (ADCC).

Can one demonstrate a positive protective effect on the
level of the whole organism, presumably depending on the
generation of cytotoxic macrophages by lymphokines released
from stimulated DH cells? For this purpose I want to go, in
some detail, into a system with which I am familiar, herpes
infections in mice. Figure 1 shows events in the pinna of
the ear of normal and of nude mice injected locally with a
dose of about 10^4 plaque-forming units of herpes simplex
virus type 1, [3]. One must draw attention to two points.
Firstly the rapid rise in swelling on day three and clearance
almost complete by day six to seven in normal mice. That is,
whatever protective mechanisms have been activated have been
effective by this stage. Now by day five antibody is just
beginning to be demonstrable by sensitive methods in the
serum, and one can say that the disappearance of virus from
the pinna of the ear is coincident with the production of
detectable antibody. There is no prima facie reason, therefore, to believe that the elimination of virus in this situation is due to anything except antibody. Secondly, I would
draw attention to the slowness of the inflammation in the
pinna of the ear of nude mice without the striking increment
of day three to four; but progressive inflammatory damage in
the infected ear nevertheless continues until the death of
the mouse, usually from spread to the nervous system, and

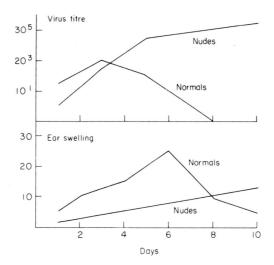

Fig. 1 Sequence of events in ears of normal and nude mice injected locally with herpes virus.

generally at about day 12 to 15. It seems reasonable, therefore, that the sudden increment in the normal mouse at day three to four is due to T-cell-mediated, specific inflammation.

I do not think it is necessary to apologize for the use of a replicating agent like a virus when demonstrating the nature of DH responses, since it is a dynamic situation in the body which we wish to analyse anyway, the situation of the destruction of a clone whether of infected cells or of aberrant ones. In the dynamic situation of virus growth and elimination one can demonstrate protection in the strict sense, which is impossible with a non-replicating antigen. Now although it is not possible to demonstrate with certainty a positive role for DH in the elimination of virus in an intact animal which is also producing antibody, it is possible to show that the absence of DH does not compromise the *eventual* clearance of virus from the ear. This can be done by tolerization of mice to DH induced by virus, by the intravenous injection of moderate doses of a non-pathogenic mutant virus or indeed of rather smaller doses, in resistant strains, of a fully pathogenic one, [4]. With this treatment we get what is known as split tolerance, that is to say all DH is completely abolished but other immune functions including antibody production are unaffected or even boosted. Elimination of live virus from the ear pinna occurs at about the same time as it occurs in the non-tolerized mouse. However one can use this model to demonstrate an effect of the DH cell in controlling the very

earliest response to viral antigen. If we transfer from a
sensitized to a normal mouse, cells from the lymph node draining the infected pinna, we transfer, as is well known, DH and
a faster elimination of infection, that is to say in two or
three days instead of six or seven days. If, however, we take
the cells from the draining lymph node of a tolerized mouse
which has been subsequently injected with live virus in the
ear some days previously, and inject these cells into the
normal mouse, there is *no* evidence of this rapid protective
effect, although cytotoxic cells and plasma cells can be
shown to be present in normal amounts in the transferred
suspension, the only cells lacking from the transferred suspension being presumably active DTH cells. Now this does suggest
that in the earliest stages of response to a self-replicating
antigen the presence of a DTH (delayed hypersensitivity T-cell)
is helpful. It is possible, in the sort of situations we considered earlier of aberrant mutant clones, that a quick DTH
response exercising this kind of control might be sufficient
to abort such dangerous clones. Tolerance of this sort can
be shown to function by way of suppressor cells as of course
in many other examples of tolerance. It is a point which
needs further investigation, almost a paradox, that these
suppressor cells in split tolerance must recognize antigen
and idiotype, and also the nature of the cell as a DTH cell;
helper cells for instance required for antibody production
are not suppressed simultaneously. It must be noted that DTH
and helper cells both carry the Lytl marker so recognition by
suppressors cannot be keyed to that marker.

   It seems that the DTH function is relatively easily tolerised compared with other immune functions. This has some
obvious biological advantages, and clearly may be relevant in
contact sensitivity situations. However, though we can see
one good reason why DH should exist, such a marginal effect
does not seem a very good reason for so sensitive and generalized a function. I feel that possible other interventions of
DH may be in the more complicated situations of the immunological network. There are four points to be considered here.
Firstly, T-cells including DTH cells, though probably not, or
not all, suppressor cells carry an idiotypic determinant.
Secondly, it is a dogma of network theory that each immune
response involves its own antithetic response (anti-idiotypic
response). Thirdly, DTH cells are in a strong position as
immunogens because they carry an in-built adjuvant function
with them, namely, the property of releasing lymphokines to
accumulate and activate macrophages. Fourthly, cells carrying
an antigenic determinant have been shown [5] to be strong
inducers of suppressor cells, if introduced intravenously,
and suppressor cells according to some are essential steps in

the network. What I am edging towards, in fact, is the
suggestion that one of the essential functions of DTH cells
is their rôle as immunogens in the network system. Suppose
they work like this, functioning as immunogens to generate
suppression in an immune response. Clearly this has to be
very strictly controlled if the immune response is to perform
a useful function. So DH cells are very easily tolerised.
One of the more extravagent but probably true deductions from
network theory is that the second generation anti-idiotype
provides a model for the original epitope of the antigen: the
antigenic stimulus may theoretically be resumed or continued
at this stage. I am unaware whether anybody has yet demonstrated the anti-anti-idiotype to be an activator of memory
cells; but so rapid is advance in this field that no doubt
someone will have shown as much before this paper appears in
print.

REFERENCES

1. Bretscher, P.A. (1979). *European J. Immunol.* **9**, 311.
2. Leung, K.N. and Ada, G.L. (1980). *Scand. J. Immunol.* **12**,
    129, 481.
3. Kapoor, A.K., Nash, A.A., Wildy, P., Phelan, J., McLean,
    C.S. and Field, H.J. (1982). *J. Gen. Virol.* **60**, 225.
4. Nash, A.A., Gell, P.G.H. and Wildy, P. (1981). *Immunology*
    43, 153, 363.
5. Claman, H.N., Miller, S.D. and Sy, M-S. (1977). *J. Exp.
    Med.* **146**, 49.

CLINICAL MANIFESTATIONS OF DRUG-INDUCED SYNDROMES

A.L. Parke

Department of Rheumatology,
Hammersmith Hospital, London, U.K.

INTRODUCTION

The incidence of adverse drug effects is almost impossible to
determine, and becomes even more difficult to assess in ambu-
lant patients as they may self-prescribe many drugs in addition to those given professionally. Cluff and Caldwell [1]
claim that hospital patients receive on average ten different
drugs, although in individual patients the number administered
may be many times this. They estimate that the probability
of an adverse drug reaction in a hospitalized patient is
about 5% if the patient receives six drugs or less, but this
number rises to more than 40% if the patient receives 15 or
more drugs [1].

Drugs are foreign chemicals and as such they may induce
immunological responses. It has been claimed that approximately 15% of adverse drug reactions are due to an allergic
response to the drug or one of its metabolites [1]. Clinical
manifestations of such allergic responses are numerous and
may involve any organ in the body, for example the clinical
features of a serum sickness-like illness may include: nausea,
vomiting, abdominal pain, rash, fever, arthritis, vasculitis,
lymphadenopathy and glomerulonephritis.

The majority of pharmacological agents are not immunogenic,
but there are certain drugs and classes of chemicals used
pharmacologically which, if given for long enough, and in
sufficient quantities, to certain susceptible individuals,
may result in the development of a drug-induced syndrome, the
clinical features of which may mimic idiopathic diseases.

In this paper the drug-induced syndromes that mimic the
connective tissue diseases will be discussed.

IMMUNOTOXICOLOGY
ISBN 0-12-282180-7

SYSTEMIC LUPUS ERYTHEMATOSUS

Clinical Features

Idiopathic systemic lupus erythematosus (SLE) is predominantly a disease of young women. This chronic inflammatory disease, characterized by exacerbations interspersed with periods of disease inactivity, can present many clinical features, but the most common are those of skin and joint disease. Initially considered to be a severe and often fatal disease, milder forms of SLE have now been identified.

Drug-induced lupus may present with clinical features similar to those of idiopathic disease, however skin, central nervous system, and renal involvement are comparatively rare (Table 1) [2-6]. Drug-induced lupus occurs in an older age group, with a mean age of 62 years for procainamide and 50.3 years for hydralazine [7], whereas that for idiopathic lupus is 29 years. Of patients who develop idiopathic systemic lupus erythematosus 30% are black [8] whereas the incidence of the drug-induced syndrome in the black population is much less [9]. One important distinguishing clinical feature between idiopathic and drug-induced lupus erythematosus is the usual prompt resolution of symptoms when the patient stops taking the offending drug.

Table 1 *Clinical manifestations of drug-induced lupus syndrome and idiopathic systemic lupus erythematosus.*

Clinical features	% positive	
	Idiopathic	Drug-induced
General malaise	>80	50
Joint involvement	>90	70-90
Rash	70	<20
Central nervous system disease	20	<5
Renal disease	40	<20
Raynaud's phenomenon	20	<5
Pleural/pericardial disease	30-50	30-50

Serological Features

The development of anti-nuclear antibodies is a major serological feature of systemic lupus erythematosus. In idiopathic disease, antibodies to various nuclear constituents have been found, but most notably antibodies to native double-stranded DNA [10]. In the drug-induced syndrome only a small percentage of the individuals that develop anti-nuclear antibodies manifest clinical symptoms. Even the development of drug-induced complement-fixing anti-native DNA antibodies (considered to be important in the pathogenesis of idiopathic systemic lupus erthematosus) may not be associated with clinical complaints [11].

In contrast to idiopathic SLE, antibodies to native double-stranded DNA are extremely rare in drug-induced lupus erythematosus. This may well explain the low incidence of renal disease in drug-induced lupus as previous studies have shown a definite association of antibodies to native double-stranded DNA with the development of glomerulonephritis [12]. Antibodies to a whole variety of other nuclear antigens have been found [13-15]; in particular anti-histone antibodies [16,17]. With procainamide-induced lupus, 96% of the sera contain anti-histone antibodies [17,18]. The incidence of hypo-complement-aemia, circulating immune complexes, and the development of anti-lymphocyte antibodies, is reduced in drug-induced lupus compared with the idiopathic disease [19].

Drugs Producing Systemic Lupus Erythematosus Syndrome

Numerous drugs have been implicated in the development of the drug-induced lupus syndrome [20], but the most important offenders and the best studied drugs are hydralazine and procainamide.

Hydralazine Approximately 24-50% of patients exposed to long-term therapy with hydralazine develop anti-nuclear antibodies, and between 8-30% develop a lupus-like syndrome [21]. Numerous factors predispose the patient to develop hydralazine lupus, and these include: the daily dosage of the drug, the total amount of drug consumed, the sex of the patient, the HLA status, and the acetylator status. A study from the Hammersmith Hospital, London, showed that of 26 patients with hydralazine-induced lupus, 25 were slow acetylators and 73% carried the HLA DR4; 21 of the patients were female and the remaining 5 males all had the HLA DR4 antigen. The most significant finding was that all females who were slow acetylators and were DR4 positive, developed hydralazine lupus [22]. This association of hydralazine-induced lupus with HLA DR4 is contrasted by the association of idiopathic SLE with HLA DR3 and DR2 [23-26].

Procainamide Slow acetylator status is also associated with procainamide-induced lupus [27]. Fast acetylators have

N-acetylated procainamide present in the plasma, and recent studies have shown that patients treated with pharmacologically active N-acetylated procainamide develop positive anti-nuclear antibodies less frequently [28]. As has been seen with hydralazine, nearly all patients with procainamide-induced lupus have anti-nuclear antibodies but these represent only a small proportion of the patients who develop drug-induced anti-nuclear antibodies [29].

Isoniazid Of patients treated with isoniazid, 22% developed anti-nuclear antibodies [30]. Reports concerning the acetylator status of patients developing isoniazid-induced anti-nuclear antibodies are conflicting [32,33].

Penicillamine Penicillamine is now well recognized as a cause of drug-induced systemic lupus erythematosus [33,34]. It is one of the few drugs associated with the development of anti-native DNA antibodies, and is capable of inducing the production of many auto-antibodies, including antibodies to striated muscle, and epidermal intercellular substance. Some of these antibodies are associated with drug-induced syndromes [35-39].

Pseudolupus Syndrome

This is a rare lupus-like syndrome that develops in up to 30% of patients taking venocuran, a drug containing pheno-pyrazone, cardiac glycosides, and horse chestnut extract [40]. It is called pseudolupus syndrome, because it is not associated with the development of anti-nuclear antibodies, but with the development of anti-mitochondrial antibodies. However, the clinical features are those of systemic lupus erythematosus.

Mechanisms

The mechanisms whereby drugs and chemicals induce these syndromes are not well understood. Various studies have shown that the incidence of these syndromes is much higher in individuals possessing certain HLA types, so it appears that there is a particular population at risk for the development of these syndromes when exposed to the appropriate stimuli. Various possible mechanisms can result in the production of auto-antibodies, and some of these have been studied with particular reference to drug-induced lupus:

1. **Cross-reactivity of drugs with nuclear antigens** Human studies to date have not shown drugs to inhibit the reaction of sera containing drug-induced anti-nuclear antibodies, with nuclear antigens [41].

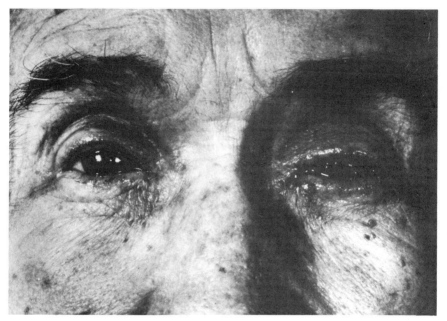

Fig. 1   Occulo-mucocutaneous syndrome associated with
practolol.

2. **Drug interaction with lymphocytes**   Drugs such as methyl-
    dopa are known to inhibit suppressor T-cell function
    directly [42], whereas hydralazine and procainamide induce
    the production of anti-lymphocyte antibodies and may
    affect lymphocyte function indirectly [43,44].

3. **"Neoantigen" formed by drugs combining with auto-antigens**
    This mechanism does not appear to play a role in the
    development of hydralazine- or procainamide-induced anti-
    nuclear antibodies [45].

Sjogren's Syndrome (Sicca Syndrome)

Sjorgren's syndrome is defined as the association of kerato
conjunctivitis sicca (dry eyes), xerostomia (dry mouth), and
a connective tissue disease, most frequently rheumatoid

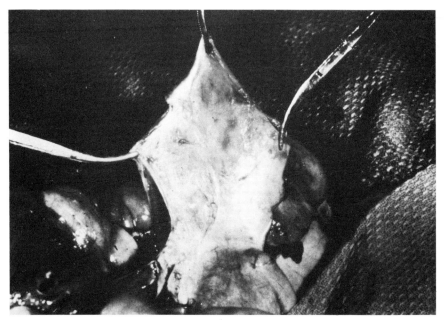

Fig. 2 Fibrous peritonitis associated with practolol. Note
the fibrous material attached to the peritoneum.

arthritis. Histologically there is a dense lymphoid infiltrate in the tissues. B-cell hyperactivity with the production of many auto-antibodies is also a feature.

Dry eyes may be associated with many conditions, e.g.
amyloidosis or sarcoidosis, and the association of dry eyes
with dry mouth, in the absence of connective tissue disease,
is called the Sicca syndrome.

The Practolol Syndrome

A specific oculo-mucocutaneous syndrome occurred as a side-
effect of the β-blocker drug, practolol. Clinically similar
to Sjogren's syndrome, this drug-induced syndrome was however
histologically and immunologically different. In the eye,
initial conjunctival changes showed hyperaemia with subsequent proliferation of vascular loops. These new blood

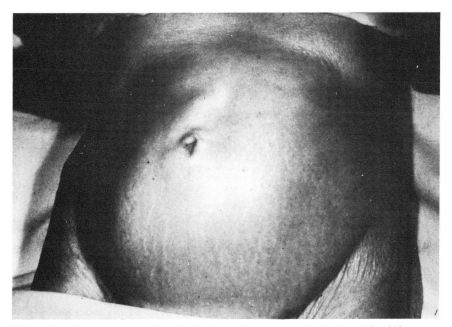

Fig. 3 Acute intestinal obstruction associated with fibrous
peritonitis following practolol administration.

vessels developed into a subconjuntival fibro-vascular sheet,
which subsequently contracted producing conjunctival scarring
and shrinkage (Fig. 1) [46]. There was no lymphoid infiltrate
of the affected tissues, as seen in the idiopathic Sjogren's
syndrome. Some patients who developed these eye changes also
developed other unwanted effects. A whole variety of skin
changes were described, but hyperkertosis of the palms, soles
and fingers, with a diffuse erythematosus, scaling, psoriasi-
form rash was a characteristic of this oculo-mucocutaneous
drug-induced syndrome [46,47]. Other associated side-effects
included deafness, tinnitus and an acute intestinal obstruction associated with the fibrous peritonitis (Figs. 2 and 3).

   Attempts to correlate the development of auto-antibodies
with this mucocutaneous syndrome were made. Wright found
that all 27 of his patients had positive anti-nuclear factors,
some in high titre, and 25 of these 27 patients also had

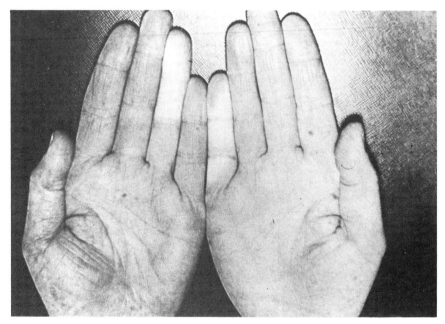

Fig. 4 Raynaud's syndrome showing vaso-constriction to the fingers.

circulating antibody to epithelial tissue [48]. Subsequent studies did not show such a close association. The reported incidence of positive anti-nuclear factor in patients treated with practolol varied from 11% to 16% for males and 24% for females [49]. Jachuk *et al*. reported that the incidence for the development of mucocutaneous complications was 10%, and 4 of the 5 patients with oculo-mucocutaneous reactions did not have positive anti-nuclear antibodies [50].

The development of a Sjogren-like syndrome has been reported to be associated with thiabendazole [51], and Sicca syndrome has been reported as a toxic reaction to busulphan therapy [52].

Raynaud's Phenomenon

This phenomenon is characterized by cold- or stress-induced

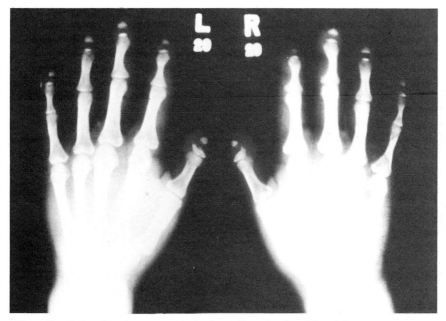

Fig. 5 Osteolysis associated with vinyl chloride exposure.
Note the loss of bone substance in the terminal digits of the
hands.

intermittent vasospasm of the peripheral circulation, resulting in white painful extremities (Fig. 4) which become
cyanosed and then hyperaemic, when the vasospasm is relieved.
In some patients this phenomenon may recur over many years,
with no further sequelae, but in others it may herald the
development of a connective tissue disease. The exact pathogenesis of this phenomenon is unknown, but many studies have
shown reduced hand and digital blood flow, in patients with
Raynaud's phenomenon [53-55]. Many treatments have been
tried in an attempt to reduce excessive sympathetic activity,
but long-term results have been disappointing [56]. More
recently encouraging results have followed infusions of
prostaglandin E_1, indicating that an imbalance of prostaglandin production may be contributory [57].
    Raynaud's phenomenon can be produced by exposure to certain

drugs. Several anti-hypersensitive drugs are capable of producing this phenomenon, but the incidence is greatest with
β-blocker drugs, being seen in up to 50% of patients [58].
The exact mechanism for the induction of vasospasm is unknown,
and it has been seen in patients treated with cardioselective
and non-cardioselective β-blocking agents [59]. Up to 37% of
patients treated with combinations of vinblastin and bleomycin
for treatment of germ cell testicular cancer, developed
Raynaud's phenomenon [60]. It is interesting to note that
neither bleomycin nor vinblastin used individually have been
associated with Raynaud's phenomenon, indicating that a
synergistic action may be necessary for this clinical side-
effect. Other drugs reported to be capable of producing
Raynaud's phenomenon in susceptible individuals include: the
contraceptive pill [61], ergotamine [62] and certain sulphonamides [63].

   This phenomenon is also a feature of vinyl chloride disease,
a systemic illness that occurs in some workers exposed to the
industrial chemical, vinyl chloride [64].

Systemic Sclerosis (Scleroderma)

In this disease there is excessive deposition of dense collagen bundles in various tissues. In the skin this results in
loss of elastic tissue, and dermal appendages, with subsequent sclerosis and thickening. In widespread systemic
sclerosis numerous organs are affected, with the development
of: arthritis, myositis, acrosclerosis, telangectasia and
calcinosis. Pulmonary fibrosis and renal insufficiency also
occur. Raynaud's phenomenon is invariably present and this
feature may precede the development of more extensive disease
by many years.

   The aetiology of systemic sclerosis remains obscure, but an
increased incidence has been reported in miners exposed to
silica dust [65], and vinyl chloride workers [64]. Clinical
features of systemic sclerosis have been described in late
sequealae of the Spanish toxic oil syndrome, and recent
studies have shown that nearly all patients developing these
late sequelae are women and that there is an association with
HLA DR3 and DR4 [66].

Vinyl Chloride Disease

The clinical features of vinyl chloride disease include:
sclerotic skin changes, Raynaud's phenomenon, osteolysis
(Fig. 5), arthralgias, myalgias, and impaired hepatic and
pulmonary function. Immunological changes have been reported in vinyl chloride disease, with: activation of the
classical complement pathway, hypergammaglobulinaemia, the

presence of mixed cryoglobulinaemia, and the presence of anti-nuclear antibodies [67]. These anti-nuclear antibodies have only been found to be present in low titre, and further studies have failed to identify anti-centromere antibodies [68]. Recent studies have found an increased incidence of HLA DR5 in these patients [68].

CONCLUSION

The aetiology of autoimmune disease remains obscure. This paper has considered many of the autoimmune diseases, and the drug-induced syndromes that mimic them. These drug-induced syndromes are *not* identical to the idiopathic disease, with both clinical and immunological differences apparent. They are however a disease model, using the most appropriate animal possible, namely, man himself.

ACKNOWLEDGEMENTS

I would like to thank Dr Carol Black for all her help and Dr Graham Hughes for his critical advice.

I would also like to thank Smith, Kline and French for their financial support during the last two years.

REFERENCES

1. Cluff, L.E. and Caldwell, J.R. (1979). Harrison's Principles of Internal Medicine, 8th edn. pp.346-352, Blakiston.
2. Alarcon-Segovia, D., Khalil, G., Wakim, K.G., Worthington, J.W. and Emmerson-Ward, L. (1967). *Medicine* **46**, 1-33.
3. Blomgren, S.E., Condemi, J.J. and Vaughn, J.H. (1972). *Am. J. Med.* **52**, 338-348.
4. Condemi, J.J., Blomgren, S.E. and Vaughn, J.H. (1970). *Bulletin on the Rheumatic Disease* **20**, 604-608.
5. Lee, S.L. and Harvey-Chase, P. (1975). *Seminars in Arthritis Rheumatism* **5**, 83-103.
6. Ladd, A.T. (1962). *N. Engl. J. Med.* **267**, 1357-1358.
7. Alarcon-Segovia, D. (1969). *Mayo Clinic Proc.* **44**, 664-681.
8. Dubois, E.L. (1969). *Medicine* **48**, 217-228.
9. Mitchell-Perry, H. (1973). *Am. J. Med.* **54**, 58-72.
10. Hughes, G.R.V. (1971). *Lancet* **2**, 861-863.
11. Hughes, G.R.V., Rynes, R.I., Gharavi, A.E. *et al.* (1981). *Arth. and Rheum.* **24**, 1070-1073.
12. Koffler, D., Sabur, P.H. and Kunkel, H.G. (1967). *J. Exp. Med.* **126**, 706-623.
13. Winfield, J.B., Koffler, J. and Kunkel, H.G. (1975). *Arth. and Rheum.* **18**, 531-534.

14. Carpenter, J.R., McDuffie, F.C., Sheps, S.G. *et al.* (1980). *Am. J. Med.* **69**, 395-400.
15. Klajman, A., Camin-Belsky, N., Kimchi, A. and Ben-Efraim, S. (1970). *Clin. Exptl. Immunol.* **7**, 641-649.
16. Tan, E.N. and Portanova, J.P. (1981). *Arth. and Rheum.* **24**, 1064-1069.
17. Fritzler, N.J. and Tan, E.N. (1978). *J. Clin. Invest.* **62**, 560-567.
18. Portanova, J.P., Rubin, R.L., Jocelyn, F.G. *et al.* (1982). *Clin. Immunol. Immunopathol.* **25**, 67-79.
19. Hess, E.V. (1981). *Arth. and Rheum.* **24**, vi-ix.
20. Weinstein, A. (1980). *Prog. and Clin. Immunol.* **4**, 1-21.
21. Harmon, E.C. and Portanova, J.P. (1982). *Clin. in Rheum. Dis.* **8**, 121-135.
22. Batchelor, J.R., Welsh, K.I., Mansilla-Tinoco, R. *et al.* (1980). *Lancet* **1**, 1107-1109.
23. Reinertson, J.L., Klippel, J.H., Johnson, A.H. *et al.* (1978). *N. Engl. J. Med.* **299**, 515-518.
24. Celada, A., Barras, C., Benzonana, G. *et al.* (1979). *N. Engl. J. Med.* **301**, 1398.
25. Gladman, D.D., Terasaki, P.I., Park, M.S. *et al.* (1979). *Lancet* **ii**, 902.
26. Black, C.M., Welsh, K.I., Fielder, A. *et al. Lancet,* in press.
27. Woosley, R.L., Drayer, D.E., Reidenberg, M.M. *et al.* (1978). *N. Engl. J. Med.* **298**, 1157-1159.
28. Lahita, R., Kluger, J., Drayer, D.E. *et al.* (1978). *New Engl. J. Med.* **301**, 1382-1385.
29. Molina, J., Dubois, E.L., Bilitch, M. *et al.* (1969). *Arth. and Rheum.* **12**, 608-614.
30. Rothfield, N.F., Bierer, W.F. and Garfield, J.W. (1978). *Ann. Intern. Med.* **88**, 650-652.
31. Godeau, P., Aukert, M., Imbert, J.-C. and Herreman, G. (1973). *Ann. Med. Interne.* **124**, 181-186.
32. Price-Evans, D.A., Bullen, M.F., Houston, J. *et al.* (1972). *J. Med. Genetics* **9**, 53-56.
33. Walshe, J.M. (1981). *J. Rheumatol.* Suppl. 7, **8**, 155-160.
34. Lee, S.L. and Chase, P.H. (1975). *Seminars in Arth. and Rheum.* **5**, 83-103.
35. Crouzet, J., Camus, J.P., Leca, A.P. *et al.* (1974). *Ann. Med. Int.* **125**, 71-79.
36. Bucknall, R.C., Dixon, A., St. Glick, E.N. *et al.* (1975). *Brit. Med. J.* **1**, 600-602.
37. Campus, J.P., Homberg, J.C., Bach, J.F. *et al.* (1976). In "Penicillamine Research in Rheumatoid Disease" (ed. E. Menthe), pp.161-165. Fabritius and Sonner, Oslo.
38. Genth, E., Genth, A., Simon, E. *et al.* (1979). 9th Europ. Cong. Rheumatology — Wiesbaden 1 (ed. Ciba-Geigy)

Basel, Abstract No.495.

39. Ameent, H.J.W., Van der Kort, J.K., Van Durgt, A.C. *et al.*
    (1978). *Dr. K. Landstrteiner Foundation Annual Report* 1,
    (ed. NEBN) Redcross, Amsterdam.
40. Grob, P.J., Muller-Schoop, J.W., Hacti, M.A. and Holler-
    Jemelken, H.I. (1975). *Lancet* ii, 144-148.
41. Carpenter, J.R., McDuffie, F.C., Sheps, S.G. *et al.* (1980).
    Am. J. Med. **69**, 395-400.
42. Kirtland, H.H., Mohler, D.N. and Horwitz, D.A. (1980).
    N. Engl. J. Med. **302**, 825-832.
43. Ryan, P.F.J., Hughes, G.R.V., Bernstein, R. *et al.* (1979).
    Lancet ii, 1248-1249.
44. Bluestein, H.G., Zvaifler, N.J., Weisman, M.H. and
    Shapiro, R.F. (1979). *Lancet* ii, 816-819.
45. Gold, E.F., Ben-Efraim, S., Faivisewitz, A. *et al.* (1977).
    Clin. Immunol. Immunopathol. **7**, 176-186.
46. Wright, P. (1975). *Brit. Med. J.* **1**, 595-598.
47. Felix, R.H., Ive, F.A. and Dahl, M.G.C. (1974). *Brit.
    Med. J.* **4**, 321-324.
48. Amos, H.E., Brigden, W.D. and McKerron, R.A. (1975).
    Brit. Med. J. **1**, 589-600.
49. Raftery, E.B. (1974). *Brit. Med. J.* **4**, 653.
50. Jachuck, S.J., Stephenson, J., Bird, T. *et al.* (1977).
    Postgrad. Med. J. **53**, 75-77.
51. Fink, A.I., McKay, C.J. and Cutler, S.S. (1979).
    Ophthalmol. **86**, 1892-1896.
52. Sidi, Y., Douer, D. and Pinkhas, J. (1977). *J.A.M.A.*
    238, 1951.
53. Peacock, J.H. (1959). *Clin. Sci.* **18**, 25-33.
54. Mendlowitz, M. and Naftchi, N. (1959). *Am. J. Card.* **4**,
    580-4.
55. Coffman, J.D. and Cohen, A.S. (1971). *New Engl. J. Med.*
    285, 259-263.
56. Baddeley, R.M. (1965). *Brit. J. Surg.* **52**, 426-430.
57. Clifford, P.C. *et al.* (1980). *Brit. Med. J.* **281**, 1031-4.
58. Marshall, A.J., Roberts, C.J.C. and Barritt, D.W. (1976).
    Brit. Med. J. **1**, 1498-1499.
59. Eliasson, K., Lins, L. and Sundqvist, K. (1979). *Acta
    Med. Scand.* Suppl. **628**, 39-46.
60. Vogelzang, N.J., Bosl, G.J., Johnson, K. and Kennedy, B.J.
    (1981). *Ann. Intern. Med.* **95**, 288-292.
61. Birnstingl, M. (1971). *Postgrad. Med. J.* **47**, 297-310.
62. Robb, L.G. (1975). *West. J. Med.* **123**, 231-5.
63. Reid, J., Holt, S., Housley, E. and Sneddon, D.J.C.
    (1980). *Postgrad. Med. J.* **56**, 106-107.
64. Veltman, G., Lange, C.E., Juhe, S. *et al.* (1975). *Ann.
    N.Y. Acad. Sci.* **246**, 6-17.
65. Rodnan, G.P., Benekek, T.G., Medsger, T.A. Jr. *et al.*

(1967). *Ann. Intern. Med.* **66**, 323-334.

66. Noriega, A.R., Gomez-Rein, O.J., Lopez-Encuentra, A. *et al.* (1982). *Lancet* **2**, 697-702.

67. Ward, A.M., Udnoon, S., Watkins, J., Walker, A.E. and Dark, S.C. (1976). *Brit. Med. J.* **1**, 936-938.

68. Black, C.M., McGreggor, A., Bernstein, R.M. *et al.* Lancet, in press.

MOLECULAR MECHANISMS
OF CHEMICAL-MEDIATED IMMUNOPATHOLOGY

D.V. Parke and G.G. Gibson

*Department of Biochemistry, University of Surrey,
Guildford, Surrey GU2 5XH, U.K.*

INTRODUCTION

Despite the rigorous safety evaluation of new drugs and other
chemicals, toxicity still continues to be manifest, especially
in certain idiosyncratic individuals. Furthermore, the nature
of toxicity manifested in man is very frequently immunological
in origin, or at least has an immunological component. The
reasons why immunological aspects of toxicity manifest themselves so frequently in man, are not hard to find as: 1) most
aspects of drug and chemical toxicity are revealed in the
development of new compounds by the comprehensive animal
safety evaluation studies, which however do not include
examination for immunotoxicity potential, and 2) because of
the high degree of immunological competency in man, humans
are particularly susceptible to immunotoxicity of chemicals.
Furthermore, it is difficult to find a suitable animal model
for man in safety evaluation studies.

CHEMICAL ANTIGENS

Lipophilic drugs and chemicals ingested into the body become
temporarily sequestered into the lipid rich components of the
body and its cells, for example the lipid membranes of the
endoplasmic reticulum of the liver cells. These lipophilic
chemicals are progressively removed from the organism by
metabolism which converts them to more hydrophilic compounds
and thereby accelerates their elimination. This metabolism
may result in the detoxication of the drugs and chemicals or,
alternatively, in their activation into reactive intermediates.
These reactive intermediates are generally electrophiles,
such as epoxides, quinones, free radicals, or alkylating
agents which ultimately bind covalently to tissue macro-

molecules, including proteins, RNA and DNA. The covalent binding to plasma and tissue proteins results in the formation of foreign proteins, which may function as circulating and bound antigens.

Drugs and other chemicals may also undergo metabolism to free radicals, which may in turn generate radicals from tissue constituents, and these secondary radicals are also capable of covalently binding to proteins and DNA. This means that the covalently-bound material need not always originate from the chemical initially ingested, e.g. after exposure of animals to higher dialkyl nitrosamines, the resultant adduct is methyl DNA and not the higher alkyl DNA.

The major pathway for the metabolism of drugs and other chemicals is that of mixed-function oxidation, the enzymes of which are located in the endoplasmic reticulum of the cells of liver, gut, lungs, kidney, etc. The major mechanism of mixed-function oxidation is cytochrome P-450-dependent, but other mechanisms of drug oxygenation are known which are mediated by the flavoprotein oxidoreductases of both endoplasmic reticulum and cytosol. It is known that different chemicals may undergo metabolism to form the same reactive intermediate, and hence could give rise to the same chemical antigen. This explains the cross-reactivity observed with many drugs and chemicals, whereby exposure to one chemical appears to induce an immune response to a number of related compounds.

Chemicals that contain an aldehyde group (glucose) or a carbonyl moiety adjacent to a hydroxy group (cortisol, 16α-hydroxyoestrone) can react non-enzymically with proteins to form Schiff base intermediates and hence antigenic proteins. Indeed, it has been proposed that the formation of covalent adducts between cortisol or 16 α -hydroxyoestrone and tissue or plasma proteins may be antigenic and result in immunological injury, as in systemic lupus erythematosus [1].

As the covalent binding of reactive intermediates to DNA is associated with mutations and with malignancy, and covalent binding of reactive intermediates to proteins is associated with immunological injury, chemicals that are associated with mutations are also likely to be associated with immunological injury and vice versa.

MOLECULAR MECHANISMS OF IMMUNOLOGICAL RESPONSE

The covalent binding of the reactive intermediates of drugs and other chemicals to plasma and tissue proteins may result in the formation of novel proteins and other macromolecules, which may act as circulating and bound antigens, resulting in the formation of immunoglobulins. The formation of bound

antibodies may result in immunological injury, and consequent
tissue necrosis on further exposure of the individual to the
initiating chemical, or sometimes to related molecules.
Immune complexes are formed in the circulation or tissues by
interaction of exogenous (bacteria, chemical-protein complexes) or endogenous (spent tissue proteins) antigens with
their corresponding antibodies, and once formed have the
ability to activate a variety of autacoids (histamine, bradykinin, 5-hydroxytryptamine, catecholamines). Circulating
immune complexes vary in size, large complexes are rapidly
eliminated by the reticulo-endothelial system and small complexes do not appreciably activate autacoids, but circulating
immune complexes of intermediate size may persist for long
periods and cause tissue injuries (glomerulonephritis,
systemic lupus erythematosus) [2].

Thus re-exposure of the sensitized individual to the chemical, or related compounds which may be metabolized to yield
the same reactive intermediate, may result in an immune reaction which will vary according to the site, but may involve
one or more of the following: inflammation, vasodilation,
pain, oedema, bronchoconstriction, ulceration (Arthus reaction), and cell death and necrosis. These physiological responses to immune reactions are initiated by a number of chemical mediators, including the autacoids (noradrenaline, histamine, 5-hydroxytryptamine and bradykinin), and the eicosanoids. Bradykinin and noradrenaline also stimulate prostaglandin synthesis, by increasing the release of arachidonic
acid from phospholipids [3]. The migration of leucocytes
through the endothelium into the tissues is a well-known
characteristic of inflammation, and the migration of lymphocytes, from various sources, shows a dose-dependent stimulation by the autacoids, 5-hydroxytryptamine and bradykinin,
and by the lymphokines, the mediators of delayed hypersensitivity [4].

Two types of histamine receptor, H_1 and H_2, are known and
are associated with the production of different eicosanoids.
In the guinea pig lung, H_1 receptors appear to be responsible for the release of thromboxane A_2, and the enhanced
response in sensitized lungs may be due to the interconversion
of H_2- into H_1-receptors [5]. Histamine receptors are found
in many tissues including the skin, gut and also leukocytes.
The role of H_2 receptors can be studied with H_2-receptor
antagonists, such as cimetidine, which has been shown to
exert various modulating effects on the immune status including, depression of cytotoxic lymphocytes with exacer-
bation of brucellosis [6], restoration of cell-mediated
immunity by inhibiting lymphocytes with modulate production
of migration inhibiting factor (M.I.F.) [7], and inactivation

of host suppressor cells with successful inhibition of tumour growth and metastasis [8].

The inflammatory response is also associated with the generation of peroxide and other species of active oxygen by monocyte macrophages and neutrophils, the physiological role of which is probably the destruction of bacteria and other infectious agents which are phagocytosed by the tissue-invading polymorphs and monocytes. Macrophages are essential to chronic inflammation and release both prostaglandins and tissue-destructive lysosomal enzymes [3].

Environmental chemicals may also result in immunosuppression. The offspring of chlordane-exposed mice exhibited severe depression of the cell-mediated immune response possibly due to a reduction in the activity or number of T effector cells as there was no effect on the T-cell-dependent humoral immune response [9].

IMMUNE GLYCOPROTEINS

The immunoglobulins are glycoproteins which are synthesized on the endoplasmic reticulum of the lymphocytes. Interferons (type 1) are gylcoproteins synthesized by most cells of the body and, in addition to their direct antiviral action, also exert a regulatory function on the immune system by modulating the various activities of lymphocytes and macrophages. Lymphokines are glycoproteins released by antigen-activated lymphocytes which also have important immune regulatory activities [10].

During inflammatory processes a leukocytic endogenous mediator (LEM) is released by cells of the reticulo-endothelial system, which induces changes in the synthesis of glycoproteins (export proteins) by the liver. This results in changes in the plasma concentration of the "acute phase proteins" - more than 100 different trauma-inducible, glycoproteins (e.g. α_1-antitrypsin, fibrinogen, haptoglobin, fibronectin, ceruloplasmin) with various biological functions directed against the destructive action of tissue inflammation. For example, α_1-antitrypsin, an antiprotease, inhibits the lysosomal enzyme activity of granulocytes, fibrinogen restricts extension of the site of inflammation, haptoglobin — as the haemoglobin complex — induces collagen synthesis at the site of inflammation, fibronectin mediates reticuloendothelial phagocytic activity [11] and ceruloplasmin is anti-inflammatory [12].

Chemical damage to the membranes of the endoplasmic reticulum, such as may occur by the interaction of free radicals and other reactive intermediates of toxic chemicals with the membranes, may cause loss of the ribosomes (RNA)

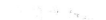

from the membranes, with impairment of glycoprotein synthesis, and impairment of the immune response. Attachment of the ribosomes to the endoplasmic reticulum membranes appears to be essential for the synthesis of glycoproteins and for the synthesis of export proteins, and in the liver is mediated by sex hormones and corticosteroids. The mediation of the attachment of the ribosomes to the endoplasmic reticulum in the leukocytes is not yet understood.

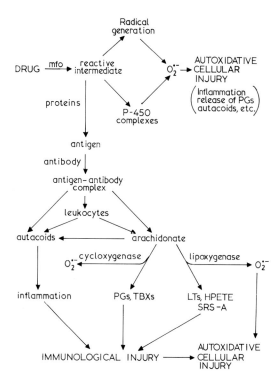

Fig. 1 **The role of eicosanoids in immunological and auto-oxidative cellular injury.** The abbreviations used are MFO: mixed function oxidative enzymes of the endoplasmic reticulum; P-450: cytochrome P-450; PG: prostaglandin; TBX: thromboxanes; LT: leukotrienes; HPETE: hydroperoxyeicosatetranoic acid; SRS-A: slow-reacting substance of anaphylaxis.

THE EICOSANOIDS

The eicosanoids are a diverse miscellany of biologically active compounds derived from C-20 unsaturated fatty acids such as arachidonic acid. They comprise the prostaglandins,

thromboxanes, and leukotrienes, formed by the oxygenation of
arachidonic acid by the cyclo-oxygenase (prostaglandins and
thromboxanes) and lipoxygenase (leukotrienes) pathways.
Arachidonic acid is released by the action of phospholipase-A
on the phospholipids of intracellular membranes, especially
those of the endoplasmic reticulum, following a complex series
of membrane reactions initiated by catecholamines, immunoglobulin complexes, IgE antigens, etc. [13,14] (see Fig. 1).
The enzymes catalysing these various reactions leading to the
biosynthesis of the prostaglandins and thromboxanes, include
the cytochrome P-450-dependent mixed-function oxidases [15,16].

Prostaglandins, together with the thromboxanes, and possibly
the leukotrienes, are synthesized in the monocyte macrophages,
but probably not by lymphocytes, and can be induced non-
specifically (phagocytosis of antigen-antibody complexes) or
specifically in response to lymphokines (from sensitized
T-cells after specific antigen stimulation) [17]. PGEs are
vasodilators and cause erythema, but do not produce oedema or
pain, although both PGE_2 and PGI_2 markedly increase the
oedema and pain responses of histamine and bradykinin, so
that in this respect prostaglandins are modulators of inflammation. PGE (cyclo-oxygenase pathway) is chemotactic for
neutrophils, but 5-HETE and the leukotriene, LTB_4, synthesized
in neutrophils by the lipoxygenase pathway, are most potent
chemotactic agents for leukocytes [18]. LTB_4 also stimulates
the release of lysozyme from neutrophils (degranulation) [19]
and, in the presence of neutrophils, produce marked increases
in vascular permeability [18]. Not only have the prostaglandins and leukotrienes roles as mediators and modulators
of inflammation, but they also function as modulators of the
immune response. Lymphocytes have specific receptors for
prostaglandins, especially PGE_1 which stimulates lymphocyte
cyclic AMP formation and inhibits T-, and possibly B-,
lymphocyte function [17]. PGEs, which may display either
pro- or anti-inflammatory effects [20], have been shown to
inhibit lymphokine formation, antibody production, lymphocyte
cytotoxicity, and can suppress both acute immune complex-
induced vasculitis and chronic adjuvant-induced polyarthritis
[21].

Certain products of the lipoxygenation of arachidonic acid,
especially 5-HETE (5-hydroxyeicosatetranoic acid) and the
leukotrienes, are unique to leukocytes and may be more important than the cyclo-oxygenase metabolites as mediators of
allergic and inflammatory states. Among these products is
the slow-reacting substance of anaphylaxis (SRS-A), the smooth
muscle contractile factor of immediate-type hypersensitivity
reactions, which has recently been identified as a mixture of
cysteine peptide derivatives of 5-HPETE (5-hydroperoxy-

Table 1 *Effect of indomethacin on metabolism of arachidonic acid in hamster isolated lungs.*

Studies were made on the effect of indomethacin (0-15 μM), infused into the pulmonary circulation, on the amounts of arachidonate and metabolites present in the pulmonary perfusion effluent following pulmonary injection of 66 nmol of ^{14}C-arachidonate.

Indomethacin: concn. (μM)	0	0.15	1.5	15
		% control		
Arachidonic acid	100 (500 pmol)	80	140	170
6-Keto-PGF$_{1\alpha}$	100 (220 pmol)	45	45	15
PGF$_{2\alpha}$	100 (120 pmol)	55	50	10
PGE$_2$	100 (140 pmol)	50	40	15
TXB$_2$	100 (700 pmol)	55	10	3
PGD$_2$	100 (65 pmol)	70	30	15
PGA$_2$	100 (115 pmol)	35	20	15

(From 24)

eicosatetranoic acid) [14,22]. In addition to the formation
of these various eicosanoids, the oxygenation of arachidonic
acid also yields active oxygen and malondialdehyde as side-
products.

The eicosanoids are, in turn, metabolically deactivated by
the cytochrome P-450-dependent mixed-function oxidases, so
that microsomal oxidative metabolism is responsible for
i) the biosynthesis of the eicosanoids, and ii) the degradation of the eicosanoids.

Corticosteroids (which inhibit phospholipase A_2) and non-
steroidal anti-inflammatory drugs (NSAIDs, e.g. salicylates,
indomethacin, ibuprofen), together with a wide variety of
natural (long-chain fatty acids) and synthetic (chloroquine,
sulphasalazine) substances, act as inhibitors or prostaglandin
biosynthesis, while other drugs (clomipramine, chloroquine,
methylxanthines) act as prostaglandin antagonists by blocking
receptors [23]. NSAIDs inhibit predominantly the cyclo-
oxygenase pathway, although indomethacin has been shown to
inhibit both cyclooxygenase and lipoxygenase pathways of
arachidonic acid metabolism in isolated hamster lungs (see
Table 1) [24]. The chromones are potent antagonists of
SRS-A [25]. Most NSAIDs inhibit both prostaglandin synthesis
and prostaglandin breakdown and it is therefore necessary to
consider the ratio of the inhibitory effects on metabolic
breakdown and synthesis; ibuprofen and flubiprofen are among
the most potent inhibitors of synthesis, and sulphasalazine
and carbenoxolone are potent inhibitors of prostaglandin
breakdown [26].

As a result of the release of arachidonic acid from phospholipids by phospholipase A, lysophosphatides, such as lysolecithins are also formed. Lysolecithins are also modulators
of inflammation and exhibit both pro-inflammatory and anti-
inflammatory properties. When injected subcutaneously, they
induce oedema, which differs from eicosanoid-reduced oedema
in not being inhibited by indomethacin [27].

Hence, in the interaction of drugs and other chemicals with
the immune system of the body, the endoplasmic reticulum
serves as the focus of the following phenomena: 1) disposition of the lyphophilic chemicals; 2) metabolic detoxication of drugs and chemicals; 3) metabolic activation
to reactive intermediates; 4) synthesis of immunoglobulins;
5) synthesis of lymphokines; 6) a source of arachidonic acid;
7) the site of activation of arachidonate to eicosanoids;
8) the site of deactivation of the eicosanoids. All of these
reactions may occur in the endoplasmic reticulum of the liver,
gut, lung, kidney and leukocytes.

Hence it is not surprising that various kinds of interactions occur between drugs and toxic chemicals and the immune
system.

OXYGEN TOXICITY

Hydrogen peroxide, superoxide anion radical and various other active forms of oxygen are generated by NADPH-dependent enzymes of the endoplasmic reticulum, and other enzymes in phagocytosing granulocytes and monocyte macrophages, to result in the destruction of infectious organisms. A similar system is probably occurring continuously within most cells to result in the regular turnover of the membranes of the endoplasmic reticulum, and possibly the lipid components of other membranes. This destructive process is controlled by a number of antioxidant mechanisms, including the enzymes superoxide dismutase, catalase and glutathione peroxidase, antioxidants such as ascorbate and α-tocopherol, and the redox buffer glutathione, which prevent this functional generation of peroxide and reactive oxygen from becoming too extended and thereby causing more extensive damage to the cell leading to possible tissue necrosis.

Scavengers of active oxygen species have been shown to decrease the inflammatory response, and α-tocopherol and propyl gallate (antioxidants) inhibit experimental granuloma formation. Catalase, but not superoxide dismutase alone, administered locally, inhibited granuloma formation, but superoxide dismutase potentiated the effect of catalase when both were administered, probably because the catalase protects superoxide dismutase against destruction by peroxide. Phenidone, an inhibitor of both the cyclooxygenase and lipoxygenase pathways of arachidonate metabolism, also inhibited granuloma formation [28]. However, superoxide dismutase administered intravenously inhibited inflammation in several experimental models, and has been shown to interact with a plasma factor to produce a potent chemotactic factor for neutrophils [29].

These natural destructive oxidation processes can however, be accelerated and augmented by the action of a foreign

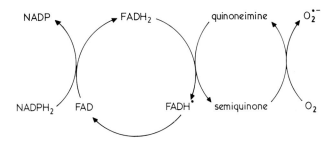

Fig. 2   Activation of tissue dioxygen by quinoneimines.

chemical. Reactive intermediates such as quinone and
quinoneimines can act as generators of superoxide and
hydroxyl radicals, and singlet oxygen, by a cyclic process
of one electron reduction by flavoprotein oxidoreductases,
followed by interaction with tissue oxygen (see Fig. 2).

INTERACTION BETWEEN THE METABOLISM OF DRUGS AND EICOSANOIDS

For more than half a century it has been considered that the
drug-metabolizing enzymes are enzymes in search of physiological substrates. In recent decades, some of these physiological substrates have been identified, for example cholesterol, steroids, non-peptide hormones, and fatty acids, but
more recently it has become apparent that oxygenation of
arachidonate, with the formation of the prostaglandins,
prostacyclins and thromboxanes, presents a whole new rationale
for the existence of the microsomal oxygenases and particularly the cytochrome P-450-dependent mixed-function
oxidases. The discovery of the leukotrienes has extended
this raison d'etre to glutathione conjugations occurring in
the cytosol. Although not all the oxygenations of arachidonate are cytochrome P-450-dependent a number of these reactions, monooxygenations and dioxygenations, do appear to be
catalysed by cytochrome P-450, although the particular cyto-
chromes concerned are probably different forms from those
concerned in the oxygenation of drugs and foreign chemicals.
Hence in the biosynthesis of the eicosanoids, a close
parallel exists with the metabolic reactions involved in the
metabolism of drugs, carcinogens, and other chemicals.

During the metabolism of arachidonate, active oxygen,
presumably the hydroxyl radical OH$^•$, is released, which may
inactivate many enzymes of the prostaglandin synthesis cascade, or may effect the co-oxygenation of xenobiotic substrates [3]. In this way, prostaglandin synthesis catalyses
the activation of paracetamol [30], and activates the carcinogens diethylstilboestrol [31], p-dimethylaminoazobenzene
(butter yellow) (see Table 2) [32], benzo(a)pyrene [33] and
several other carcinogenic polycyclic dihydrodiols [34]. The
products of co-oxygenation differ from those normally formed
in the liver by cytochrome P-450-dependent mixed-function
oxidation, in that they are more highly reactive, toxic and
carcinogenic. The mechanism for this co-oxygenation involves
a novel form of mixed-function oxygenation, by which arachidonate is oxygenated by molecular oxygen to the hydroperoxides
PGG$_2$ and 5-HPETE; these are then further metabolized to the
corresponding hydroxy derivatives with loss of active oxygen,
probably hydroxyl radicals, which subsequently hydroxylate
xenobiotics non-enzymically. The reason for the greater

Table 2 *Covalent binding of metabolites of* ^{14}C-*p*-*dimethyl-aminobenzene to exogenous DNA by prostaglandin synthetase in vitro.*

	Pig bladder microsomes		Sheep vesicular microsomes	
	DNA	Protein	DNA	Protein
	(nmol/g)		(nmol/g)	
Microsomes only	3	10	8	7
Microsomes + NADPH	60	100	8	7
Microsomes + cumene hydroperoxide	430	1400		
Microsomes + arachidonate	800	1400	4100	4300
Denatured microsomes + arachidonate	20	80	7	7

(From reference 32)

formation of reactive intermediates is that the arachidonate-dependent oxygenation appears to parallel cytochrome P-448-dependent oxygenation in that sterically-hindered, as well as sterically non-hindered, positions in the xenobiotic molecules ("bay regions") are oxygenated, whereas cytochrome P-450 appears able only to insert oxygen in unhindered positions. When a xenobiotic (carcinogen) becomes oxygenated at a sterically-hindered position, epoxide hydrase, and possibly other detoxicating enzymes, are unable to accept these reactive intermediates as substrates, leaving the latter to interact non-enzymically with glutathione and tissue macromolecules. Immunological injury, with the accelerated release of the eicosanoids may therefore result in the co-oxygenation and activation of carcinogens, with consequent increase in the risk of malignancy.

Prostaglandins are deactivated by ω-(C-20) and ω-1-(C-19) hydroxylation, and eventually are excreted in the urine as dicarboxylic acids. Inducing agents of the cytochrome P-450-dependent monooxygenases, such as benzo(a)pyrene and Aroclor, appear to increase only the 19-hydroxylation of prostaglandins [35].

Immunosuppresant drugs, such as indomethacin, markedly inhibit many facets of prostaglandin biosynthesis, and consequently neutralize other physiological roles of prostaglandins, in addition to suppressing their immunological functions. Among these other physiological functions of prostaglandins is their cytoprotective action on the gastric and intestinal mucosa, probably by enhancing the micro-circulation and stimulating the secretion of mucus [36]. So, following administration of indomethacin and other NSAIDs for treatment of rheumatoid arthritis, depletion of mucus and gastrointestinal inflammation and ulceration can occur, which may be prevented or treated by administration of prosta-glandins.

Prostaglandin biosynthesis is one of the factors involved in the failure of the immune system to reject neoplasia. For although PGE_2 is an important mediator of inflammation, it is also a feedback inhibitor on the immune response, including T-cell function and antibody production [37], and prosta-glandins E_2 and $F_{2\alpha}$ markedly enhanced 3-methylcholanthrene-induced squamous cell carcinoma in mice [38]. Inhibitors of prostaglandin synthesis (indomethacin) cause marked retard-ation in the growth of transplanted mouse tumours [37] and NSAIDs may therefore have a role in anticancer therapy.

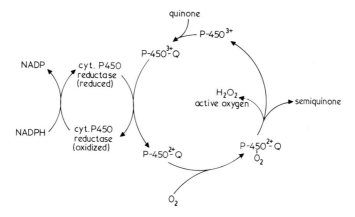

Fig. 3 Cytochrome P-450-mediated oxygen activation

INTERACTION BETWEEN THE METABOLISM OF DRUGS AND OXYGEN TOXICITY

The formation of ligand complexes from the interaction of reactive intermediates with cytochrome P-450, and the co-valent binding of reactive intermediates to the cytochrome, are known to result in autoxidative reactions, probably by a modulation of the cytochrome P-450 catalytic cycle, to gener-ate superoxy anion or hydrogen peroxide (see Fig. 3). This generation of peroxide and reactive oxygen by the cytochrome P-450 mixed-function oxidation mechanism leads to destruction

of the endoplasmic reticulum, and particularly denaturation
of cytochrome P-450 to cytochrome P-420 and its eventual
oxidation by haem oxygenase.

Reactive intermediates of certain xenobiotics, such as
nitro compounds (e.g. the 5-nitrofurans), quinoneimines (e.g.
anthracycline antibiotics, and intermediate metabolites of
aromatic compounds) may also generate active oxygen by a
cyclic process involving one-electron flavoprotein reduction
with the formation of free radical nitroso compounds and
semiquinones which then subsequently interact with tissue
oxygen to generate hydroxyl radicals and superoxy anion [39].

The microsomal flavoprotein NADPH-cytochrome P-450 reduc-
tase is one such enzyme that catalyses one-electron reductions of quinones to semiquinones with the concomitant cyclic
generation of active oxygen radicals whereas, in contrast,
the cytosolic flavoprotein DT-diaphorase catalyses a two-
electron reduction of quinones to hydroquinones, which are
then detoxicated by conjugation and do not lead to the
activation of oxygen [40]. These other mechanisms for the
generation of reactive oxygen, subsequent to the formation of
reactive intermediates from drugs and other chemicals, may
result in some of the characteristics of immunological injury
becoming manifest, without any direct involvement of the
immune response. Hence there are two alternative pathways
for autoxidative cellular injury resulting from toxic chemicals, namely:

1. Chemical ⟶ reactive intermediate ⟶ covalent
    antigen ⟶ immune reaction ⟶ autacoids + active
    oxygen

2. Chemical ⟶ reactive intermediates ⟶ direct
    generation of H_2O_2 and active oxygen.

REFERENCES

1. Bucala, R., Fishman, J. and Cerami, A. (1982). *Proc.
    Natl. Acad. Sci. U.S.A.* **79**, 3320-3324.
2. Ritzmann, S.E. and Daniels, J.C. (1982). *Clin. Chem.*
    28, 1259-1271.
3. Kuehl, F.A. Jr. and Egan, R.W. (1980). *Science* **210**,
    978-984.
4. Paegelow, I. and Lange, P. (1982). In "Trends in
    Inflammation Research",2. (eds. H. Bekemeier and R.
    Hirschelmann), pp.255-262, *Agents and Actions*, Suppl.,
    10, Birkhäuser, Basel.
5. Berti, F., Folco, G.C., Nicosia, S., Omini, C. and
    Pasargiklian, R. (1979). *Br. J. Pharmacol.* **65**, 629-633.
6. Thornes, R.D. (1982). *Lancet* **2**, 217.

7. Daman, L.A. and Rosenberg, E.W. (1977). *Lancet* **2**, 1087.
8. Osband, M.E., Shen, Y.-J., Shlesinger, M., Brown, A., Hamilton, D., Cohen, E., Lavin, P. and McCaffrey, R. (1981). *Lancet* **i**, 636-638.
9. Spyker-Cranmer, J.M., Barnett, J.B., Avery, D.L. and Cranmer, M.F. (1982). *Toxicol. Appl. Pharmacol.* **62**, 402-408.
10. De Maeyer, E. and De Maeyer-Guinard, J. (1981). *C.R.C. Critical Rev. Immunology* **2**, 167-188.
11. Mosher, D.F., Proctor, R.A. and Grossman, J.E. (1981). *Adv. in Inflammation Res.* **2**, 187-207.
12. Schade, R., Götz, F., Porstmann, B., Friedrich, A. and Nugel, E. (1982). In "Trends in Inflammation Research" 2, (eds. H. Bekemeier and R. Hirschelmann), pp.213-231, *Agents and Actions*, Suppl., **10**, Birkhäuser, Basel.
13. Goetzl, E.J. (1981). *Med. Clin. N. Amer.* **65**, 809-828.
14. Wolfe, L.S. (1982). *J. Neurochem.* **38**, 1-14.
15. Oliw, E.E., Guengerich, F.P. and Oates, J.A. (1982). *J. Biol. Chem.* **257**, 3771-3781.
16. Capdevila, J., Marnett, L.J., Chacos, N., Prough, R.A. and Estabrook, R.W. (1982). *Proc. Natl. Acad. Sci. U.S.A.* **79**, 767-770.
17. Goldyne, M.E. and Stobo, J.D. (1981). *C.R.C. Crit. Rev. Immunology* **2**, 189-223.
18. Ford-Hutchinson, A.W. (1981). *J. Roy. Soc. Med.* **74**, 831-833.
19. Bokoch, G.M. and Reed, P.W. (1981). *J. Biol. Chem.* **256**, 5317-5320.
20. Bonta, I.L. and Parnham, M.J. (1982). *Int. J. Immunopharmacol.* **4**, 103-109.
21. Kinkel, S.L., Ogawa, H., Conran, P.B., Ward, P.A. and Zurier, R.B. (1981). *Arthritis and Rheumatism* **24**, 1151-1158.
22. Ohnishi, H., Kosuzume, H., Kitamura, Y., Tamaguchi, K., Nobuhara, M., Suzuki, Y., Yoshida, S., Tomioka, H. and Kumagai, A. (1980). *Prostaglandins* **20**, 655-666.
23. Metz, S.A. (1981). *Med. Clin. North America* **65**, 713-757.
24. Uotila, P., Männisto, J., Simberg, N. and Hartiala, K. (1981). *Prostaglandins Med.* **7**, 591-599.
25. Chand, N. (1979). *Agents and Actions* **9**, 133-140.
26. Moore, P.K. and Hoult, J.R.S. (1982). *Biochem. Pharmacol.* **31**, 969-971.
27. Giessler, A.J., Bekemeier, H., Hirschelmann, R. and Bakathir, H.A. (1982). In "Trends in Inflammation Research" 2, (eds. H. Bekemeier and R. Hirschelmann), pp.195-211, *Agents and Actions*, Suppl., **10**, Birkhäuser, Basel.
28. Bragt, P.S., Bansberg, J.I. and Bonta, I.L. (1980).

Inflammation **4**, 289-299.

29. McCord, J.M., Wong, K., Stokes, S.H., Petrone, W.F. and English, D. (1980). *Acta Physiol. Scand.* Suppl. **492**, 25-30.

30. Moldeus, P., Anderson, B., Rahimtula, A. and Berggren, M. (1982). *Biochem. Pharmacol.* **31**, 1363-1368.

31. Bennett, S., Marshall, W. and O'Brien, P.J. (1982). In "Prostaglandins and Cancer: First International Conference" pp.143-148. Alan R. Liss, New York.

32. Vasder, S., Tsuruta, Y. and O'Brien, P.J. (1982). In "Prostaglandins and Cancer: First International Conference" pp.155-158. Alan R. Liss, New York.

33. Sivarajah, K., Anderson, M.W. and Eling, T.E. (1978). *Life Sci.* **23**, 2571-2578.

34. Guthrie, J., Robertson, I.G.C., Zeiger, E., Boyd, J.A. and Eling, T.E. (1982). *Cancer Res.* **42**, 1620-1623.

35. Kupfer, D., Miranda, G.K., Navarro, J., Piccolo, D.E. and Theoharides, A.D. (1979). *J. Biol. Chem.* **254**, 10405-10414.

36. Miller, T.A. and Jacobson, E.D. (1979). *Gut* **20**, 75-87.

37. Ceuppens, J. and Goodwin, J. (1981). *Anticancer Res.* **1**, 71-78.

38. Lupulescu, A. (1978). *J. Natl. Cancer Inst.* **61**, 97-106.

39. Holtzman, J.L. (1982). *Life Sci.* **30**, 1-9.

40. Lind, C., Hochstein, P. and Ernster, L. (1982). *Arch. Biochem. Biophys.* **216**, 178-185.

REGULATION OF HYPERSENSITIVITY REACTIONS

D. Parker and J.L. Turk

Department of Pathology, Royal College of Surgeons of England, Lincoln's Inn Fields, London WC2A 3PN, UK

The immunological response of an individual to a particular antigen is the resultant of interacting forces that are mediated through a number of different cell types, each with its own particular function. Research during the past twenty years has succeeded in identifying many of these cells, mainly through the identification of specific cell membrane antigens and their use as cell surface markers. Cell types identified in this way have been correlated with particular functions in the evaluation of the immune response.

Antigen-specific immune responses mediate their reactions either through B-lymphocytes releasing antibody (immunoglobulin) into the serum, or by the release, into the circulation, of specifically reactive T-lymphocytes. The T-lymphocytes carry on their surface peptide chains that are programmed according to their specific amino-acid sequence to react with a particular antigen. This carries the same antigenicity (idiotype) as the variable amino-acid region of the immunoglobulin molecule that is programmed to react with the same antigen. There is, therefore, considerable homology between the antigen reactive site of the "specifically sensitized T-lymphocyte" and the immunoglobulin molecule directed against the same antigen. The third key cell is the macrophage, which plays an important role in the induction of the immune response. Antigens, which are taken up by macrophages, show increases in immunogenicity of up to 10,000 fold. This role in antigen presentation is taken over in the skin by a specialized form of mononuclear phagocyte — the Langerhans cell. In addition to their role in the induction of the immune response, macrophages are important as effector cells, particularly in T-lymphocyte-mediated responses. In this function they respond to a family of pharmacological mediators, of mainly T-lymphocyte origin, known as lymphokines.

IMMUNOTOXICOLOGY
ISBN 0-12-282180-7

Copyright © 1983 by Academic Press London
All rights of reproduction in any form reserved

Control of the immune response may be undertaken by
T-lymphocytes, B-lymphocytes or by macrophages, although the
primary function of these cells is as effector cells. Helper
and suppressor cells, whose main function is to regulate the
immune response, have been identified as specific subgroups
of T-lymphocytes by the presence of particular membrane
markers. In the mouse, suppressor T-cells (T_S) can be distinguished from effector T-cells by the presence of specific
Lyt antigens. Control by B-lymphocytes may be through antibody producing a phenomenon similar to immunological enhancement. Macrophages can act as regulators through cytophilic
antibody, on the cell surface, which may also compete for
antigen. Specific regulation of the immune response may
depend on competition between antigen-reactive sites of different affinity on lymphocytes or antibodies. If the balance
between effector and regulatory mechanisms is disturbed, the
result will be either an increase or a decrease in the immune
response.

It is the purpose of this paper to discuss various ways in
which the immunoregulatory balance can be disturbed by immunosuppressive agents and particularly by the drug cyclophosphamide. In the balance between effector and suppressor
cells, immunopotentiation can be produced by depression of
suppressor cells as much as by increasing effector cell
activity. Evidence will be presented suggesting that the
suppressor T- or B-lymphocytes, which regulate delayed hypersensitivity reactions, differ from effector cells in that
they are derived from a population of rapidly dividing precursor cells that are susceptible to treatment with cyclophosphamide given before or around the time of immunization.
These immunoregulatory mechanisms are a clear feature of not
only the normal immune response but also of some forms of
immunological tolerance, antigenic competition and desensitization.

EFFECT OF CYCLOPHOSPHAMIDE ON NORMAL IMMUNE REACTIONS

Delayed Hypersensitivity

Our initial observations were that guinea pigs pretreated with
cyclophosphamide (300 mg/kg) would give enhanced contact hypersensitivity responses to 2,4-dinitrofluorobenzene (DNFB) and
4-ethoxy-methylene-2-phenyl oxazolone [1]. This confirmed an
earlier observation that repeated treatment with lower doses
of the drug before sensitization had a similar effect [2].
These reactions were not only increased in intensity but were
prolonged in time. Similar studies on animals immunized with
ovalbumin in Freund's incomplete adjuvant (Jones Mote type
of delayed hypersensitivity) showed that the development of

enhanced delayed hypersensitivity also occurred in reactions
to a soluble antigen [3]. Enhancement of delayed hypersensitivity to microbial antigens could be demonstrated using
tularaemia vaccine [4] and *M. tuberculosis* [5]. Others, using
mice, have shown enhanced delayed hypersensitivity reactions
to sheep erythrocytes, as well as contact sensitivity [6,7,8]
following the same protocol. The effect of cyclophosphamide
as an immunopotentiating agent was shown to be proportional
to the extent of the control exerted on the immune response
by the suppressor cells that were regulating it. Thus, the
stronger the regulation, the greater the potentiation produced
by cyclophosphamide [9].

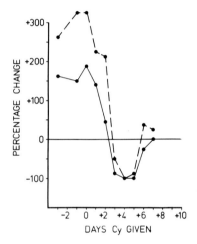

Fig. 1 **Effect of cyclophosphamide (300 mg/kg) given before
or after sensitization.** Skin reactivity at 24 hours ————,
48 hours ------.

Figure 1 shows the effect of 300 mg/kg cyclophosphamide,
given before or after sensitization with DNFB, on skin reactivity at 24 and 48 hours after skin testing on day 8. It
can be seen that maximum potentiation is achieved when the
drug is given between the third day before immunization and
the first day after. If the drug is given later, between the
third and fifth days after immunization, the response is depressed due to a temporary effect on the T-effector cells
which go into a proliferative phase, maximal during these
three days [10]. A study of the effect of this dose of
cyclophosphamide on T-lymphocyte proliferation in the draining lymph node shows that T-cell proliferation is maximally
depressed, on days 4 and 5 after sensitization, by the drug
given on days 2 and 3 respectively (Fig. 2). This indicates
that effector T-lymphocytes are maximally sensitive to

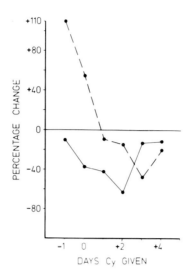

Fig. 2 Effect of cyclophosphamide (300 mg/kg) given before
or after sensitization. T-lymphocyte proliferation in draining lymph node on day 4 ———, day 5 ------.

cyclophosphamide during their proliferating phase. They
appear to be most susceptible to the drug given 48 hours
before the period of maximum DNA and RNA synthesis, when they
can be visualized as "large pyroninophilic cells" in the
paracortical area of the draining lymph node. However, if
cyclophosphamide is given one day before sensitization, when
enhanced skin reactivity is produced on day 8, there is a
massive increase in T-cell proliferation five days after
sensitization indicating that these cells have been released
from normal immunoregulatory control.
   Histological and cytological studies of the action of
cyclophosphamide on lymphoid tissue of guinea pigs and mice
have indicated that the drug has its greatest effect on
B-lymphocytes, with a relatively sparing effect on T-lymphocytes. This has been confirmed by the use of Thy-1 antigen,
as a membrane marker [11,12]. In addition, mice show an
increased lymphocyte proliferative response to PHA *in vitro*
after cyclophosphamide pre-treatment [13]. Studies on the
effect of cyclophosphamide on lymphocyte turnover, using
radioactive labels, have indicated that the effect of the
drug is greatest on cells that have recently incorporated
^{125}I-UDR indicating a preferential effect on the more rapidly
turning over population of lymphocytes [14]. Thus, it can be
inferred that the preferential action of cyclophosphamide on
suppressor cells is because they are derived from a more

rapidly turning over population of precursor cells than the
effector cells, whose precursors turn over less rapidly.

The enhanced Jones-Mote type of delayed hypersensitivity
reaction in guinea pigs treated with one large dose of cyclophosphamide three days before immunization, has been shown to
be due to the elimination, by the drug, of a specific population of suppressor cells [15]. When spleen or peritoneal
exudate cells (PEC), from untreated guinea pigs immunized
with ovalbumin in Freund's incomplete adjuvant, were transferred into similarly immunized but cyclophosphamide-pretreated
animals, the enhanced delayed hypersensitivity reaction was
suppressed. This suppression was found to be antigen-specific.
Further work indicated that B-lymphocytes might be responsible
for the suppressor activity as sensitized spleen cells could
be depleted of these suppressor cells by passage down a column
of degalan beads coated with anti-immunoglobulin antibody [16].
More recently we have shown that these suppressor cells are
unaffected by treatment with anti-T-cell serum and complement
[17] demonstrating that, in the spleen, the T-lymphocyte is
not the cell responsible for the suppressor cell activity.

However, it was thought possible that, despite the fact that
the degalan columns were run at 40°C, macrophages may have
been retained on these columns and these could be the cells
responsible for the specific suppression. In addition, recent
work in mice indicated that macrophages may be responsible for
some specific and non-specific suppression [18]. Large numbers of macrophages were isolated from the PEC of guinea pigs
immunized with dinitrophenyl-bovine gamma globulin (DNP-BGG),
by density gradient centrifugation on Percoll. This population was shown to consist of 95% macrophages and to be in-
capable of producing macrophage inhibitory factor, although
it did respond to lymphokine. In addition, it was not
possible to transfer passively tuberculin-type-hypersensitivity
with this fraction. On assaying for suppressor cell activity,
the macrophage population showed as much suppression as the
total PEC (Table 1A). However, in contrast to the suppression
induced by the PEC that of the macrophages was not antigen-
specific (Table 1B). In addition, macrophages from non-
immunized guinea pigs were found to suppress the skin reactions in the recipient animals, which had been immunized with
DNP-BGG in Freund's incomplete adjuvant eight days earlier
(Table 1C). As this non-specific suppression by macrophages
was found not to be due to Percoll contamination, it would
seem that PEC from sensitized animals contain both suppressor
lymphocytes and suppressor macrophages. However, the former
are antigen-specific whereas the suppressor macrophages show
no antigen-specificity and are also present in the PEC from
non-immunized guinea pigs. It is suggested that PEC from

Table 1 *Non-specific suppression of delayed skin reactions by Percoll separated macrophages*

	Number of recipients	Hours after skin test	
		24	48
(A) Cells from DNP$_{50}$BGG sensitized animals			
No cells	20	8.2 ± 3.4	7.1 ± 3.3
Total PEC	9	4.9 ± 2.4*	5.0 ± 2.7
Macrophages	12	4.5 ± 2.6**	6.5 ± 2.9
(B) Cells from ovalbumin-sensitized animals			
No cells	6	6.4 ± 3.6	6.1 ± 4.1
Total PEC	5	5.8 ± 1.9	5.6 ± 2.9
Macrophages	6	2.2 ± 1.8†	3.1 ± 1.7
(C) Cells from non-immunized animals			
No cells	14	7.9 ± 2.5	7.7 ± 2.6
Macrophages	5	4.2 ± 1.5**	3.4 ± 1.0**

Results expressed as mean increase in skin thickness (10^{-1} mm) ± S.D. following intradermal injections of DNP$_{50}$BGG into animals sensitized eight days previously with DNP$_{50}$BGG in Freund's incomplete adjuvant and given 250 mg/kg cyclophosphamide three days before sensitization.

* $p < 0.02$; ** $p < 0.01$; † $p < 0.05$.

sensitized guinea pigs contain both suppressor lymphocytes, suppressor macrophages and effector macrophages. This latter population would balance the non-specific suppressor macrophages in the sensitized PEC, which would explain why the total PEC population shows no greater suppression than that induced by the separated macrophages.

Antibody Production

With a number of antigens, pretreatment of guinea pigs with cyclophosphamide will cause a significant depression of the antibody response. This is in keeping with the histological appearance of depletion of B-lymphocytes from lymph follicles, germinal centres and at the cortico-medullary junction of lymph nodes. However, pretreatment with cyclophosphamide may expose a latent potential to produce antibody in an animal that does not normally respond to that antigen [19]. Animals immunized with $DNP_{50}BGG$* do not normally make antibody to BGG, but, after cyclophosphamide pretreatment, anti-BGG antibody can be detected. This indicates that the failure of normally immunized animals to produce anti-BGG antibodies is not directly due to the antigenic determinants being hidden by the concentration of DNP groups on the surface of the BGG molecule, but to the generation of suppressor cells that block the development of the response. In general, Arthus reactivity is blocked in cyclophosphamide-pretreated animals even when there is an increase in antibody levels. A similar stimulatory effect on only the IgG_1 antibody formation to the DNP group was found in guinea pigs immunized with $DNP_{20}BGG$ by Drössler et al. [20] and given 10 mg/kg cyclophosphamide daily for seven days after immunization. These workers also found that 6-mercaptopurine had the same effect.

More recently we have investigated the effect of cyclophosphamide given either three days before, on the day of, or three or seven days after immunization with DNP_{47}-BGG in Freund's incomplete adjuvant, on the anti-hapten and anti-carrier IgG_1 and IgG_2 antibody synthesis (see Fig. 3). IgG_2 antibody was assayed by passive haemolysis, and IgG_1 homocytotropic antibody by passive cutaneous anaphylaxis. In this study there was no detectable anti-BGG humoral immune response in any of the groups. Cyclophosphamide, given three days before immunization, induced a temporary enhancement of anti-DNP IgG_1 antibodies but suppressed the IgG_2 antibody. The IgG_1 anti-DNP antibody levels in the serum were not altered in guinea pigs given cyclophosphamide on the day of

---

* (50 mol DNP per mol of bovine gamma-globulin)

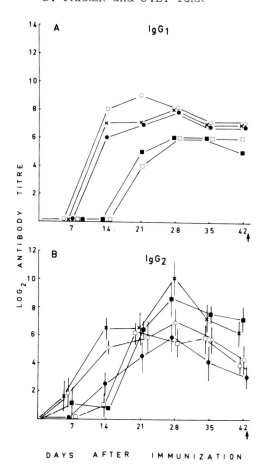

Fig. 3 **Anti-DNP antibody titres after immunization.** Anti-
DNP antibody titres (IgG$_1$ in A and IgG$_2$ in B) after immunization with DNP$_{47}$-BGG in Freund's incomplete adjuvant (x——x)
and treatment with 250 mg/kg on day -3 (o——o), day 0 (●—●)
day +3 (□—□) and day +7 (■—■).

immunization, but the IgG$_2$ antibodies were suppressed.
Cyclophosphamide given either three or seven days after
immunization suppressed both subclasses of anti-hapten antibody. In contrast DNP-BGG specific IgE antibody was not
detected in the control or pretreated guinea pigs but was
found in those given cyclophosphamide on the day of, three or
seven days after immunization. These results demonstrate
that whereas cyclophosphamide given at these times has no
effect, or suppresses the anti-hapten IgG$_1$ and IgG$_2$ antibodies,

the IgE antibody synthesis is stimulated. From these data it would appear that the kinetics of the antibody subclasses are very different.

EFFECT OF CYCLOPHOSPHAMIDE ON MODELS OF IMMUNOLOGICAL UNRESPONSIVENESS

Reversal of Immunological Tolerance

The demonstration that cyclophosphamide pretreatment could increase contact reactivity and certain forms of delayed-type hypersensitivity by elimination of suppressor cells led to a study of the action of this drug in certain models of immunological unresponsiveness.

Guinea pigs, treated with 500 mg/kg of 3,5-dinitrobenzenesulphonic acid (DNBSO$_3$) twice at 14-day intervals before attempted sensitization with 2,4-dinitrochlorobenzene (DNCB), are completely unresponsive to DNCB [21]. However, if they are treated with cyclophosphamide (250 mg/kg) three days before attempted sensitization, they become responsive [22]. In this model, cyclophosphamide-pretreatment was able to reverse completely the tolerant state, as once tolerance had been shown to be broken, the animals remained responsive. However, if one allowed a 14-day gap between the cyclophosphamide-pretreatment and attempted sensitization, the animals were subsequently found to remain responsive. Thus, the effect of the cyclophosphamide was a temporary one and after a limited time the population of suppressor cells was able to regenerate. It was also shown that tolerance induced by feeding DNCB could be reversed by cyclophosphamide in a similar manner [23]. However, the tolerance induced by feeding was not as complete as that induced by intravenous injection, as when such tolerant animals were treated with cyclophosphamide before attempted sensitization, the resultant sensitivity was far greater than that found after reversal of tolerance induced by DNBSO$_3$. The level reached was that found when normal animals were treated with cyclophosphamide before sensitization. This could indicate that the tolerance induced by feeding is completely reversible, whereas that induced by intravenous injection might be a combination of reversible suppressor cell action, with perhaps some degree of irreversibility resulting from clonal elimination.

Another form of specific tolerance to DNCB is that which can be induced by the epicutaneous application of the cross-reacting dinitrothiocyanatobenzene. This also involves the preferential induction of suppressor cells which act both centrally and peripherally, and this also can be reversed by treatment with cyclophosphamide before attempting sensitization [24].

Antigenic Competition

In antigenic competition the suppression of the immune response to a given antigen is accomplished by the administration
of a second antigen at the same time [25]. Both the cellular
and humoral immune response to the first antigen may be significantly depressed if compared with the response observed
when the antigen is administered on its own. Immunization of
guinea pigs with ovalbumin (OA) in addition to *M. tuberculosis*
results in depression of tuberculin PPD (purified protein
derivative) skin test reactivity. This antigenic competition
was even more marked if the animals were skin tested with OA
at the same time as PPD. If the guinea pigs were given
cyclophosphamide three days before immunization, or one day
after, there was a significant enhancement of the delayed
hypersensitivity reaction to PPD in animals immunized with
OA as well as *M. tuberculosis*. The action of the drug was to
minimize the effect of the antigenic competition (Fig. 4) [5].
Bovine gamma-globulin (BGG) could be shown to have a similar
depressing effect on tuberculin sensitivity, which was also
reversed by cyclophosphamide. The reversal of antigenic

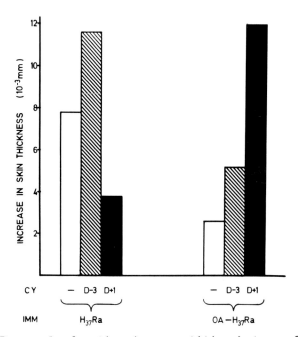

Fig. 4 Reversal of antigenic competition between OA and PPD
by cyclophosphamide. Guinea pigs immunized with Freund's
complete adjuvant containing *M. tuberculosis* H$_{37}$Ra, with and
without OA, skin tested with PPD at 8 days.

competition indicates the likelihood that this phenomenon
develops as a result of a positive immunoregulatory mechanism
involving suppressor cells.

Desensitization

If animals are immunized with a soluble protein such as
ovalbumin or bovine gamma-globulin in Freund's adjuvant and
then given a large injection (2 mg) of the protein, they
become temporarily anergic. The animals fail to respond to
an intradermal challenge with either the protein used for
desensitization (specific desensitization) or another immunizing antigen (non-specific desensitization) [26]. PPD
is also capable of desensitizing guinea pigs immunized with
M. tuberculosis. Cyclophosphamide given three days before
immunization failed to affect specific desensitization induced by OA, BGG or PPD, however, if given one day after
immunization, it was not possible to induce specific desensitization. The induction of non-specific desensitization
was prevented in all three antigenic systems if cyclophosphamide was given either three days before or one day after
immunization. These findings [27] show that non-specific
desensitization differs from specific desensitization (Table
2), and indicate that a suppressor cell, activated by

Table 2 *Differentiation of cyclophosphamide sensitive
suppressor mechanisms by effective dose and time of administration*

Type	Effective dose of cyclophosphamide (mg/kg)	Days of injection that give maximum effectiveness
Delayed hypersensitivity	50–300	D-3 → D+1
Tolerance	250	D-3
Antigenic competition	300	D+1
Desensitization	300	
- Antigenic specific		D+1
- Non-specific		D-3 → D+1
Arthus reaction	10	D-3 → D+1

Cyclophosphamide was administered in one single intra-
peritoneal injection.
D-3 = three days before sensitization
D+1 = one day after sensitization

immunization and susceptible to cyclophosphamide, might be
partially responsible for specific desensitization. This
suppressor cell is presumably different from that involved in
the normal control of the delayed hypersensitivity reaction,
as the precursors of these latter cells are far more sensitive
to cyclophosphamide. The precursors of the suppressor cells
involved in specific desensitization are not susceptible to
cyclophosphamide as this phenomenon is only affected by the
drug given after immunization.

SUMMARY

Cyclophosphamide given before immunization causes greatly increased delayed hypersensitivity skin reactions. Increased
cell-mediated immunity is associated with depletion of
B-lymphocytes from lymphoid tissue and with the elimination,
by cyclophosphamide, of a specific population of suppressor
cells. In the guinea pig, replacement studies showed that
these depleted cells were not T-lymphocytes and had immunoglobulin adherent to their surface, a characteristic of
B-lymphocytes. Delayed hypersensitivity reactions increased
by cyclophosphamide include chemical contact sensitivity, the
tuberculin reaction, delayed hypersensitivity to tularaemia
vaccine and the Jones-Mote reaction to soluble protein antigens. Treatment with cyclophosphamide can also increase the
antibody response to some antigens, but depress the response
to others. In addition, it has been found to reverse immunological tolerance where this form of unresponsiveness is due
to suppressor cells. Cyclophosphamide can also enhance the
immune response following depression by antigenic competition
or desensitization.

REFERENCES

1. Turk, J.L., Parker, D. and Poulter, L.W. (1972).
    Immunology **23**, 493-501.
2. Maguire, H.C. and Ettore, V.L. (1967). *J. Invest. Derm.*
    48, 39-43.
3. Turk, J.L. and Parker, D. (1973).   *Immunology* **241**, 751-758.
4. Ascher, M.S., Parker, D. and Turk, J.L. (1977). *Infect.*
    and Immunity **18**, 318-323.
5. Dwyer, J.M., Parker, D. and Turk, J.L. (1981).   *Immunology*
    42, 549-560.
6. Kerckhaert, J.A.M., Berg, J. and Willers, J.M.N. (1974).
    Annls. Immun. Inst. Pasteur **125c**, 415-426.
7. Lagrange, P.H., Mackaness, G.B. and Miller, T.E. (1974).
    J. Exp. Med. **139**, 1529-1539.
8. Sy, M-S., Miller, S.D. and Claman, H.N. (1977). *J. Immun.*
    119, 240-244.

9. Scheper, R.J., Parker, D., Noble, B. and Turk, J.L. (1977). *Immunology* **32**, 265-272.
10. Turk, J.L. and Stone, S.H. (1963). In "Cell Bound Antibodies" (Eds B. Amos and H. Koprowski), pp.51-60, Wistar Inst. Press, Philadelphia.
11. Turk, J.L. and Poulter, L.W. (1972). *Int. Arch. Allergy* **43**, 620-629.
12. Poulter, L.W. and Turk, J.L. (1972). *Nature New Biol.* **238**, 17-18.
13. Stockman, G.D., Hein, L.R., South, M.A. and Trentin, J.J. (1973). *J. Immunol.* **110**, 271-282.
14. Turk, J.L. and Poulter, L.W. (1972). *Clin. Exp. Immunol.* **10**, 285-296.
15. Katz, S.I., Parker, D., Sommer, G. and Turk, J.L. (1974). *Nature* **248**, 612-614.
16. Katz, S.I., Parker, D. and Turk, J.L. (1974). *Nature* **251**, 550-551.
17. Ota, F., Parker, D. and Turk, J.L. (1979). *Cell. Immunol.* **43**, 263-270.
18. Lichtenstein, A., Murahata, R., Sugasawara, R. and Sighelboim, J. (1981). *Cell. Immunol.* **58**, 257-268.
19. Noble, B., Parker, D., Scheper, R.J. and Turk, J.L. (1977). *Immunology* **32**, 885-889.
20. Drössler, K.J., Klima, F. and Ambrosius, H. (1981). *Immunology* **44**, 61-66.
21. Frey, J.R., De Weck, A.L. and Geleick, H. (1964). *J. Invest. Derm.* **42**, 41-47.
22. Polak, L. and Turk, J.L. (1974). *Nature (Lond)* **249**, 654-656.
23. Polak, L., Geleick, H. and Turk, J.L. (1975). *Immunology* **28**, 939-942.
24. Sommer, G., Parker, D. and Turk, J.L. (1975). *Immunology* **29**, 517-525.
25. Ben Efraim, S. and Liacopoulos, P. (1967). *Nature* **213**, 711-713.
26. Dwyer, J.M. and Kantor, F.S. (1973). *J. Exp. Med.* **137**, 32-41.
27. Parker, D., Dwyer, J.M. and Turk, J.L. (1981). *Immunology* **43**, 191-196.

MECHANISMS OF HYPERSENSITIVITY

D.R. Stanworth

*Rheumatology and Allergy Research Unit,
University of Birmingham, Vincent Drive, Birmingham B15 2TJ, UK*

INTRODUCTION

Considerable progress has been made in the last 20 to 30 years in our understanding of the mechanisms underlying hyper-sensitivity responses. I propose, first, to compare briefly the effector elements implicated in the four main types of hypersensitivity reaction, paying some attention to the role of the initiating agent (foreign/toxic substance) in directing the allergic response along a particular pathway. Then, I shall focus in more detail on immediate-type allergy of the asthma/hay fever type, not only because this has been one of the major interests of my laboratory for a number of years, but also because a substantial amount is now known about the manner in which the immunological interaction between sensi-tizing antibody and antigen (allergen) at the target cell surface leads to the release of pharmacological mediators. Finally, I shall suggest how certain agents could bring about so called anaphylactoid reactions of the immediate-type; where there is no reason to suppose that IgE sensitizing antibody (or indeed, in some cases, any class of anaphylactic antibody) is involved.

COMPARISON OF THE PRINCIPAL DIFFERENCES DISTINGUISHING THE IMMUNOLOGICAL BASIS OF THE MAIN TYPES OF HYPERSENSITIVITY RESPONSE

As pointed out by Gell and Coombs [1], the responses which can occur when a pre-sensitized host is re-exposed to the offending antigen can be conveniently divided into four main types (I-IV). These are listed in Table 1, where I have indicated the nature of the antibody and principal target cells involved, and whether complement activation can also be implicated.

IMMUNOTOXICOLOGY
ISBN 0-12-282180-7

Table 1 *Classification of main hypersensitivity responses* (Based on Gell and Coombs [1])

Type	Effector System			Clinical Manifestations
	Antibody	Cells	Complement	(Examples)
I Immediate	Cytophilic IgE/IgG (? IgG4)	Mast cells, Basophils	−	Hay fever, Extrinsic asthma
II Antibody-dep. cytotoxic	IgG v cell surface Ag.	Macrophages, Polymorphs, K. cells	$\pm$	Autoimmune haemolytic anaemia
III Complex mediated	Ab. (IgG/IgM) -Ag. complexes	Polymorphs, Platelets	+	Farmer's lung
IV Delayed	−	Lymphocytes (T)	−	Contact dermatitis

From the clinical manifestation standpoint, allergic reactions are usually of the first (I) or fourth (IV) types. The former (immediate-type) characteristically involves the production of a cytophilic, mast cell-sensitizing antibody of the IgE class, although in some situations, IgG rather than IgE anaphylactic antibodies appear to be involved, as I shall discuss later. In contrast, the latter (delayed-type) appears to be mediated through lymphocytes (T), without the involvement of antibody of any class. Non-cytophilic antibody, usually of the IgG class, is, however, intimately concerned with the mediation of hypersensitivity reactions of the other two types (II and III). Moreover, unlike the cytophilic IgE antibodies predominant in immediate-type (I) hypersensitivity reactions, the IgG antibodies responsible for these types of hypersensitivity response are cytotoxic; either directly (being formed against target cell surface antigens), or indirectly (via the formation of tissue damaging antibody-antigen complexes).

It is important to recognize, however, that this clear-cut division of the various types of hypersensitivity response is a convenient form of classification, and does not necessarily imply that a particular individual will demonstrate exclusively one or another such response. On the contrary, there is growing evidence, from both clinical and animal studies, that more than one type of hypersensitivity response can occur concurrently. For instance, serum sickness (type III response), which can result from exposure of humans to heterologous antiserum, is usually accompanied by a transitory production of IgE antibody (i.e. a type I response) against the offending protein. In addition, there have been recent reports in the literature that the histamine released during type I responses (as a result of the IgE antibody-allergen interaction, to be discussed in more detail later), is capable of "switching off" on-going delayed type (IV) hypersensitivity responses by interaction with histamine receptors on the effector T-lymphocytes.

Of greater relevance to the present discussion are the factors which direct towards a particular type of hypersensitivity response, in suitably genetically-predisposed individuals. Obviously the initial sensitizing agent plays a decisive role. A major class of potentially toxic agents, namely drugs, are of particular interest in this respect. In immunochemical terms, such substances can usually be regarded as "haptenic", rather than immunogenic, or "sensitogenic" to employ a term that I coined myself [2] to signify an agent capable of primary sensitization in its own right. Consequently, a prior requisite for sensitization by such substances is combination with a suitable carrier, usually a protein of

Table 2 *Potential hypersensitivity responses to an immunotoxic agent*

Foreign Substance ⟶ Antibody Formation

Hapten ⟶ Host Protein
    (e.g. Serum albumin)

Cytophilic Ab (IgE/IgG)   I
  ⟶ Sensitization of tissue mast cells
    — Ag ⟶ Vasoactive amines.

"Precipitating" Ab (IgG/IgM)   III
  — Ag → Complex deposition
    ⟶ Cl. Activation ⟶ Chemotaxis
      Polymorphs. ⟶ Lysosomal enzymes.
      ⟶ Platelet aggregation → Vasoactive amines.

Hapten ⟶ Host Cells   II
    e.g., erythrocytes,
    platelets
Auto-Ab. (IgG) v Surface Ag
    ⟶ Lysis

    dermal cells ⟶ Cell Response   IV
T.Lymphocytes
    —— Ag ⟶ Lymphokines

endogenous or exogenous origin. The requirements in this
respect for initiation of hypersensitivity responses of the
four different types, confirmed by the results of experimental
sensitization studies, are indicated in Table 2. Thus, in
order for a foreign low molecular weight substance to be
capable of eliciting an IgE antibody response it will be necessary for it to combine with a suitable carrier protein, such
as a host plasma protein, or an exogenous protein (e.g., a
bacterial protein, used in the production of the drug).
Alternatively, if the drug-carrier conjugate is able to elicit
the production of relatively high circulating levels of a
"precipitating" antibody (say of the IgG class), there is
scope for the formation (in relative antigen excess) of
soluble antibody-antigen complexes, which get deposited in
preferred sites (e.g., in the glomerular membrane, in the
joints or in the skin) resulting (a few hours after re-
exposure to antigen) in a characteristic type III response.
In the skin this is, of course, manifested as an oedema and
erythematous response known as an Arthus Reaction.

   In contrast, for a foreign low molecular substance to
initiate a hypersensitivity response of the other two types
(II and IV), there is a requirement for interaction with host
cellular elements. An example of a type II clinical hypersensitivity response initiated in this manner, which is frequently quoted in text books, is the elicitation of a mild
attack of generalized purpura with thrombocytopaenia resulting from the intra-dermal injection of a small dose (1.4 x
10^{-6} g) of sedormid into a highly sensitized patient [3].
Other drugs are capable of initiating similar types of response, sometimes as a result of their interaction with the
patient's erythrocyte membrane constituents, resulting in the
induction of an autoimmune haemolytic anaemia. On the other
hand, repeated application of a drug to the skin can result
in a contact dermatitis (i.e., type IV) response, attributable
to its binding to epidermal proteins. In view of my earlier
comments, it is interesting to note that Asherson and colleagues [4] have shown that the experimental induction of
contact sensitivity in mice, as a result of painting their
skin with picryl chloride (a frequently used experimental
delayed sensitizing agent), leads also to IgE (as well as IgG
and IgM) antibody production. Nevertheless, despite this
observation, there is evidence that inoculation via the dermal
route tends to favour the development of a T-lymphocyte response, which is a pre-requisite for a delayed-type hypersensitivity reaction.

   In addition, therefore, to the form of the potential sensitizing agent, the route of its administration is of some consequence in influencing the type of hypersensitivity response

that might ensue. As far as immediate type (I) hypersensitivity responses are concerned, IgE antibody production
appears to occur by inhalation of allergen or by oral presentation (where in some cases, a metabolic product could prove
to be the effective sensitizing agent, and where immunological
processes occurring within the gut could exert some control).
In this connection, it is interesting to note that in contrast
there is some evidence that injection of foreign proteins
appears to favour production of anaphylactic antibody of the
IgG class. It should be mentioned that even parenteral administration of foreign protein (e.g.,ovalbumin) to appropriate
animal species (certain strains of rats, mice etc.), can lead
to the experimental production of IgE antibodies, provided
that suitable adjuvants are employed. In this connection, it
could be significant that incomplete adjuvants (e.g., Al(OH)$_3$)
favour IgE antibody production in mice and rats, whereas a
complete (e.g., Freund's adjuvant) would, of course, favour
production of high levels of IgG antibodies. Such experimental findings could be of relevance to understanding the factors influencing clinical sensitization, where there is a
suspicion that depot agents, and even the aggregation of drugs
themselves (e.g. penicillin) contribute to their sensitizing
capacity. Certainly, at the later antigen-challenge stage of
a hypersensitivity response, there is good reason to suppose
that a monovalent (unaggregated) low molecular weight substance lacks allergenic capacity (a point to which I shall
return in the next section, in discussing IgE mediated responses in more detail).

Any consideration of the requirements for primary sensitization should also not neglect this having occurred to some
cross-reacting substance, a possibility which is often difficult to exclude. This is suspected, for instance, in some
cases of antibiotic (e.g., penicillin) sensitization, where
the initial exposure could have been to other types of mould
(e.g., cephalosporins) in the atmosphere. Moreover, it is
important not to fail to recognize the chemical relationships
that exist between many different drugs as the primary sensitizing agent may not necessarily be among those only available on prescription.

MOLECULAR BASIS OF IMMEDIATE-TYPE HYPERSENSITIVITY RESPONSES

IgE Mediated Responses

The various factors which are known to influence IgG antibody
production are listed in Table 3. In addition to those
already mentioned in the previous section, like the form of
the sensitogen and its route of administration, genetic predisposition is of prime importance. Even in animal (e.g.,

Table 3 *Factors influencing immediate-type hypersensitivity responses*

---

1) Genetic status of host.

2) Immunological status of host — at both cellular and humoral levels.

3) Hormonal status of host.

4) Mode of exposure to sensitizing substance (sensitogen) — particle size, dose, adjuvanticity, route of administration.

5) Nature of potential sensitogen.

6) Concomitant immunological stimuli — e.g. from parasite infections.

---

mice, rats) sensitization studies, one can demonstrate "good" and "bad" responder strains [5]; and, interestingly, the latter can be converted to the former by treatment (e.g., X-ray irradiation, anti-thymocyte serum administration) which "knocks out" the animal's T-suppressor cell population. Translating these experimental observations to the clinical level, the suggestion is that atopic individuals possess an impaired T-suppressor cell function, which is responsible for their failure to regulate IgE antibody production against certain sensitogens. If such people could be identified by a pre-screening test of some sort, it might be possible to anticipate a potential tendency to respond adversely, to a particular pharmaceutical agent (or, natural, allergen). However, much more basic immunological research is needed before this stage can be reached.

In 1968 Bennich *et al.* [6] discovered a myeloma form of the class of immunoglobulin (IgE) of which reaginic antibodies proved to be representative [2,7] and the successful allergenicity in pre-sensitized individuals was demonstrated. As already mentioned, the valency of such substances can sometimes change spontaneously, as a result of self-aggregation or by combination with a suitable carrier. Moreover, as work currently in progress in my own laboratory on the experimental production (in rats, mice and rabbits) of IgE antibodies directed against radiographic contrast media is beginning to show, not only is it necessary to conjugate such compounds to suitable carrier proteins to render them allergenic as well as sensitogenic, but different types of contrast media (i.e., non-ionic as opposed to ionic) appear to differ in their structural requirements in these respects. There is obviously

much to learn about the manner in which these and other
pharmaceutical agents could combine with host proteins under
clinical conditions.

Returning to the role of IgE antibodies in mast cell
triggering, in recent years we have been interested particularly in defining the nature of the signal responsible for
transduction of the primary "message". One school of thought
suggests that all that is required is to cross-link the mast
cell Fc receptors in some way (a requirement that can be met
artificially by use of specific anti-receptor antibody). In
contrast, we have obtained interesting evidence for the active
involvement of the cross-linked IgE antibody in transmission
of the triggering "message" via, we think, a specific Fc
effector site, which in some way, activates a "second receptor" on the mast cell membrane (see Figs. 1 and 2). Initial

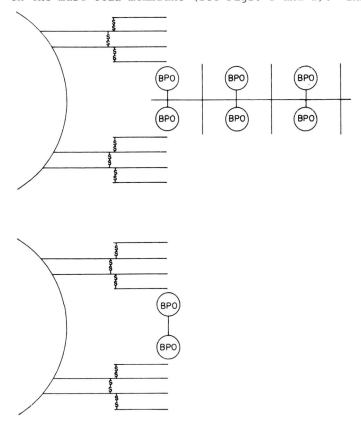

Fig. 1 Diagrammatic representation of the manner in which
IgE anaphylactic antibody molecules bind to target mast cells,
and subsequently interact with specific antigen (allergen).
BPO = benzyl penicillinoyl group.

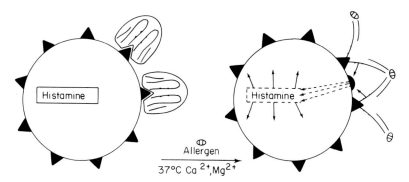

Fig. 2 Postulated manner in which the cross-linking by
allergen of mast cell bound IgE antibody could lead to the
activation of a "second receptor", by an antibody Fc located
effector site.

structure—activity studies [8] on model polypeptide (synthetic ACTH derivatives, and melitin cleavage fragments),
using an *in vitro* rat peritoneal mast cell assay, defined the
principal features of such an effector site. Consequently,
a careful examination of the primary sequence of the human
ε-chain [9], pointed to its likely location within the Fc
region of the IgE antibody molecule. We have subsequently
synthesized peptides representative of this sequence (i.e.,
Arg-Lys-Thr-Lys-Gly-Ser-Gly-Phe-Phe-Val-Phe) and shown octa-,
nona- and deca-peptides to be potent releasers of histamine
selectively (i.e., non-cytotoxically), by a process which in
many ways resembles the IgE antibody-allergen mediated one
from isolated rat mast cells [10]. In other words, we have
reason to suppose that such synthetic agents, in mimicking
the crucial role of IgE antibodies in mast cell triggering,
are "short-circuiting" the regular two-stage process by
avoiding the primary need of binding of sensitizing antibody
to Fc receptors.

   Encouragingly, a prediction of the 3-dimensional structure
of the domain (Cε4), in which the putative effector site is
located by application of a modified Chou and Fasman procedure [19], indicates that it is in an accessible region of
the molecule from which it might be brought into juxtaposition
with the postulated "second receptor" as the result of an
antibody conformational change resulting from allergen cross-
linking. Thus, in summary we envisage (see Fig. 3) that the
role of the IgE antibody in immediate type hypersensitivity
reactions can be likened to a "pro-hormone" which pre-
sensitizes the tissue mast cells by combining with ("address-
ing") specific Fc receptors, but which does not gain full
hormonal status until the cell-bound IgE antibody molecules

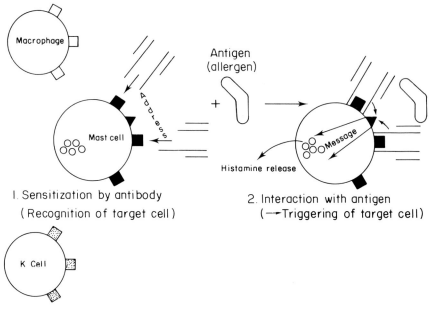

.Fig. 3   Postulated mechanism of immunological triggering of
mediator release from mast cells.

have been cross-linked by specific allergen. This results in
conveyance of the stimulatory message, via the basic Fc effector sites, culminating in changes in mast cell membrane phospholipids, leading to an increase in permeability with the
influx of calcium ions (which act as "second messengers", and
are responsible for bringing about exocytosis of the mast
cell granules).

    Research work now in progress in our laboratory is aimed at
producing peptide derivatives of the IgE antibody Fc receptor
sequence which are antagonistic towards allergen-induced
mediator release from antibody-sensitized mast cells and
which, therefore, are potentially new anti-allergy compounds.

IgG Type Anaphylactic Antibodies

The production of anaphylactic antibodies of the IgG class as
a result of the experimental sensitization of animals of many
species is now well established. As is seen in Table 4, these
show important differences from IgE antibodies in both their
biological and chemical properties.

    Similarly, IgG anaphylactic antibodies have been demon-
strated more recently in the sera of allergic patients
(sensitive to foods, drugs, and other allergens) and have
been referred to by Parish [11] as short term sensitizing
(STS)-antibodies, as they are detected by passive cutaneous

Table 4 *Comparison of properties of IgE and IgG anaphylactic antibodies*

Property	IgE	IgG
Skin sensitization time (optimum)	50–80 h	2–4 h
Persistence in skin	4 weeks	1–2 days
Turnover in humans (half-life)	21 days	2 days
Placental transmission	–	+
Complement (Clq) activation	–	–
Response to heat (56°C/1 h) treatment	labile	stable

anaphylaxis (PCA) testing in sub-human primates following much shorter periods of preliminary sensitization (i.e., 2 to 4 hours) than is necessary in IgE-mediated PCA responses.

Following our demonstration [12] that a human myeloma protein of the IgG4 sub-class was capable of inhibiting the latter type of PCA response (i.e., that mediated by IgE antibodies), we suggested that tissue mast cells might also contain Fc receptors for IgG anaphylactic antibodies, as well as IgE ones. More recently we [15] and other investigators, have obtained further experimental evidence that such antibodies could be of the human IgG4 sub-class and could have some unique clinical significance. For instance, we have shown raised serum IgG4, as well as IgE, levels in many patients with asthma; parallel rises in both antibody levels appearing to be much more prevalent in the sera of those patients showing symptoms of eczema associated with their asthma [13]. Furthermore, we have since obtained evidence of raised levels of IgG4 antibodies directed against certain common inhalant allergens in the sera of allergic patients whose IgE levels are normal and who have failed to respond to conventional chemotherapy (e.g., Intal treatment), but who show a late onset response (in contrast to an early, IgE mediated, one) as a result of bronchial provocation with specific allergen [14]. Although the mode of action of these human IgG anaphylactic antibodies is far from understood (as discussed recently elsewhere [15]), there is good reason to suppose that they act differently to IgE antibodies in eliciting mediator release. In this connection, it might be worth mentioning that quite

apart from possessing one pair of constant domains less than
IgE antibody molecules within their Fc regions, human IgG4
molecules do not include a sequence similar to the one within
the IgE Fc region to which mast cell triggering action has
been attributed (as discussed earlier).

ANAPHYLACTOID RESPONSES

It is important to note that not all allergic reactions of
the immediate-type are mediated by anaphylactic antibody,
despite their showing similar clinical manifestations to the
IgE antibody responses discussed in the previous section.

Table 5 *Examples of pseudo-allergic (anaphylactoid) reaction
systems*

Agent	Examples	Possible Effector Mechanism
Colloid volume substitutes.	Dextran.	IgG2 Ab-Ag complex $\longrightarrow$ Clq activation. (? $\longrightarrow$ platelets).
Radio-graphic contrast media.	Acetrizoate, diatrizoate, ioxathalamate.	Alternative complement pathway (C3) changes $\longrightarrow$ C3a, C5a anaphylatoxins.
Basic polypeptides.	ACTH 1-24 polymyxins.	Triggering of mast cell "second receptor".

These (examples of which are listed in Table 5) are usually
referred to as anaphylactoid, or pseudo-allergic, reactions.
These are mediated by such agents as colloid volume substitutes (e.g., dextran and gelatin), basic polypeptide drugs
(like polymyxin B and ACTH) and radiographic contrast media.
It was shown many years ago [16] that the injection (i.p.)
of dextran into non-sensitized rats evokes an anaphylactoid
reaction; presumably as a result of the formation of anaphylatoxic complement cleavage products (C3a and C5a) with histamine releasing ability. The possibility has obviously
arisen as to whether the allergic reactions exhibited by
those patients who react adversely to the clinical administration of dextran are attributable to a similar mechanism.
The extensive studies carried out by Hedin and colleagues
[17] in Sweden in recent years have provided an alternative
explanation. They have demonstrated the presence of anti-
dextran antibodies of the IgG2 sub-class, the only one of
the four human IgG sub-classes which is non-cytophilic to

heterologous as well as homologous mast cells, in high titres
in the sera of such patients. These antibodies appear to be
responsible for initiating vasoactive amine release via activation of the classical complement pathway i.e., by a type III
allergic reaction.

It should be pointed out that, at least theoretically,
either classical or alternative complement pathway activation
can lead to the formation of basic C3a and C5a polypeptide
cleavage fragments, which are capable of initiating histamine
release by direct action on mast cells *in vitro*. There is
also evidence to indicate that certain drugs exert their adverse effects through the non-immunological formation of such
anaphylatoxins. For instance, evidence has been obtained in
our own, and other, laboratories to suggest that radiographic
contrast media might bring about the adverse reactions attributed to these tri-iodinated substituted benzoic acid compounds in this manner. Although these substances can be
shown to effect certain changes to the complement C3 system
in vitro, these appear to differ from the C3 degradation processes associated with activation of the alternative pathway
by endotoxins and zymosan. For example, by application of a
simple haemolytic method of measuring C3 activation, developed
recently in our laboratory [18], we can demonstrate contrast
media-induced consumption of this complement component *in
vitro*, but, by inclusion of rat peritoneal mast cells in the
system, we have not succeeded in obtaining direct evidence
of the formation of anaphylatoxic sub-components.

It would, of course, be tempting to suppose that the
anaphylatoxic C3a and C5a sub-components — like the basic
polypeptides (e.g., ACTH and melitin) used in our structure-
activity studies, referred to earlier, act directly on the
postulated "second receptor" on the mast cell plasma membrane
(discussed earlier, and depicted in the diagrams in Figs. 2
and 3). However, as discussed in detail elsewhere [20],
present available experimental evidence indicates that this
is unlikely. Nevertheless, it is quite conceivable that
certain polypeptide drugs such as synacthen (ACTH 1-24 peptide) and polymyxin B do indeed exert adverse effects by
acting directly on the second receptor. However, this still
leaves the problem of explaining why only a minute number of
all patients to which such drugs are administered respond
adversely.

SUMMARY

An attempt has been made to illustrate the wide variety of
mechanisms underlying human hypersensitivity responses.

Although mention has been made of IgG anaphylactic antibodies, attention has been focussed particularly on IgE

antibody-mediated responses of the asthma — hay fever type, because more is probably known about their mechanism than those of any of the other main types of hypersensitivity response. Moreover, it is indicated that our own recent work on the synthesis of histamine-releasing peptides, representative of human ε-chain sequences, offers an explanation of the precise role of the antibody in the elicitation of mediator release and this could lead eventually to the development of more effective forms of anti-allergy compound. Our studies also point to a possible mode of action of certain substances (such as basic polypeptide antibiotics) implicated in non-immunologically mediated, pseudo-anaphylactic, responses.

Brief reference has also been made to the probable mechanisms underlying the modes of action of other types of pharmaceutical substance (such as radiographic contrast media) responsible for eliciting anaphylactic-like responses. In this area much detailed laboratory and clinical investigative work remains to be undertaken. However, even when this has been accomplished, there will still be the problem of explaining why such a very small number of patients react adversely to these foreign proteins.

REFERENCES

1. Gell, P.G.H. and Coombs, R.R.A. (1963). (Eds). "Clinical Aspects of Immunology", Blackwell Scientific Publications, Oxford.
2. Stanworth, D.R. (1973). "Immediate Hypersensitivity: The Molecular Basis of the Allergic Response". Frontiers of Biology Series, Vol.28. North Holland Research Monographs Frontiers of Biology, North Holland/American Elsevier.
3. Acroyd, J.F. (1954). *Clin. Sci.* **13**, 409-423.
4. Thomas, W.R., Watkins, M.C. and Asherson, G.L. (1978). *Immunology* **35**, 41-7.
5. Katz, D.H. (1978). *Immunological Rev.* **41**, 77.
6. Bennich, H., Ishizaka, K., Johnasson, S.G.O., Rowe, D.S., Stanworth, D.R. and Terry, W.D. (1968). *Bull. World Health Org.* **38**, 151.
7. Stanworth, D.R., Humphrey, J.H., Bennich, H. and Johnasson, S.G.O. (1968). *Lancet* **ii**, 17.
8. Jasani, B., Stanworth, D.R., Mackler, B. and Krell, G. (1973). *Int. Archs. Allergy Appl. Immun.* **45**, 74-81.
9. Bennich, H. and Von. Bahr-Lindstrom, H. (1974). *Prog. Immunol. Vol.* **II**, 1, pp.49-58, North Holland, Amsterdam.
10. Stanworth, D.R., Kings, M., Roy, P.D., Moran, J.M. and Moran, D.M. (1979). *Biochem. J.* **180**, 665-8.
11. Parish, W.E. (1970). *Lancet* **ii**, 591-2.
12. Stanworth, D.R. and Smith, A.K. (1973). *Clin. Allergy* **3**, 37-41.

13. Gwynn, C.M., Morrison Smith, J., Leon Leon, G. and Stanworth, D.R. (1979). *Clin. Allergy* **9**, 119-123.
14. Gwynn, C.M., Ingram, J., Almosawi, T. and Stanworth, D.R. (1982). *Lancet* **i**, 254-256.
15. Stanworth, D.R. (1982). Immunochemical aspects of human IgG4. In "Non Reaginic Anaphylactic and/or Blocking Antibodies" (Ed. G. Halpern), Clin. Reviews in Allergy. (in press).
16. Voorhees, A.B., Baker, J. and Pulaski, E.J. (1951). *Proc. Soc. exp. Biol. Med.* **76**, 254-6.
17. Hedin, H., Kraft, D., Richter, W., Scheiner, O. and Devey, M. (1979). *Immunobiology* **156**, 289.
18. Riches, D.W.H. and Stanworth, D.R. (1980). *Immunology Letters* **1**, 363-6.
19. Chou, P.Y. and Fasman, G.D. (1974). *Biochemistry* **13**, 222-245.
20. Stanworth, D.R. (1980). Oligopeptide-induced release of histamine. In "Pseudo-Allergic Reactions: 1. Genetic Aspects and Anaphylactoid Reactions" (Eds. P. Dukor, P. Kallos, H.D. Schlumberger and G.B. West). pp.56-107, Karger.

CHEMICAL ASPECTS OF HYPERSENSITIVITY

J. Morley, C.P. Page and F.M. Cunningham

*Department of Clinical Pharmacology,
Cardiothoracic Institute, Fulham Road, London SW3 6HP, UK*

INTRODUCTION

Hypersensitivity is manifest as a disproportionate increase
in the response to a stimulus and is commonly detected as a
reduced threshold to the stimulus. The concept of hypersensitivity can readily be appreciated by consideration of
skin reactions to proteins (e.g. ovalbumin or gammaglobulin).
In an unsensitized animal such proteins elicit modest plasma
protein extravasation, even when relatively large quantities
are injected intradermally. The bases for this limited response are several, including non-specific mechanisms, such as
mast cell degranulation induced by a high proportion of basic
charges on the surface of protein molecules, as well as more
specific actions such as generation of kinins (e.g., by plasma
kininogenase present in gammaglobulin fractions). The inflammatory activities of such proteins are not usually subjected
to detailed analysis in non-sensitized animals, but it is
reasonable to consider that the relevant contribution to
extravasation, by various mechanisms, will be peculiar to an
individual protein.

By way of contrast, the response to intradermal injection
of these same proteins (or any other antigen) in a sensitized
animal, is determined by a group of well defined processes
(e.g., mast cell degranulation, complement activation, lymphocyte activation) which are initiated only subsequent to recognition of the antigen, and at antigen concentrations that are
insufficient to evoke a non-specific host response. In this
way, responses to diverse allergens conform to a common pattern, which provides the basis for classification of allergic
reactions. It follows therefore that such responses are
likely to be both quantitatively and qualitatively dissimilar
from those produced in non-sensitized animals. Hypersensitivity may exhibit both immediate and delayed components.

IMMUNOTOXICOLOGY
ISBN 0-12-282180-7

Clsssically, hypersensitivity is thought to result from the
interaction of antigen, with either circulating antibodies
(Arthus type), sensitized mast cells or basophils (Anaphylactic type), or lymphocytes (Delayed type). The mechanisms
underlying such hypersensitivity reactions can be arranged
into two broad categories, namely, cytotoxicity, and mediator
release.

CYTOTOXICITY

Cell death initiates a secondary response in the host.
Initially, this takes the form of invasion by phagocytic
cells to remove cellular debris and this cellular infiltration
may be succeeded by initiation of repair processes. Tissue
damage is accompanied by inflammatory symptoms, as is well
established in experimental pathology (e.g., the inflammatory
response to thermal, mechanical or electromagnetic stimuli).
The mechanisms responsible for cell death may be physiological,
as in infarction, or immunological, when there is selective
destruction of target cells. For example, antibody-mediated
cytotoxicity effects cell death by perforation of the target
cell membrane following complement activation at the site of
antibody localization. Antibody-dependent cell-mediated cytotoxicity, as well as lymphocyte cytotoxicity, are complement-
independent processes, in which the primary cause of cell
death has yet to be defined [1].

MEDIATOR SECRETION

When cytotoxic mechanisms would be inappropriate, the host
response to antigen is that of mediator secretion, whereby the
recognition system triggers cellular activation and the secretion of biologically active materials. A variety of chemical
mediators have been implicated in hypersensitivity reactions
and these may conveniently be considered by reference to their
cellular origin.

Mast Cells and Basophils

Mast cell and basophil involvement has been demonstrated in
anaphylaxis which typically depends upon allergen recognition
by IgE or IgG bound to the surface of these cells. The binding of antigen to such sensitized cells initiates a sequence
of events leading to the exocytosis of intracellular granules,
with release of their constituents on contact with the extra-
cellular environment. Granule constituents include the biogenic amines (histamine and serotonin), the mucopolysaccharide,
heparin, vasoactive intestinal polypeptide, and a number of
enzymes which, by weight, comprise the major portion of the

granules. It has been proposed that the secretory process is dependent upon successive methylation of membrane phospholipids, thereby altering membrane fluidity. This process is associated with the activation of phospholipase A_2, and release of arachidonic acid from membrane phospholipids. Arachidonic acid is rapidly metabolized via cyclo-oxygenase or lipoxygenase enzymes to form prostaglandins, thromboxanes or hydroxy-fatty acids. During mast cell activation, prostaglandin D_2 is the predominant arachidonic acid metabolite released.

Conspicuous consequences of mast cell degranulation are oedema and vasodilation, which in man are manifest as a wheal and flare response. This type of reaction is faithfully reproduced by histamine, but as antihistamines fail to fully inhibit anaphylactic responses a single mediator concept is untenable. Prostaglandin D_2, like PGE2, will potentiate responses due to histamine or kinins, but this effect cannot be of major consequence as non-steroidal, anti-inflammatory drugs only modestly affect anaphylaxis. SRS-A release was long attributed to mast cell degranulation, but with the characterization of the active constituents, leukotrienes, has come an appreciation that other cell types are a more likely source of these materials. Kininogenase activation during degranulation implicates kinins in hypersensitivity responses, but the extent to which these materials can account for acute responses involving mast cells remains unestablished. Recently, it has been shown that rat mast cells are able to release a peptide (inflammatory factor of anaphylaxis) that can induce a cellular infiltration, indicating that mast cells may also be involved in delayed hypersensitivity reactions [2]. The secretory process of the mast cell have recently been reviewed [3].

Macrophages

Macrophages are well established as participants in delayed type hypersensitivity reactions and in the latter phase of Arthus and anaphylactic responses. These cells are not usually considered to be participants of acute allergic reactions, as they are recruited to sites of allergic and other inflammatory responses only after a delay of some hours. However, as it can be shown that alveolar macrophages respond to anti-IgE antibodies by secretory activity [4], the possibility should be considered that in situ macrophages may participate in acute responses to bronchial provocation with antigen.

Macrophages exhibit the capacity to secrete a wide range of biologically active materials. Their ability to secrete

lysosomal enzymes (e.g., lysozyme and beta-glucuronidase) is
associated with phagocytosis and digestion of invading pathogens and cellular debris. Additionally, these cells have an
abundance of phospholipase A_2 and, as the predominant poly-
unsaturated fatty acid in their cell membranes is arachidonic
acid, this cell type is a rich source of prostaglandins,
thromboxanes and leukotrienes. More recently, such cells
have been shown also to secrete another phospholipid mediator,
unrelated to arachidonic acid, 1-0-alkyl-sn-glyceryl-3-
phosphorylcholine, (PAF-acether).

The potent inflammatory properties of prostaglandins,
leukotrienes and PAF-acether are appropriate to mediators of
oedema and erythema, whilst the ability of leukotrienes and
PAF-acether to effect neutrophil and mononuclear cell accumulation is suggestive of a role in cellular inflammation. In
the specific context of delayed hypersensitivity, macrophages
produce Interleukin I, an obligatory co-factor for lymphocyte
activation. The secretory processes of macrophages have been
extensively reviewed elsewhere [5].

Lymphocytes

Lymphocytes are evident in responses of delayed hypersensitivity, and cell transfer experiments have established them
as the primary agencies of such reactions. T-lymphocytes,
following activation, produce lymphokines which exhibit a
range of biological activities, irrespective of the presence
of antigen. Crude lymphokine preparations exhibit a spectrum
of biological effects and purification and bioassay techniques
reveal heterogeneity of biological activity in such preparations. The extent to which lymphokine activities can be
ascribed to specific substances remains uncertain and awaits
purification of biologically active fractions to high specific
activity. The possibility still remains that some of the
biological actions of lymphokines are attributable to low
molecular weight mediators bound to plasma proteins [6].

The properties of lymphokines are more pertinent to reactions of delayed hypersensitivity than are the properties of
the low molecular weight mediators. *In vivo*, lymphokines
produce increased vascular permeability and erythema on intradermal injection and these skin reactions exhibit a neutrophil-
rich cellular infiltration. Lymphokines also cause activation
of macrophages, thereby increasing host resistance to invading
pathogens. *In vitro*, lymphokines are potent chemotactic
agents for neutrophils and mononuclear cells and cause lymphocyte activation. This mitogenic activity of lymphokines for
lymphocytes is now attributed to a specific agency, Interleukin II, whose primary role seems to lie in amplification

of lymphocyte activation. The cytotoxic effects of lymphokines are due to lymphotoxin, a highly unstable complex composed of five subunits. These subunits are constituents of
lymphokine preparations, which, until the lymphotoxin complex
is formed, exhibit only modest toxicity. The physiology and
biochemistry of lymphokines has been extensively reviewed
elsewhere [7].

Neutrophils

Neutrophil infiltration is a characteristic feature of Arthus
responses, and neutrophils are also prominent in the initial
phase of delayed hypersensitivity reactions. These cells may
also participate in anaphylactic responses [8]. Histamine,
PAF-acether, cationic proteins, arachidonic acid metabolites
and toxic oxygen radicals are all released from neutrophils,
as a result of cell activation by cytotaxins, such as the
complement peptide C5a, rather than via antigen recognition.
These substances can cause tissue injury, increased vascular
permeability and altered haemodynamics, thus suggesting the
involvement of neutrophils in hypersensitivity reactions.
  Recently, it has been postulated that neutrophils must be
present for cytotaxin-mediated increases in plasma protein
extravasation to occur in a variety of target organs [9,10],
indicating the importance of these cells in such processes.
Since increased plasma protein extravasation is controlled by
alterations in two variables (blood flow and vascular permeability), it is of interest that neutrophils can produce a
potent vasodilator substance, vasoactive intestinal polypeptide
(VIP) [11], which is more potent than PGs at potentiating increased plasma protein extravasation caused by inflammatory
mediators [12]. This indicates that one mechanism by which
neutrophils may contribute to increased vascular permeability
is through the release of potent vasodilator substances. The
involvement of neutrophil derived mediators in inflammatory
processes has recently been reviewed [13].

Platelets

Platelets have classically been considered in the context of
their role in haemostasis [14]. However, platelet activation
has recently been demonstrated in anaphylactic reactions [15,
16]. Like mast cells and basophils, platelets often undergo
a release reaction during activation, which produces an abundance of chemical mediators, including the biogenic amines,
histamine and serotonin, arachidonic acid metabolites, predominantly thromboxane A_2, and various enzymes [6]. Platelets,
like neutrophils, are not thought to be activated directly by
antigen recognition.

It is of interest that one of the mediators released from
activated platelets, PAF-acether, mimics many aspects of
immediate hypersensitivity (e.g., bronchoconstriction and
acute inflammatory responses). However, unlike other chemically defined mediators, PAF-acether is capable of inducing
both acute and delayed inflammatory responses following intradermal injection in man [17]. The time course of the response is reminiscent of antigen-induced responses in sensitized individuals [18]. As PAF-acether is released in such
situations [15,16], it may contribute to the delayed responses observed clinically after antigen exposure. In bronchial asthma, allergic individuals who exhibit a dual response
following allergen exposure become hyper-reactive to diverse
stimuli for some time afterwards. Hyper-reactivity is associated with the expression of a delayed response, hence PAF-
acether formation should be considered as a potential basis
for bronchial hyper-reactivity. As it has been shown that
PAF-acether is cytopathic towards vascular endothelium, this
activity may underlie the delayed response observed following
administration of this mediator. The role of platelets and
mediators originating from platelets has recently been
reviewed [6].

DISCUSSION

A plethora of biologically active materials are released
from, or generated by, the various cellular elements that
participate in allergic inflammation. It has been conventional to associate particular cell types with classes of
allergic reaction (e.g., lymphocytes in delayed hypersensitivity, neutrophils in Arthus responses and mast cells in
anaphylactic reactions). Although such associations are well
established, they do not preclude a central role for other
cell types in these responses. For instance, in delayed
hypersensitivity reactions, lymphocyte activation has an
obligatory dependence upon macrophage activation; furthermore,
the initial response to antigen in delayed hypersensitivity
is characterized by a substantial infiltrate of neutrophils
and basophils. It is apparent, therefore, that a wide range
of mediators may contribute to the inflammatory responses
which characterize allergic reactions. If a hierarchy of
mediator release can be established, this can provide a logical (and possibly effective) basis for therapeutic intervention
by selective antagonists. If, on the other hand, a variety of
mediators are released in parallel, then the prospects for
therapeutic intervention by selective antagonists are limited.
Such hierarchies have yet to be established with certainty
for all classes of allergic response; perhaps the best defined

hierarchy is that of Interleukin regulation of lymphocyte activation with cyclosporin-A providing an example of a highly selective anti-allergic agent. In cytotoxic processes, a hierarchy is inescapable, since non-specific endogenous inflammatory processes are activated subsequent to cytotoxin-induced cell death. For this reason, mediators with cytotoxic activity (e.g., lymphotoxin and PAF-acether) may be accorded a primary role in inflammatory processes, implying that antagonism of the effects of these substances could have substantial therapeutic advantage.

ABSTRACT

Hypersensitivity responses are manifest as a consequence of changed cellular behaviour (e.g., erythema and induration of skin reactions). Selective changes in cell behaviour can be attributed to the release, or generation, of pharmacologically active materials (mediators) following allergen recognition, with the release of histamine and generation of prostaglandins or lymphokines providing classical examples. Alterations in cell behaviour can also take place as a consequence of cell death by antibody-mediated cytotoxicity or the action of cytotoxic lymphocytes, including natural killer cells. It is now evident that certain mediators, by being cytotoxic, combine both processes.

REFERENCES

1. Sanderson, C.J. (1981). *Biol. Rev.* **56**, 153-197.
2. Oertel, H.L. and Kaliner, M. (1981). *J. Immunol.* **127**, 1398-1402.
3. Lewis, R.A. and Austen, K.F. (1981). *Nature* **293**, 103-108.
4. Joseph, M., Tonnel, A.B., Capron, A. and Dessaint, J.P. (1981). *Ag. Act.* **11**, 619-621.
5. Morley, J. (1981). In "Lymphokines", (Ed. E. Pick) Vol.4, 377-394, Academic Press, London.
6. Henson, P.M. and Ginsberg, M.H. (1981). Research Monographs in Cell and Tissue Physiology — Platelets in Biology and Pathology (Ed. J.L. Gordon), Vol.2 Elsevier/ North-Holland Biomedical Press, Amsterdam, pp.249-308.
7. Hanson, J.M., Rumjanek, V.M. and Morley, J. (1982). *Pharmacol. Ther. [B]* **17**, 164-198.
8. Atkins, P.C., Norman, M., Weiner, H. and Zweiman, B. (1977). *Ann. Intern. Med.* **86**, 415-418.
9. Heflin, A.C. and Brigham, K.L. (1981). *J. Clin. Invest.* **68**, 1253-1260.
10. Wedmore, C.V. and Williams, T.J. (1981). *Nature* **289**, 646-650.
11. O´Dorisio, M.S., O´Dorisio, T.M., Cataland, S. and

Balcerzak, S.P. (1980). *J. Lab. Clin. Med.* **96**, 666-672.

12. Williams, T.J. (1982). *Brit. J. Pharmacol.* **77**, 505-509.

13. Repine, J.E., Bowman, C.M. and Tate, R.M. (1982). *Chest* **81**, 47-50.

14. Pinckard, R.N., Halonen, M., Palmer, J.D., Butler, C., Shaw, J.O. and Henson, P.M. (1977). *J. Immunol.* **119**, 2185-2193.

15. Knauer, K.A., Lichtenstein, L.M., Franklin Adkinson Jr, N. and Fish, J.E. (1981). *N. Engl. J. Med.* **304**, 1404-1407.

16. Owen, R.T. (1979). *Drugs of Today* **15**, 489-516.

17. Basran, G.S., Page, C.P., Paul, W. and Morley, J. *J. Clin. Allergy* (in press).

18. Dolovich, J., Hargreave, F.E., Chalmers, R., Shier, K.J., Gauldie, J. and Bienenstock, J. (1973). *J. Allergy Clin. Immunol.* **52**, 38-46.

CLINICAL DIAGNOSIS OF DRUG HYPERSENSITIVITY

J. M. Dewdney

*Beecham Pharmaceuticals, Research Division,
Biosciences Research Centre, Yew Tree Bottom Road,
Epsom, Surrey KT18 5XQ, UK*

INTRODUCTION

Clinical diagnosis of drug allergy is an exercise in differential diagnosis. Few objective tests are available and, in most cases, diagnosis is based on presumptive evidence alone.

This situation is far from satisfactory. It is important to the future care of patients who have experienced adverse drug reactions to try to establish the underlying pathogenesis as this has significant therapeutic implications. Moreover, until diagnostic accuracy is improved, there is no sound basis for statistical surveys of allergic drug reactions and most incidence figures are undoubtedly over-estimations [1-3].

The inherent dangers in applying presumptive logic to the diagnosis of drug allergy are illustrated by reference to the penicillins. These antibiotics are essentially non-toxic and possess few pharmacological actions which could lead to adverse reactions. It is well known, however, that penicillins can introduce antigenic determinants into macromolecules *in vivo* and thus initiate a specific immune response which may lead to clinically important adverse reactions [4]. An adverse reaction of an allergic-type in a patient receiving a penicillin will thus, on probability reasoning alone, be viewed as allergy and this may be so even if, as in the hospitalized patient, many other drugs are being co-administered. The hazards are clear. Under these circumstances the true incidence of penicillin allergy cannot be determined and the allergenic potential of a co-prescribed drug may be overlooked.

Objective tests are required. Priority given to the development of tests, and to the extent to which detailed diagnosis is justified, depends on national health care

IMMUNOTOXICOLOGY
ISBN 0-12-282180-7

strategy, but the cost-benefit ratio of such an undertaking
may not be favourable. The magnitude of the problem is
addressed in this paper and an outline diagnostic procedure
is proposed.

CLASSIFICATION OF ADVERSE DRUG REACTIONS

Conventional classification of adverse drug reactions attempts
to distinguish those which can be explained on the basis of
the pharmacological actions of the drug and those which are
of an aberrant or idiosyncratic nature and are thus patient-
orientated. Drug allergy falls within this second group
(Table 1).

Table 1 *Classification of adverse drug reactions*

Adverse reaction reflects pharmacology of drug	Overdosage	Patient responsiveness may influence magnitude of response but response dictated by direct and indirect drug actions
	Side-effect	
	Secondary effect	
Adverse reaction reflects aberrant patient response	Intolerance	Pharmacokinetic and metabolic abnormalities
	Idiosyncrasy	Allergic reactions
		Pseudo-allergic reactions
		Other aberrant responses

Based on Brown [22]

Simplistic classifications of this kind help to focus
attention on the characteristics of each type of adverse
reaction, although it is only of help in taking the first
step towards diagnosis. The most difficult reactions to distinguish from drug allergy are the pseudo-allergic reactions,
in which the signs and symptoms of allergic disease are
mimicked through non-immunological pathways. Some, such as
the histamine releasing properties of the aminoglycosides,
arc better classified under secondary effects [5]. Others
seem to have their origins in a hypersensitivity on the part
of the patient to pharmacological mediators of the allergic
response [6].
    The more detailed characteristics of drug induced allergic
responses are given in Table 2.

Table 2 *Characteristics of allergic drug reactions*

Clinically based characteristics	Response unrelated to pharmacological actions of drug
	Response occurs only after prior exposure
	Response provoked by chemically related structures
	No dose-response relationships apparent
	Clinical response consistent with established pathology of allergic dysfunctions
Laboratory based characteristics	Changes in immune parameters indicative of a state of specifically altered reactivity; may be manifest in any immunological class, in cell reactivity or in complement factors

It is clear that the clinician, faced with the task of categorizing an adverse reaction, must be fully informed on the pharmacology of the drug, not only its main therapeutic actions but also its side-effects and secondary effects, and not only within but also outside its recommended therapeutic dosage limits. Demonstration of altered immune responsiveness will be difficult and, therefore, diagnosis has to depend, in the majority of cases, on this careful analysis of both drug and patient.

It should perhaps be stressed that before even this level of sophisticated analysis is attempted it is the *sine qua non* of drug allergy that it is a drug-induced reaction. Many investigators fail to establish, beyond reasonable doubt, that the adverse response seen is drug related rather than being a feature of the patient's disease state.

Many attempts have been made to improve the reliability of assessment of the causal relationship between drug and effect. Both the adverse drug reactions scoring system (ASS) and the adverse drug reactions probability scale (APS), are of value. Each involves answers to a set of questions probing clinical response, temporal relationships of drug administration and effect, dose responses, blood levels and alternative aetiology [7-9]. These are time-consuming tasks but, in the absence of facile laboratory tests to help diagnosis, they are well justified.

DIAGNOSTIC PROCEDURES

If there are reasonable grounds for believing that the adverse
reaction is indeed drug-induced, and presumptive evidence indicates an allergic aetiology, detailed investigation may be
justified.

Strategy to be adopted depends on the circumstances. *In
clinical medicine,* diagnosis is orientated to an individual
patient and is of importance because of future therapy. In
some cases, alternative therapy can be substituted but the
choice of that alternative therapy needs some knowledge of the
nature of the adverse reaction. If the adverse reaction were
of the allergic aetiology, then only drugs of similar structural type would be as equally contraindicated as the original
drug. If the adverse reaction were of other aetiology it is
possible that the patient was unduly intolerant to a pharmacological class of drugs, for example, all β-blocking drugs and
even structurally quite different replacements could be
hazardous. *In occupational medicine,* the priorities and
strategies may be very different. Diagnosis tends to be
group-orientated in the first instance with comparisons made
between exposed, affected individuals and exposed but non-
affected individuals.

It is not difficult to see why many of the diagnostic procedures one would wish to apply in the therapeutic area are
more effective when used in the industrial environment [10].
In the latter, highly reactive chemicals are handled and many
of these will prove to be protein reactive and thus to behave
as haptens capable of stimulating specific immune responses.
Examples of such chemicals include toluene diisocyanate and
trimellitic anhydride. Such reactive chemicals clearly have
no place in a therapeutic context. Group analysis allows
another important aspect of diagnosis to be evaluated, that
of the functional significance of a specific immune response.
Drug specific antibody may be of functional significance or
may represent an epiphenomenon, and studies in industrial
environments frequently allow decision on this point.
Finally, the route of exposure is different in the two
situations. Industrially, exposure is usually by contact
with skin or through inhalation of dusts, both of which provide opportunities for diagnostic provocation studies as
discussed below.

Diagnostic procedures which may be considered can be classified as those involving the patient directly, that is,
provocation tests, and those which are performed *in vitro*
using blood donated by the patient.

PROVOCATION TESTING

Provocation testing may be a legitimate procedure to be employed in the diagnosis of adverse drug reactions and, provided due consideration is given to the potential hazards, it
can give valuable information [11]. Provocation testing is
used most frequently to diagnose allergic drug reactions.

Table 3 *Provocation testing in the diagnosis of allergic
drug reactions*

Method	Immunological Basis	Reagents Required
Skin tests: 　Prick 　Scratch 　Intradermal	Histamine release from IgE sensitized mast cells As above, plus Arthus reactions	Parent drug may be useful; drug-hapten covalently bound to carrier preferred
Patch tests	Covalent binding of drug or metabolite to protein and provocation of delayed hypersensi- tivity reaction	Parent drug or chemical
Inhalation tests	IgE- and IgG-mediated bronchoconstriction or nasal airways change	Parent chemical if non-irritant. Of value primarily in industrial medicine
Oral tests	Unknown. Possibly IgE in gut mucosa and release of mediators or absorp- tion of drug and interaction with antibody at distant site	Parent drug

The main methods used are outlined in Table 3. Parent drug
or reactive chemical can be used in all these tests and this
is a significant advantage in that special reagents are un-
necessary. If antigenic determinants are known, as in the
case of β-lactam antibiotics, then more effective reagents

can be prepared for skin testing by reaction of drug with a
non-immunogenic carrier such as poly-L-lysine.

Additional information can be obtained in provocation tests
by the use of anti-allergy drugs; inhibition of a provoked
reaction by, for example, disodium cromoglycate provides
additional, although not conclusive, evidence of an allergic
aetiology [12].

Further comment on the patch test is justified. It represents perhaps, the most widely used diagnostic procedure in
industrial medicine and, by specialist dermatologists, in
clinical medicine. The immunological basis of the reaction
induced is one of delayed hypersensitivity, with cellular
infiltration, by mononuclear cells and basophils, into the
dermis and epidermis, increased vascular permeability and
local activation of the clotting system. It is used primarily
to diagnose contact hypersensitivity and is of unquestioned
value [13].

It is worth noting that in this test the initiating event
is the formation of an immunogen comprising autologous carrier
and antigenic determinant derived from the drug. Under the
conditions of the patch test, this initial event leads to a
cell-mediated immune response, whilst the same stimulus provokes antibody formation to a drug or its metabolites. This
is the hapten theory of drug immunogenicity. What, therefore,
the patch test tells us, in addition to its diagnostic significance, is that the drug is, a priori capable of forming
antigenic determinants and thus could be a potential initiator
of other immune effector mechanisms including drug allergy.

SPECIFIC IMMUNE RESPONSIVENESS - IN VITRO ASSAYS

It has proved difficult to establish reliable in vitro assays
to detect specific immune responsiveness to drugs. Some
investigators have found that techniques based on cellular
responsiveness to the parent drug, or to a reagent derived
from it, give reliable results. The most studied are the
lymphocyte transformation test and techniques based on the
release of histamine from peripheral white blood cells. The
latter is claimed to be of value in diagnosis of IgE-mediated
drug reactions but not all workers find it reliable. Opinion
is also divided on the lymphocyte transformation test; at best
it will indicate a drug-specific immune response though the
functional significance of the response is unclear [14,15].

The same question of functional significance arises over the
detection of drug-specific immune responses by measurement of
IgG and IgM antibody. Experience in the field of penicillins
suggests that whereas low levels of IgM antibody are of no
real significance, IgG antibody may be of biological importance

and may be critical to the development of certain types of
drug allergy, for example, haemolytic anaemia, thrombocytopenia or immune complex disorders. However, as with the
proliferative response of lymphocytes, the presence of drug
specific antibodies of any immunoglobulin class indicates that
the drug is capable of generating an immune and thus an allergic response and this is a valuable finding.

A number of assays are available for the measurement of IgM
and IgG antibody. The direct Coombs antiglobulin reaction is
one of some interest in relation to drug-mediated adverse
reactions. The test detects the presence of antibody on the
surface of red blood cells by a detector system comprising
broad spectrum or class specific antibodies raised in animals.

Thus it is possible to detect IgG antibody on the surface of
erythrocytes in cases of penicillin-induced haemolytic anaemia.
It is important to perform careful controls however. Some
drugs, and within the antibiotics field cephalothin is an
example, cause the non-specific adsorption of not only immunoglobulins but other serum proteins to the red cell. Clearly
this has no allergic or immunological implications but the
phenomenon could lead to a misdiagnosis. The use of an antibody reagent specific for serum albumin or trypsin will
identify this type of problem in the Coombs test, as is exemplified by the reactivity of β-lactam antibiotics in Table 4
[4].

Table 4 *Antibiotics and the direct Coombs test*

Antiserum	Antibiotic Class		
	Penicillins	Cephalothin	Other Cephalosporins
Broad spectrum anti-globulin	+++	+++	+++
Anti-IgG	+++	+++	+++
Anti-IgM	(+)	+++	Negative
Anti-C_3	+	+++	+
Anti-albumen or anti-trypsin	Negative	+++	Negative

(+) Only occasional positive results recorded

Of more direct diagnostic significance is the presence of
IgE antibody of drug-related specificity. The radioallergo-
sorbent test has proved to be of value particularly in penicillin allergy although many studies, including our own, draw
attention to the complexity of reagents required [16-18].

It should be noted that only for very few allergic reactions
to drugs has it proved possible to demonstrate specific IgG
antibodies. This may reflect our lack of knowledge of the
appropriate drug-derived antigenic determinants or may be a
true reflection of the comparative infrequency of IgE-
mediated reactions.

GENERAL IMMUNOLOGICAL EFFECTS

In view of the difficulties experienced in demonstrating drug-
specific immune responses, it is worth considering whether
useful information could be obtained by measuring changes in
general immunological parameters temporally related to the
adverse reaction.

Two approaches are worth further appraisal. It has been
shown that the concentration of total IgE immunoglobulin may
be elevated in patients experiencing drug allergic reactions
[19,20]. Only in certain circumscribed conditions, however,
can this finding be used in diagnosis. It is of particular
value in the non-atopic individual who will have levels of
total IgE within normal physiological ranges for the local
area and from whom it is possible to obtain sequential blood
samples before and immediately following drug provocation.
Occasionally blood samples are available for an individual
patient who experiences an adverse drug reaction. More frequently they are not and if the measurement of total IgE is
to be of value, it is necessary to carry it out in association
with drug provocation. Clearly this is a significant limita-
tion on the usefulness of the procedure but there are circumstances where it could be of value [21].

The second type of investigation worth considering is the
measurement of alterations in complement components. No such
changes will be seen in IgE-mediated allergic reactions but
it can be anticipated that there will be complement depletion
in certain immunologically-mediated adverse reactions, such
as haemolytic anaemia and immune complex deposition syndromes.

CONCLUSIONS

In the present state of knowledge, the clinical diagnosis of
drug allergy depends more on careful analysis of clinical
history, drug pharmacology and the characteristics of adverse
drug reactions than on measurement of specific immune
responsiveness.

Table 5 *Diagnosis of allergic drug reactions: proposed outline procedures*

Question	Procedure
Is adverse reaction drug related?	Prepare ASS or APS algorithms
Is adverse reaction allergic in origin?	Check pharmacology of drug
	Check response characteristics as in Table 2
Is detailed diagnosis justified?	In clinical medicine, consider alternative therapy
	In occupational medicine, consider removal of patient from exposure
Is provocation challenge justified?	Route of challenge may be oral, inhalation, topical or parenteral. Consider potential hazards and the need for controls
Can changes in general immunological parameters be detected?	Sequential changes in total IgE immunoglobulin
	Changes in complement factors
Can a specific immunological response be detected by serum or cell based assays?	Check drug structure, protein, reactivity, literature
	If antigenic determinants known or predictable prepare reagents for antibody measurement - priority, IgE by RAST. Consider cell tests

Demonstration of specific immune responses can be time-consuming and expensive and may only be considered worthwhile in certain circumstances where no alternative therapy can be offered to the patient.

Provocation testing has considerable merit and can be effectively combined with cellular or antibody assays to demonstrate changes in responsiveness or of antibody titre in sequential samples taken at times appropriate to the provocation testing.

Research is needed on two fronts. We need to understand

better the role of reactive metabolites in generating immune
responses to drugs as this will allow the preparation of
reagents for use in diagnosis based on knowledge of antigenic
determinants. We need also to ask whether it is possible to
identify "at risk" patients on the basis of aberrant handling
and metabolism of xenobiotics, or on a genetically determined
basis.

Meanwhile, adoption of the type of procedure outlined in
Table 5 may help clarify this important area of diagnostic
difficulty.

REFERENCES

1. Levy, M., Lipshitz, M. and Eliakim, M. (1979). *Am. J.
    Med. Sci*. **277**, 49-56.
2. Van Arsdel, P. (1982). *J.A.M.A*. **247**, 2576-2781.
3. Eaton, K.K. (1982). *Clinical Allergy* **12**, 107-110.
4. Dewdney, J.M. (1977). In "The Antigens, Vol.IV" (Ed. M.
    Sela), pp.73-245. Academic Press, New York.
5. Dewdney, J.M. (1980). In "Pseudo-Allergic Reactions"
    (Eds. P. Dukor, P. Kallos, H.D. Schlumberger and G.B. West).
    Vol.1, pp.273-293. S. Karger, Basel.
6. Pseudo Allergic Reactions (Eds. P. Dukor, P. Kallos,
    H.D. Schlumberger and G.B. West). Vol.1 (1980) and 3
    (1982). S. Karger, Basel.
7. Hutchinson, T.A., Leventhal, J.M., Kramer, M.S., Karch,
    F.E., Lipman, A.G. and Feinstein, A.R. (1979). *J.A.M.A*.
    242, 633-638.
8. Naranjo, C.A., Busto, U., Sellers, E.M., Sandor, P.,
    Ruiz, I., Roberts, E.A., Janecek, E., Domecq, C. and
    Greenblatt, D.J. (1981). *Clin. Pharmac. Ther*. **30**, 239-
    245.
9. Busto, U., Naranjo, C.A. and Sellers, E.M. (1982). *Br.
    J. Clin. Pharmac*. **13**, 223-227.
10. Dewdney, J.M. and Edwards, R.G. (1980). *Chemistry in
    Britain* **16**, 600-605.
11. Kauppinen, K. (1972). *Acta Derm. (Kyoto)* **52** Suppl 68,
    1-89.
12. Davies, R.S., Hendrick, D.J. and Pepys, J. (1974).
    Clinical Allergy **4**, 227-247.
13. Adams, R.M. (1969). In "Occupational Contact Dermatitis"
    (Eds.
14. Amos, H. (1976). "Allergic Drug Reactions" In "Current
    Topics in Immunology Series" (General Editor, J.L. Turk).
15. Amos, H. (1981). In "Immunological and Clinical Aspects
    of Allergy" (Ed. M. Lessof). Chapter 11, pp.389-406.
    MTP Press Limited, England.
16. Juhlin, L., Ahlstedt, S., Andal, L., Ekstrom, B., Svard,

P.O. and Wide. L. (1977). *Int. Archs. Allergy appl. Immunol.* **54**, 19-28.

17. Kraft, D., Berglund, A., Rumpold, H., Roth, A. and Ebner, H. (1981). *Clinical Allergy* **11**, 579-587.
18. Edwards, R.G., Spackman, D.A. and Dewdney, J.M. (1982). *Int. Archs. Allergy appl. Immunol.* **68**, 352-357.
19. Wide, L. and Juhlin, L. (1971). *Clinical Allergy* **1**, 171-177.
20. Couteaux-Dumont, C., Poncelet-Maton, E. and Radermecker, M. (1974). *Rev. franc. Allergol.* **14**, 71-76.
21. Lindemayr, H., Knobler, R., Kraft, D. and Baumgartner, W. (1981). *Allergy* **36**, 471-478.
22. Brown, E.A. (1955). *J.A.M.A.* **157**, 814-819.

ALLERGIC REACTIONS OF THE RESPIRATORY TRACT TO LOW MOLECULAR WEIGHT CHEMICALS

J. Pepys

Brompton Hospital, London, U.K.

INTRODUCTION

Respiratory tract reactions to chemical agents in occupational, and now increasingly in non-occupational environments, present the clinician with the question as to whether these are due to their irritant or allergenic effects or both. "Allergy" as defined by von Pirquet can be summarized as the "acquired, specific, altered capacity to react" and is based on immunological sensitization. The nature of the reactions elicited depend upon the different types of allergy, Types 1 to 4, and are determined by the relevant antibodies. Whilst these have their own characteristics, more than one type of allergy may be present and in the case of Type III allergy, an introductory Type I reaction is a feature of its development. Thus, the same tissue and clinical responses are elicited by all agents in which the same particular form or forms of allergy are present. Non-immunological effects on the other hand have features characteristic for the particular agent.

In practice, an allergic mechanism can be assumed where there shall have been a period of symptomless exposure, that is the period of sensitization. Once sensitized, reactions are elicited by minimal and often minute exposures, far less than the amounts required for sensitization. This is a feature of allergic reactions, distinguishing them from irritant effects. Finally, only a proportion of exposed subjects are affected in this way. This is usually low, except for highly allergenic substances such as the halide salts of platinum. In many of the examples of allergy to chemical agents to be cited, an allergic mechanism was assumed, to be confirmed by the later demonstration of appropriate specific antibodies.

IMMUNOTOXICOLOGY
ISBN 0-12-282180-7

OCCUPATIONAL ASTHMA

Asthma arising at work often provides a penetrating model for
the study in immunochemical terms of sensitization to well-
defined chemical substances, and in clinical terms since the
exposure history can be established and subsequent events
monitored. It is common for affected subjects to have a
period of exercise-induced asthma, suggestive of developing
sensitization, before clinical asthma appears. This in turn
tends to come on late in the day or in the early hours of the
next morning, or immediately on exposure, reflecting patterns
of asthmatic reaction found in controlled exposure tests.
The relationship of asthma to work can be shown by the use of
a peak flow meter or gauge, with readings taken frequently
and regularly, two-hourly for example, over days or weeks, in
which periods at and away from work can show the role of the
occupational exposures [1]. The next step, after a diagnosis
of occupational asthma is made or suspected, is to make a
specific etiological diagnosis in often complex exposures to
many substances [2,3].

Etiological Diagnosis in Occupational Asthma

Many chemicals are either irritant, toxic or too potently
allergenic for provocation testing in the same way as the
common allergens. These problems have been overcome by our
development of simulated, occupational type exposures under
controlled conditions [2-4]. The tests are identical to, or
as close as possible to, the occupational exposures, thus
representing what actually happens. The exposures in turn
are of a limited order, sometimes as little as one or a few
breaths of a fume or vapour, or of a few minutes duration.
All in all the tests correspond to a very brief part of the
subjects ordinary daily exposure of many hours at work.
   The results of such tests show that asthma, defined as
widespread airways obstruction, reversible spontaneously or
by treatment, comprises a heterogeneity of patterns of
bronchial reaction. They are divided into (1) Immediate
asthmatic reactions. These are familiar, coming on within
minutes and lasting $1\frac{1}{2}$ to 2 h. The causal relationship
between exposure and symptoms is obvious and the reactions
are mediated by Type I allergy, based mainly on IgE antibodies
and also on IgG-STS antibodies and probably in some instances
on both. (2) Non-immediate asthmatic reactions. These are
less familiar, though probably even more important than the
immediate reactions. There are three patterns of non-
immediate asthma, (a) a reaction coming on after 1 h and
lasting about 5 h, (b) a reaction, the commonest so far,
coming on slowly and progressively after several hours and

lasting for about 24 h and likely to be clinically evident at
the end of the day; this reaction has features compatible with
a Type III reaction and, like it, is readily blocked by corticosteroids; it is also followed by days or weeks of bronchial
hyper-reactivity to non-specific stimuli, unlike the immediate
reaction, (c) a reaction coming on about 16 h after the test
and manifest in the early hours of the morning; this reaction
is remarkable in that it can recur at the same time for many
nights after a single test exposure [5]. It probably reflects
a combination of the reaction to the agent and circadian
rhythms, in which the lowest levels of plasma catecholamines
and highest levels of histamine are present at this time. It
is important in provocation testing to ensure that the subject
is not reacting in this way to previous exposures at work.
It must also be taken into account in assessing the effects
of cessation of work as a guide to occupational asthma.

The non-immediate reactions may be accompanied by systemic
responses, such as fever, malaise and myalgia. They are also
poorly responsive to bronchodilators, in contrast to the
immediate reaction which is usually completely reversed.
Sodium cromoglycate can block immediate reactions whatever
the cause and can also block the 5-8 h reaction. Corticosteroids have little effect on the immediate reaction, but
effectively block the 1-5 and 5-8 h reactions.

An association of immediate and 5-8 h reactions is commonly
found and is referred to as a "dual reaction". There are
however many patients showing combinations of the various
patterns of asthma.

The bronchial provocation tests are made under controlled
conditions preferably in hospital in a small cubicle, when
the patient's ventilatory performance has been found to be
stable over a period of several days. In tests for agents
met as dusts, the material is mixed in carefully determined
amounts with well-dried lactose. The mixture is then poured
from one receiver to another so that the subject inhales the
dust as if at work, the lactose itself being used as the
control. The exposure in all the tests is made for periods
of 30-60 sec. to start with, increasing up to 5 min. or
longer where necessary, with careful monitoring for possible
reactions throughout.

Tests for fumes or vapours are made by creating these from
the source materials as ordinarily used, for example, as
varnishes or after heating, as in soldering and other processes. Individual chemical components of the exposure
situation are tested in turn with only one test made on any
one day. Examples, mainly from our own experience, of
reactions to dusts, vapours and fumes will be given to illustrate the points cited and to show some of the "spin-offs"
from such studies.

ASTHMA DUE TO CHEMICAL DUSTS

Platinum halide salts. The halide salts of platinum, encountered mainly in the refining of platinum, are amongst the
most highly allergenic substances known for man. They are
also histamine liberators. In sensitized subjects skin prick
tests with solutions of tetrachlorplatinate and hexachlorplatinate salts can elicit wealing reactions at concentrations
of 10^{-9} g/ml [6]. The volume introduced by the prick test has
been calculated at 3×10^{-6} ml, thus giving in this case an
absolute skin test dose of about 10^{-15} g, that is of the
order of 100,000 to 200,000 molecules. In practice the prick
test concentrations go up to 10^{-3} g/ml, which was found in
intra-cutaneous tests to give reactions due to histamine
liberation [7]. The differences between concentrations giving
allergic reactions and those giving non-specific reactions
are greater than 10^3, illustrating the characteristically low
allergenic dose.

The availability of a well-defined inorganic platinum salt
made it possible to assess the eliciting capacity of a range
of platinum salts containing from one to six chlorine atoms
[6]. It was found that this was directly related to the
number of halide ligands. Information of this sort is
not known for other more complex allergens and should be

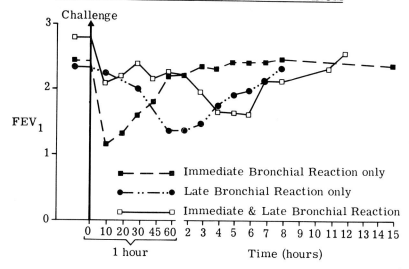

BRONCHIAL REACTIONS ON 'INHALATION' TESTING WITH THE COMPLEX SALTS OF PLATINUM

Fig. 1 Immediate, non-immediate and dual asthmatic reactions
to halide salts of platinum.

studied further, for example, in immediate type allergy to
chloramine-T [8] and amprolium chloride [9], in both of which
chlorine ligands are present.

Immunological evidence in support of an allergic mechanism
has been provided by development of a RAST for specific IgE
antibody in man [10] and in the rat in which a model for the
induction of IgE antibody production to the platinum halide
salt has now been developed. Passive transfer tests in man
with the sera of sensitized workers have shown the presence
of both heat labile, IgE antibody and heat-stable IgG-STS
antibody to the platinum halide salt. These latter findings
were confirmed by PCA tests in the monkey [11].

A clinical point of practical importance is the finding that
atopic subjects, as defined, i.e. by the development of IgE
antibodies to common environmental allergens, demonstrable by
skin prick tests, and with or without symptoms related to
this, become sensitized more rapidly in a higher proportion
than non-atopics. Pre-employment screening by prick tests
with three or four common environmental allergens is used to
identify and exclude these subjects. Serial prick tests with

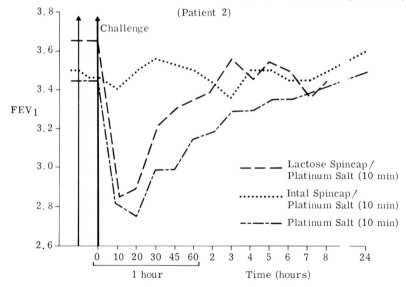

'INHALATION' TESTS WITH AMMONIUM HEXACHLORPLATINATE WITH &
WITHOUT PRETREATMENT WITH INTAL & INTAL PLACEBO (LACTOSE)

Fig. 2 Immediate asthmatic reaction to ammonium hexachlorplatinate and blocking by sodium cromoglycate.

Patient 2

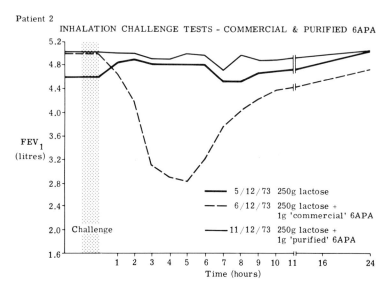

Fig. 3 Non-immediate asthmatic reactions to commercial and not to purified 6-aminopenicillanic acid (6-APA).

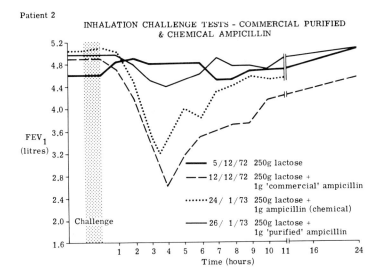

Fig. 4 Non-immediate asthmatic reactions to commercial but not to purified ampicillin.

a platinum halide salt are also used to identify the development of sensitivity and is taken as a guide to cessation of
exposure, if possible before symptoms have appeared.

Bronchial provocation tests by the dust exposure method
elicited immediate, non-immediate and dual asthmatic reactions (Fig. 1) [12]. The immediate reaction was blocked by
prior inhalation of sodium cromoglycate (Fig. 2).

Antibiotic dusts. The discriminating capacity of the bronchial provocation tests is shown by the findings in a group of
subjects engaged under identical conditions at the same time
in the manufacture of penicillin and ampicillin [13].
Figures 3 and 4 show that in one worker non-immediate asthmatic reactions were elicited by commercial preparations of
6-aminopenicillanic acid (6-APA) and ampicillin but not by
highly purified preparations. This showed that an impurity
was responsible for the reactions and since these were identical for both 6-APA and ampicillin, that it was probably the
same impurity. The non-immediate asthmatic reaction was
blocked by prior inhalation of beclomethasone diproprionate,
suggestive of a Type III or Type III-like allergy mechanism.

Figures 5 and 6 in another of the subjects show identical
non-immediate reactions to the commercial and purified 6-APA
preparations, coming on after 16 h, that is, in the early

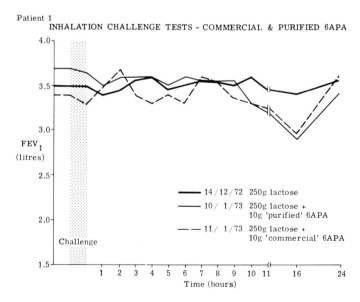

Fig. 5 Non-immediate asthmatic reactions at 16 h to both
commercial and purified 6-APA.

hours of the next morning. Tests with the commercial and
purified ampicillin elicited a non-immediate reaction after
1 h, followed by a second prolonged reaction after 3 h, and
with a further fall at 16 h. The difference between the
6-APA and the ampicillin is the linking of phenylglycine to
the 6-APA nucleus. Phenylglycine is a known cause in its own
right of occupational asthma. These results show differences
in the allergens in the two patients and very informative
immunochemical findings. The latter patient without any
further exposure also had a recurrent nocturnal asthmatic
reaction in the early hours of the next day.

Further tests were made on the affected group of workers
by giving the antibiotics orally. Figure 7 shows that non-
immediate asthmatic reactions were elicited, identical to
those with the provocative tests, accompanied by gastrointestinal and skin reactions.

In yet another worker from a different factory, sensitivity
to a macrolide antibiotic, spiramycin, was found (Fig. 8)
[14]. This patient gave a prolonged non-immediate asthmatic
reaction. He improved, but not completely, on changing his
employment; and the adverse reaction cleared up completely
when his wife, employed in the same factory as a secretary,
also left. The symptoms recurred some months later and
appeared to the patient to be related to eating eggs.

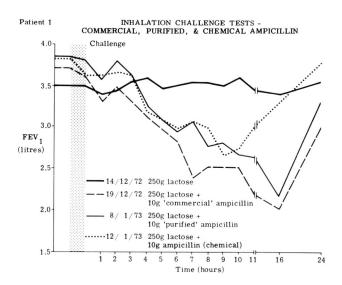

Fig. 6 Non-immediate asthmatic reactions to both commercial
and purified ampicillin.

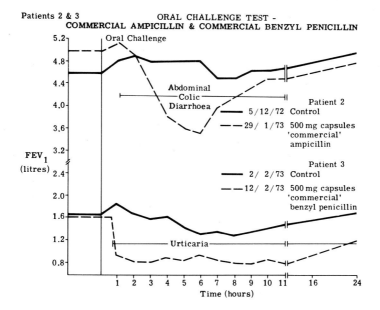

Fig. 7 Non-immediate asthmatic and other reactions to oral ingestion of ampicillin and benzylpenicillin in workers with occupational asthma.

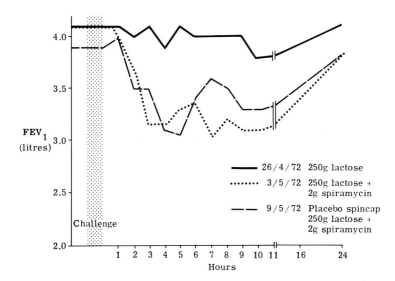

Fig. 8 Non-immediate asthmatic reactions to spiramycin.

Spiramycin is fed to egg-laying poultry as an antibiotic. It
is found in egg white in concentrations of 3 ppm and was
partly responsible for his symptoms.

Carmine. Two workers handling carmine, from *Coccus cactus,*
in the manufacture of cosmetics both gave non-immediate
asthmatic reactions in the provocation test. Also they gave
identical reactions on drinking Campari or cochineal, both of
which contain carmine [15]. The possibility that the allergen is an organic acid, such as carminic acid, needs to be
explored in view of the role of vegetable acids in asthma due
to colophony and western red cedar (to be discussed).

Piperazine. Two workers manufacturing piperazine gave non-
immediate asthmatic reactions to it, capable of being blocked
by 3-hourly inhalation of sodium cromoglycate (Fig. 9) [16].

Cotton dyes. Asthma in cotton workers handling anthracene
and anthraquinone dyes has been shown to be of an immediate
nature, with positive skin and provocation tests [17].
Specific IgE antibody was shown by dyeing paper discs with
the unconjugated dyes for the RAST, showing that haptens may
suffice for the purpose of demonstrating antibodies and also
for skin and other reactions.

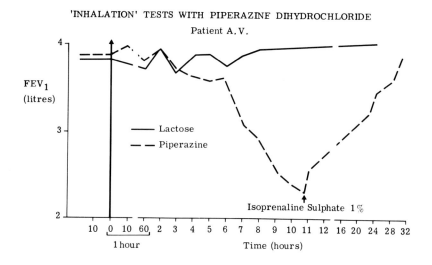

Fig. 9 Non-immediate asthmatic reaction to piperazine.

Wood dusts. Asthma due to wood dusts can be elicited by exposure to the specific dusts. In the case of western red cedar, plicatic acid has been identified as the cause and IgE antibodies have been shown against it [18].

ASTHMA DUE TO FUMES

Colophony. About 20% of workers engaged in the electronics industry, in which colophony (pine-resin) bonded solders are used (Fig. 10), have been found to develop asthma [19]. Its use as a hot melt glue can also cause asthma (Fig. 11). Occupational type provocation tests, in which the whole material and its components are heated as in the soldering process, have shown that the colophony fumes are responsible [20]. A few breaths of the fume, otherwise inhaled for many hours each day, can suffice for the test. Reactions can be immediate, non-immediate, or both, and can be blocked by sodium cromoglycate. Heating of abietic acid, a component of colophony can elicit the reactions and possibly other acids, such as piniaric acid could also play a part. A previous report attributing, without proof, the asthma to aliphatic aldehydes, formaldehyde, has been shown by these tests to be

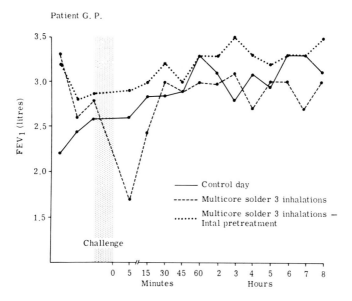

Fig. 10   Immediate asthmatic reactions to Multicore solder bonded with colophony. Blocking of reaction by sodium cromoglycate.

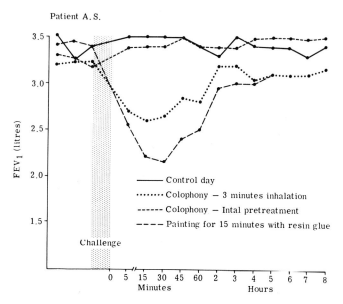

Patient A.S.

FEV$_1$ (litres)

——— Control day
········· Colophony — 3 minutes inhalation
------ Colophony — Intal pretreatment
———— Painting for 15 minutes with resin glue

Challenge

0 5 15 30 45 60   2   3   4   5   6   7   8
       Minutes   Hours

Fig. 11 Immediate asthmatic reactions to colophony fumes
from soldering and to emanations from use as a hot melt glue.

incorrect. This illustrates the essential value of such
tests for the precise identification of the causal agent.
   Some affected workers also develop asthma in pine forests,
where the pine resin is being extruded and where the causal
agents are probably being inhaled. In an atopic asthmatic
subject, not exposed occupationally to colophony, in whom an
attack of asthma developed in a pine forest, the occupational
type test with colophony and abietic acid elicited an
asthmatic response. Asthma occurring in pine forest exposure
has long been a puzzle as the pine pollen does not appear to
be the cause. The above findings suggest that it is the
emanations which may be responsible. Atopy, as defined, is
significantly related to the development of asthma in these
workers.

ASTHMA DUE TO DI-ISOCYANATE EMANATIONS

Immediate and non-immediate asthmatic reactions can be
elicited in affected workers by occupational type exposures
for brief periods to the various di-isocyanate preparations,
TDI, HDI, MDI and NDI (Figs. 12, 13) [21,22]. TDI atmospheric
concentrations as low as 0.001 ppm can suffice, far below
irritant concentrations and TLV levels recommended for prevention of occupational illness. A cogent example of the

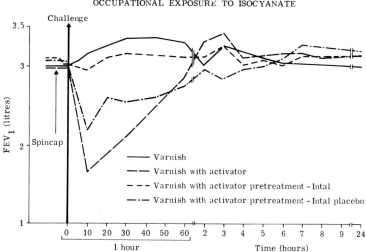

Fig. 12   Immediate asthmatic reaction to polyurethane resin with toluene di-isocyanate.   Blocking of reaction by sodium cromoglycate.

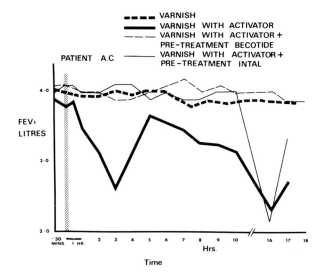

Fig. 13   Non-immediate asthmatic reactions to toluene di-isocyanate.   Blocking of reactions by sodium cromoglycate, except for 16 h reaction.

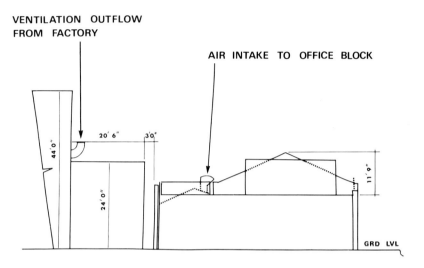

Fig. 14 Sensitization to toluene di-isocyanate of workers in office block by exhaust fumes from polyurethane foam factory.

potential influence of industrial emanations on the general environment is provided by workers sensitized to TDI from an adjoining factory [23]. The exhaust fumes were drawn into the factory through the ventilation system (Fig. 14). Proof of the sensitivity was provided by the bronchial provocation tests.

The presence of specific IgE antibodies is claimed by several workers, though requiring further confirmation [24, 25]. Sensitization of experimental animals with the production of IgE and other antibodies to di-isocyanate is reported.

ASTHMA DUE TO EPOXY RESIN ACTIVATORS

The highly reactive chemicals used in the manufacture of epoxy resins are candidates from allergic sensitization as shown by the findings with exposure to: phthalic anhydride as a fume, a powder and crystals; and to trimellitic anhydride and triethylenetetramine [25].

Phthalic anhydride. Figure 15 shows an acute immediate asthmatic reaction to one breath of fume from a phthalic anhydride epoxy resin in a highly sensitive worker. A previous diagnosis of probable TDI sensitivity was disproved by appropriate testing. Non-immediate asthmatic reactions

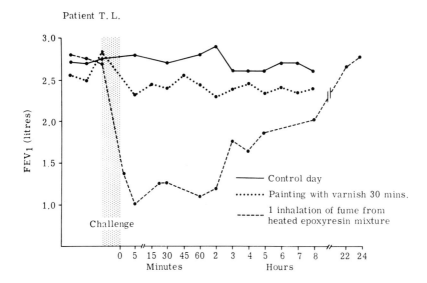

Fig. 15   Immediate asthmatic reaction to heated epoxy resin containing phthalic anhydride.   No reaction to varnish-containing toluene di-isocyanate.

were elicited in other subjects exposed to this material in dust and crystal form.

   Positive immediate skin test reactions and RAST for specific IgE antibody have been found against phthalic anhydride [26].   Sensitization of experimental animals with the production of IgE antibody has also been reported.

Trimellitic anhydride.   Rhinitis, asthma and pneumonitis can be elicited by trimellitic anhydride exposure in sensitized subjects.   Provocation tests elicit immediate and non-immediate reactions, the latter with a "flu-like" syndrome [25,27].   Specific IgE and IgG antibodies and lymphocyte reactions have been found.   The IgG antibody appears to be particularly related to the non-immediate reactions.

Triethylenetetramine.   Figure 16 shows the non-immediate asthmatic reaction to a relatively prolonged occupational type exposure test, and corresponds with the clinical history [25].

ASTHMA DUE TO AMMONIUM PERSULPHATE

In two young female hairdressers asthmatic reactions, immediate in one (Fig. 17) and non-immediate in the other,

Patient A.W.

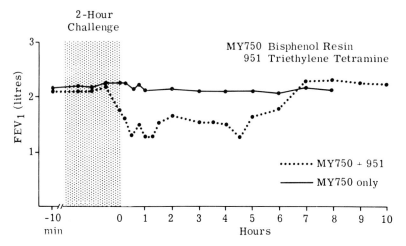

Fig. 16   Non-immediate asthmatic reaction to triethylenetetramine.

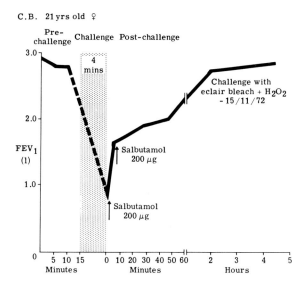

Fig. 17   Immediate asthmatic reaction to ammonium persulphate.

were elicited by brief occupational type exposures to the mixing with a pestle and mortar of a bleach (Eclair) with H_2O_2 [28]. The eleven unnamed powdered ingredients of this material were produced for testing, which showed that ammonium persulphate was the causal agent. In the patient giving the immediate asthmatic reaction a drop of ammonium persulphate solution on unbroken skin elicited a typical immediate wealing reaction which took several minutes longer to develop than the usual Type I wealing reaction. These findings provide yet another example where the known chemical nature of the agent could make it possible by simple skin prick tests to identify precisely the reacting determinants.

CONCLUSIONS

Respiratory allergic diseases due to chemical agents will be one of the most important topics for clinical and immuno-chemical advances in coming years. Occupational circumstances provide what is virtually a designed experimental situation and the relevance to non-occupational environments is also very evident. Advances in immunological tests will make epidemiological studies more feasible, though the observations of individual patients under controlled conditions will remain an essential key to identifying new problems as they arise.

REFERENCES

1. Burge, P.S., O'Brien, I.M. and Harries, M.G. (1979). *Thorax* **34**, 317-323.
2. Pepys, J. and Hutchcroft, B.J. (1975). *Amer. rev. Resp. Dis.* **112**, 829-859.
3. Pepys, J. (1977). *Amer. rev. Resp. Dis.* **116**, 573-588.
4. Pepys, J. and Davies, R.J. (1978). In "Allergy, Principles and Practice" (eds. E. Middleton Jr., C.E. Reed and E.F. Ellis). 1st edn. Vol.2, pp.812-842.
5. Newman Taylor, A.J., Davies, R-J., Hendrick, D.J. and Pepys, J. (1979). *Clin. Allergy* **9**, 213-220.
6. Cleare, M.J., Hughes, E.G., Jacoby, B. and Pepys, J. (1976). *Clin. Allergy* **6**, 183-195.
7. Roberts, A.E. (1951). *Arch. Ind. Hyg.* **4**, 549-559.
8. Kern, R.A. (1939). *J. Allergy* **10**, 164-165.
9. Greene, S.A. and Freedman, S. (1976). *Clin. Allergy* **6**, 105-108.
10. Cromwell, O., Pepys, J., Parish, W.E. and Hughes, E.G. (1979). *Clin. Allergy* **9**, 109-118.
11. Pepys, J., Parish, W.E., Cromwell, O. and Hughes, E.G. (1979). *Clin. Allergy* **9**, 99-108.
12. Pepys, J., Pickering, C.A.C. and Hughes, E.G. (1972). *Clin. Allergy* **2**, 391-396.

13. Davies, R.J., Hendrick, D.J. and Pepys, J. (1974). *Clin. Allergy* **4**, 227-247.

14. Davies, R.J. and Pepys, J. (1975). *Clin. Allergy* **5**, 99-107.

15. Burge, P.S., O'Brien, I.M., Harries, M.G. and Pepys, J. (1979). *Clin. Allergy* **9**, 185-190.

16. Pepys, J., Pickering, C.A.C. and Landon, H.W.G. (1972). *Clin. Allergy* **2**, 189-196.

17. Alanko, K. (1978). *Clin. Allergy* **8**, 25-31.

18. Tse, K.S., Chan, J. and Chan-Young, M. (1982). *Clin. Allergy* **12**, 249-258.

19. Burge, P.S., Edge, G., Hawkins, R., White, V. and Newman Taylor, A.J. (1981). *Thorax* **36**, 828-834.

20. Fawcett, I.W., Newman-Taylor, A.J. and Pepys, J. (1976). *Clin. Allergy* **6**, 577-585.

21. Pepys, J., Pickering, C.A.C., Breslin, A.B.X. and Terry, D.J. (1972). *Clin. Allergy* **2**, 225-236.

22. O'Brien, I.M., Harries, M.G., Burge, P.S. and Pepys, J. (1979). *Clin. Allergy* **9**, 1-6 and 7-15.

23. Carroll, K.B., Secombe, C.J.P. and Pepys, J. (1976). *Clin. Allergy* **6**, 99-104.

24. Bernstein, I.L. (1982). *J. Allerg. Clin. Immunol.* **70**, 24-31.

25. Fawcett, I.W., Newman-Taylor, A.J. and Pepys, J. (1977). *Clin. Allergy* **7**, 1-14.

26. Maccia, C.A., Bernstein, I.L., Emmett, E.A. and Brooks, S.M. (1976). *Amer. rev. Resp. Dis.* **113**, 701-704.

27. Patterson, R., Zeiss, C.R. and Pruzansky, J. (1982). *J. Allerg. Clin. Immunol.* **70**, 19-23.

28. Pepys, J., Hutchcroft, B.J. and Breslin, A.B.X. (1976). *Clin. Allergy* **6**, 399-404.

USES AND LIMITATIONS OF MODELS
FOR PREDICTING HYPERSENSITIVITY

G.E. Davies

Imperial Chemical Industries PLC,
Central Toxicology Laboratory,
Alderley Park, Nr Macclesfield, Cheshire SK10 4TJ, UK

In the context of our present discussion, laboratory models
of allergy are used for two purposes: i) to identify (and
quantify) potential allergenicity of drugs and industrial
chemicals and ii) to identify the allergen responsible for a
given clinical case of allergy. I will deal separately with
each of these two aspects restricting my remarks to general
principles rather than to a consideration of the technical
details of various models which will be dealt with by the
other speakers in this session.

POTENTIAL ALLERGENICITY

From a practical viewpoint it is important that we should
carefully consider our objectives in seeking to identify
chemical allergens.
   Although it is important to devise tests that will maximize
our chances of detecting allergenic chemicals, our major concern is the possibility that the test-substance will induce
allergy in the user in the form and strength used, and with
the frequency and duration of contact expected. Demonstration
of immunogenicity under extreme conditions of testing is insufficient. It can be postulated that suitable experimental
conditions could reveal immunogenicity in virtually *any* substance and one may go so far as to assert that virtually all
compounds are allergenic in that they have sensitized, or will
sensitize, someone, somewhere.
   A Task Force of the European Chemical Industry [1] considered
the problems posed by the EEC Sixth Amendment to the 1967
"Directive on the Classification Packaging and Labelling of
Dangerous Substances" which directed that some chemicals should
be classified as requiring the "R-phrase", "may cause

IMMUNOTOXICOLOGY
ISBN 0-12-282180-7

sensitization by skin contact". The Directive did not attempt
to define a sensitizer. The ECETOC Task Force, after a considerable effort, was able to give only general guidance restricting their consideration to industrial chemicals, specifically excluding formulations for direct consumer uses. They
recommended "an adjuvant-type of test" in the guinea pig but
allowed (with provisos) "alternative tests": they went on to
state that "if in an approved test on 20 animals, three or
more give a positive result on the first epidermal challenge,
irrespective of the severity, the R-phrase will be required".
The recommendation was further qualified by allowing that
"...it may be necessary to supplement this result by further
tests on sensitization, or skin penetration, relevant to the
physico-chemical properties of the substances". The report
emphasized that the testing and labelling indicated sensitization potential but not risk and went on to point out that
chemicals classified as potential human sensitizers were used
in the chemical industry and by its customers, with due precautions.

The popularity of the Magnusson and Kligman Maximization
Test [2] is illustrated by a survey carried out by the ECETOC
Task Force which showed it to be used by 10 out of 14 responding companies. It is important to appreciate that the Maximization Test is a test of potential allergenicity; it is not
an estimate of risk. The authors themselves say of the test:

> The results emphatically do not indicate the likely
> prevalence of human sensitization. The antigenic
> stimulus is far greater than is possible under the
> conditions of normal use...there is one result which
> is predictive...that is when no animal becomes sensi-
> tized. This indicates an allergenicity potential so
> feeble that no imaginable human exposure is likely to
> be attended by a significant incidence of sensitization.

This explicit qualification is often ignored. All this is of
course of little help when we need to know something about
the "likely prevalence of human sensitization", and no firm
guidance is available.

A distinction must be made between hazard and risk. Hazard
might be regarded as what *could* happen and risk as what *will*
happen. Animal tests, then, indicate hazard: experience
indicates risk.

For diluted and formulated products it seems only sensible
that the tested concentration should bear some relationship
to that actually used: ten times the user concentration has
been found by experience to be a reasonable strength to use
[3]. As I have already stated, the size of the exposed population and the circumstances of exposure (deliberate or

accidental) must also be taken into account. All of this can
be summarized by the following "equation":

Risk of individual sensitization = f (Inherent Allergenicity),
(size of exposed population), (frequency of exposure), (exposure concentration).

It is sometimes claimed that, because low molecular weight
chemicals can be coupled to protein, and it can then be shown
that the conjugate can be used to raise antibodies to the
small molecule, then it follows that the coupled chemical is
allergenic. This is nonsense. Virtually any small molecule
can be rendered immunogenic by such procedures, and this
represents the basis of α-sera preparation used in many immuno-
assay procedures.

I have dealt exclusively with tests for contact (Type 4)
allergy. The reasons for this will emerge from the remaining
papers. Tests for other types of allergy are even less satisfactory. As in many other fields of endeavour the need is
for more basic research: little has changed since I considered
the problem 20 years ago! [4].

An additional consideration, therefore, is to define what
incidence of allergy is acceptable and this in turn will depend on the purpose for which the material is intended and
the size of the exposed population — an acceptable incidence
for a life-saving drug must be higher than that for a less
essential compound and the numbers of affected individuals
will relate to the number exposed.

There seem to be three aspects of the problem: i) how do
the responses in test animals (usually guinea pig) relate to
responses in man? ii) how likely are individuals to respond?
iii) what level and pattern of exposure is involved? No
standardized approach is possible: each case must be considered on its merits as will be exemplified by the following
hypothetical situation.

Test Material Compound X is a biocide intended for widespread industrial and domestic use and marketed either in the
final product (e.g., in paint), or as a concentrated solution
for dilution by the user (e.g., as a household disinfectant),
or already formulated (e.g., in a cosmetic). It is graded as
a sensitizer in animal tests. We thus have three levels of
exposure with their accompanying hazards and risks (Table 1).
Exposed to the neat material are the synthetic chemist, and
his assistants, who first prepared the compound, the process
worker who manufactured the material on a large scale and the
formulator who prepared the concentrated solution or formulations. The chemist will probably be unaware of the allergenic potential, at least before animal tests are carried
out, but will be an experienced worker and will naturally

Table 1

	Concn.	Exposed population	Period	Hazard[*]	Risk[†]
Chemist	Neat	1-3	Days – weeks	Unknown	Minimal
Process worker	Neat	1-10	Months – years	Known	Minimal
Formulator	Neat – 20%	1-10	Months – years	Known	Minimal
Painter	0.1%	100 – 1000	Months – years	Known	Low
Diluter of disinfectant	20% – 0.1%	100 – 1000	Months – years	Known	Low
User of disinfectant or cosmetic	1-100 ppm	10^4	Months – years	Unknown	Nil to very low

[*] Hazard as defined by test in guinea pigs

[†] Chance of clinical sensitization

adopt safe working practices. The process operative will
have been informed of the hazard and will take suitable precautions to minimize exposure, as will the formulator. In all
three instances the risk of sensitization will be related to
accidental spillage or the normal level of exposure in use.
The painter will be handling diluted material under less controlled conditions and the exposed population will be higher;
there may therefore be greater risk of sensitization in this
group. Finally, the user of the diluted disinfectant, or the
cosmetics, or the occupant of the painted house, may have
virtually no risk of becoming sensitized because of the low
concentration to which they are exposed, although the actual
risk may well depend on a number of factors impossible to define, not least of which would be the sensitizing potency
(for man) and the size of the exposed population.

IDENTIFICATION OF ALLERGENS

We are on slightly firmer ground when we consider the use of
models for the identification of allergens responsible for
clinical cases of allergy, but even here the current state of
affairs is far from satisfactory. Two series of models are

available — those identifying antibodies and those concerning lymphocyte functions.

Estimations of specific IgE antibodies have been used with considerable success in the identification of complex allergens, such as those derived from pollens or house-dust mites but, with the noteworthy exception of penicillin 5 , there is much less information on their use in the identification of chemical haptens of low molecular weight. Where the chemical is sufficiently reactive to function as a hapten in its own right and to conjugate directly with proteins (e.g., acid anhydrides [6]) then the tests may be expected to work perfectly well. Failure to identify the allergen correctly is frequently attributable to the fact that the actual sensitizing moiety is a metabolite, but there are instances where the explanation of anomalous results is unclear or where the reports are not in agreement (e.g., with isocyanates [7,8].

The literature on this problem is large and further elaboration on this occasion is undesirable but I would plead for continued research, particularly with regard to the nature of antigenic conjugates formed *in vivo* from metabolites and autogenous macromolecules.

Lymphocyte transformation tests for the identification of chemical allergens are notoriously variable. Parker [5] has stated that "the value of *in vitro* assays for cellular immunity in the diagnosis of drug allergy is not well enough substantiated to merit their routine use for this purpose".

There are no "Conclusions" to this paper. They must follow from the remaining contributions. If I am to leave a "message" it would simply be that we should maintain our present pragmatic attitude and should oppose the application of any rigid scheme which would remove our ability to treat each case according to its merits.

REFERENCES

1. European Chemical Industry Ecology and Toxicology Centre (1980). Skin Sensitization: paper prepared by an ECETOC Task Force.
2. Magnusson, B. and Kligman, A.M. (1970). "The Identification of Contact Allergens by Animal Assay". Thomas, Springfield, Illinois.
3. Ritz, H.L. and Buehler, E.V. (1975). In "Conference on Sensitization Testing and its Relevance to Humans". (Int. Federation of Societies of Cosmetic Chemists, Basle.
4. Davies, G.E. (1962). *Proc. Roy. Soc. Med.* **55**, 11-14.
5. Parker, C.W. (1980). In "Clinical Immunology" (Ed. C.W. Parker), Vol.2, pp.1219-1260. W.B. Saunders Co., Philadelphia.

6. Zeiss, C.R., Patterson, R., Pruzansky, J.J., Miller, M.M.,
    Rosenberg, M. and Levitz, D. (1977). *J. Allergy Clin.
    Immunol*. **60**, 96-103.
7. Karol, M.H., Sandberg, T., Riley, J. and Alarie, Y. (1979).
    J. Occup. Med. **21**, 354-358.
8. Butcher, B.T., O'Neil, C.E. and Salvaggio, J.E. (1980).
    J. Allergy Clin. Immunol. **65**, No.3, Abs.17.

EXPERIMENTAL CONTACT SENSITIVITY

E.V. Buehler

*Proctor and Gamble Co., Miami Valley Laboratories,
P.O. Box 391, Southern 5, Cincinnati, Ohio 45239, U.S.A.*

For toxicologists who are actively involved in safety testing
and risk assessment, the ideal animal model should accurately
predict the biological response of humans after any contact
with potentially hazardous materials. Unfortunately this
goal is seldom approached. Therefore, the toxicologist must
design and execute experiments that will define to a higher
degree of accuracy the inherent toxicity of the chemical. If
the biological response of the model can be defined and
understood, and if the relevant information is available for
comparable human responses, then the extrapolation to the
human situation, although not always precise, can be made
with a measure of assurance. Finally, and perhaps most
importantly, it is essential that follow-up on human exposures
be in sufficient detail so that the variations in biological
response can be further defined. In this way the precision
and accuracy of the safety assessment can be checked.

I am not going to discuss the methodology of guinea pig and
human testing nor will I compare results to the other models
available. There are other sources for that information
[1-4]. Rather I will present, very briefly, some theoretical
and practical aspects of sensitization testing, present a
brief over-view of the models that we use, and finally propose a series of experiments that can be conducted to provide
more substantive data for safety assessment. Since my experiences are primarily with the guinea pig I will stress this
aspect of testing. The major point I will try to make is
that both models, guinea pig and human, can effectively
define the sensitization potential of individual chemicals
and formulations. In addition, they can provide quantitative
data that can be compared to other materials already in
commerce. This exercise in comparative toxicology does not
differ in any important way from other toxicological

IMMUNOTOXICOLOGY
ISBN 0-12-282180-7

evaluations. These data, however, cannot be used by themselves to "predict" the occurrence, the incidence or the severity of contact dermatitis when and if the materials are introduced into commerce. The number of subjects and the exposure conditions will vary considerably. As in all other areas of toxicology, it is also necessary to collect and recycle all relevant human experience, and to depend on the knowledge and experience of the toxicologists to assess the "relative" risk and safety of newly identified sensitizers. It is perhaps appropriate to regard these prospectively conducted studies as prophetic since it would seem almost inevitable that allergens will sensitize if exposure occurs under the right set of conditions.

It is a fact that a substantial number of humans can and do develop adverse reactions to otherwise innocuous compounds after repetitive exposures to skin. These adverse reactions may be mild, severe, or even incapacitating. Paradoxically they are caused by the same immunological responses that have evolved to protect the organism from potentially harmful environmental agents.

The reaction produced is eczematous. It is this type of reaction that is the second most prevalent skin reaction seen in dermatology practice; the first being adolescent acne. In the industrial setting, skin problems are the *most* prevalent of the occupationally-related disorders. There are many causes of eczema, delayed contact hypersensitivity being only one. The industrial physician and/or the clinician will attempt to define the aetiology in individual cases. If the appearance of the clinical state persists after empirical treatment, and if the patient's clinical history does not result in diagnosis, the dermatologist may resort to diagnostic patch testing.

Table 1 shows some selected results from a diagnostic patch test study by dermatologists in the North American Contact Dermatitis Group [5]. The materials utilized for testing represent those from a typical testing tray. The results substantiate earlier but less extensive studies. Nickel is recognized and accepted as the most prevalent cause of contact dermatitis followed by the topical anaesthetics, dichromate and Balsam of Peru. It should be obvious, however, that these percentages are not applicable to the total population. These particular subjects were selected from either private or clinical practices. Individual dermatologists were permitted to exclude certain materials from the tray in individual cases. The purpose of the exercise was to select significant allergens for standard testing trays. There is no indication in the report whether positive reactions were diagnostic for the aetiology or whether avoidance of the test

Table 1 *Patch test reactivity to common sensitizers.*

Substances	Results % Reactivity
Nickel sulfate 2.5%	13
Potassium dichromate 0.5%	7.8
Neomycin sulfate 20%	4.7
Ethylenediamine hydrochloride 1%	6.0
Thimerosal 0.1%	6.5
Ammoniated mercury 1%	4.6
Paraben mixture 15%	3.5
Formaldehyde 2%	3.4
Paraphenylenediamine 1%	6.1
Turpentine peroxides 1%	2.2
Wool wax alcohols 30%	2.7
Thiram 1%	5.0
Mercaptobenzothiazole mixture 1%	3.0
Caine mixture 8%	8.4
Naphthyl mixture 1%	1.4
Carba mixture 3%	2.9
Epoxy resin 1%	2.8
Paraphenylenediamine mixture 0.6%	2.2
Balsam of Peru 25%	7.2

From Rudner, E.J. *et al.* (1975). Contact Dermatitis 1, 277.

materials led to a resolution of the diseased state. Neither
is it stated whether or not there were multiple reactions
noted in different individuals. It is well known that highly-
sensitized individuals become non-specifically hyper-reactive.
To the diagnostician this is the "Angry Back Syndrome" [6].
Certainly there were a substantial number of patients, in
this case, who did not respond to any of the materials since
the percentages do not add up to 100%. For further perspective
it must be realized that dermatologists are constantly search-
ing for new sensitizers and there are speciality trays for a
whole variety of types of sensitizers, for example the
preservatives and perfumes. Fisher [7], lists the patch test
concentration and vehicle for testing over 800 materials.
    One should note the relative concentrations of the indi-
vidual test materials. They are selected for testing at the
highest possible non-irritating concentration, but it is surprising that these concentrations tested under occlusive
dressing for 24 to 48 h are required to diagnose clinical
patients who are responding adversely to casual contacts with
these sensitizers. Eczematous reactions to metallic jewellery

Table 2 *Exposure and reactivity to senstizers*

| | | % Reactive | |
Test material		Normals	Clinicals
20% Neomycin	(1.5)*	1.1	6.3
5% Benzocaine	(0.85)	0.17	1.6
2.5% Nickel sulfate	(1.0)	5.8	11.0
1% Ethylenediamine HCl	(0.15)	0.43	3.1

*Relative exposure rates.   From Prystowsky, S.D. *et al.*
(1979).   Arch. Dermatol. 115, 959.

due to nickel, and induction of neomycin sensitivity by first-
aid cream are illustrative.   The point is that dermatologists
use these kind of data to evaluate the problem of sensitization in the human population.

   They consider the patch test to be diagnostic and will
treat patients accordingly.   Table 2 presents some abstracted
data and illustrates a problem with this assumption.   In this
case, [8] both clinic patients and normal subjects were tested
for reactivity to the indicated allergens.   There were 127
clinic patients and 1,152 normal subjects.   The numbers in
parentheses are anecdotal data on exposure rates based on a
personal history questionnaire.   They indicate that everybody
was exposed to nickel while only 15% could recall exposure to
ethylenediamine.   It is instructive that there is a detectable incidence of reactivity to these sensitizers by normal
subjects who were experiencing *no* dermatoses.   The authors
employed use tests on some of the clinical patients with
positive patch tests.   They were able, on occasion, to correlate exposure rates and severity of reactions to put the
clinical problem into perspective.   Finally, they calculated
a "relative risk" factor.   For example, it was apparent that
more women than men were reactive and clinically responsive
to nickel and that pierced ears increased the prevalence by
about seven times.   This report is extremely interesting and
informative and I believe the approach used could be the key
to future studies that might make risk assessment of immunologic phenomena more substantive.

   Very briefly, I would like to review the theoretical
aspects of delayed contact hypersensitivity (Fig. 1).   The
diagram represents the essence of the two dominant pathways
of the immune response.   It is recognized that lymphocytes
are the cells that generate the immune response.   These cells
can be roughly classified as B or T cells based on their
surface characteristics and how they are processed as stem

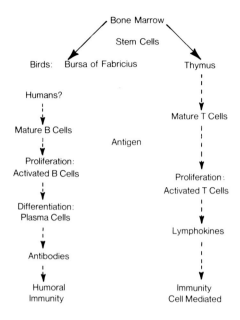

Fig. 1 **The dominant pathways of the immune response.**

cells. The earliest work, in chickens, demonstrated that the
Bursa of Fabricius was the organ for differentiating the
cells responsible for circulating antibody. Therefore, these
were designed as B cells. The human correlate is probably
processed in bone marrow. The end cell in the process is the
plasma cell and it actively produces antibody. Rodent work
has clearly established the thymus as the processing organ
for cell mediated hypersensitivities. The end cell, in this
case is a lymphocyte that produces a number of mediators,
called lymphokines, that produce the disease state. In
actuality, the immunological system is an interacting one and
the functions of the cells are many and varied (Table 3).
The cells can not only be induced to produce antibody and
lymphokines, but can interact with each other and with macrophages producing a biodynamic and homeostatic response. In
the case of homeostatis, "suppressor cells" are the key to
regulation of the immune system and can even produce the
phenomenon known as tolerance. The intricacies and subtle-
ties of this system have only recently been examined more
fully and there remains much to be learned.
     It is apparent, however, that species differences in
responsiveness of the immune system exist. Most of the work
on the B and T cells has been elucidated in the mouse

Table 3 *Cellular components of the immune response.*

---

1. Macrophage — Langerhans cell

2. Thymus (T) derived lymphocytes

    a) effectors
    b) helpers
    c) suppressors
    d) cytotoxic (killer)

3. Bursal equivalent (B) lymphocytes

    a) T-dependent
    b) T-independent

---

followed by comparative or confirmatory studies in humans; for example, the work related to homograft rejection and tissue transplantation. In extrapolating this information to delayed contact dermatitis one must remember that the mouse can produce delayed reactivity by the fourth day and can be non-responsive on the tenth. The guinea pig retains the hypersensitive state longer, but apparently not as long as man.

The sequence of events (Fig. 2) that leads initially to the induction of delayed contact sensitization and then is repeated on a magnified scale during elicitation is outlined. It is dogma to the immunologist than antigens must have a

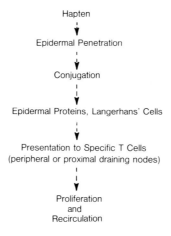

Fig. 2 The induction phase of contact sensitization.

molecular weight of approximately 10,000 in order to be antigenic; that is, to have the specificity and the ability to
induce the immune response. It is, therefore, a requirement
that low molecular weight chemicals react with skin protein
in order to become allergenic. It is also, at least, semi-
dogmatic that the immune system will differentiate "self"
from "non-self", and will respond only to foreign protein.
Theoretically, this haptenic interaction is sufficient to
alter "self into non-self". The site(s) of this interaction
and the details of this very important chemical reaction have
not been identified. It is clear, however, that the specificity of the immune reaction in delayed contact hypersensitivity is directed not only to the three dimensional
aspects of the hapten, but also to portions of the protein.
In fact, the data show that the longer the immune system is
stimulated the broader this specificity becomes. Another
point to stress is that the effect of the Langerhans' cell,
or skin macrophage, on the interactions of the lymphocytes,
as well as the mechanism for lymph node involvement in proliferation and recirculation, are also incompletely understood.

Skin is the target organ in delayed contact hypersensitivity
and although the skin of mammals has much in common there are
basic differences among the various genera and species. For
example the epidermis of the guinea pig appears to be thicker
and the dermis is disordered and resistant to the formation
of vesicles. Furthermore, the dermis is repeatedly penetrated by hair shafts and is separated from underlying fat by
the *panniculus carnosus*. Human skin on the other hand is
more complex, having less hair at most sites, but containing
both eccrine and apocrine sweat glands. The undulating rete
papilla of the epidermis is superimposed on a much more
ordered dermis.

There are additional and significant differences in anatomy
on different portions of the body. This translates into wide
variations in physical properties, such as, penetrability,
and also susceptibility to irritating agents. Other factors
such as ageing and pigmentation can also have dramatic
effects. In addition to these differences in skin, the
immunology of homograft rejection tells us that there are
tissue, genus, species and individual antigenic differences
in skin protein. Each of these proteins, whether in epidermis or dermis, has the potential to react with hapten, and
become antigenic. It is this inherently complex array of
possible hapten/protein interactions that will continue to
delay the development of specific *in vitro* tests to quantify
the delayed reaction.

At the present time it is necessary that the assessment of

delayed contact hypersensitivity, both qualitatively and
quantitatively, be based on a gross observation of the resulting lesion. Microscopic histopathology, for all practical
purposes, cannot differentiate between irritation and sensitization and *in vitro* techniques are insensitive. It is
obvious, however, that the specific nature of lymphokines
and/or the nature of the skin are sufficiently different that
the gross reactions seen on the two models are not directly
comparable. The guinea pig's response is limited to erythema
and occasionally oedema. The human's response is more complex
and can result in papular/vesicular responses that are capable
of spreading beyond the area of contact in the case of the
most severe reactions.

Table 4 *Experimental variables in detecting inherent aller-*
genicity

Genetics

    Human - resistant/susceptible
    Guinea pigs - strains 2 and 13

Route of exposure

    Injection
    Topical
    Occlusive patch

Skin

    Morphology
    Transplant antigens
    Area

Biological properties

Vehicles

    Solubility, penetration

Exposure

    Concentration, time, number

Grading

Table 4 lists some other experimental variables inherent in
the models and covers some points already stressed. The
human genetics involved are not well understood, except that
it is obvious that there is sharp distinction between a susceptible group and a resistant group. For example, strain 2
and strain 13 are inbred in guinea pigs that differ only in
their ability to respond immunologically to two different

and specific dipeptides [9]. Within these susceptible populations, however, the usual rules for toxicology probably
apply. There is a dose response relationship and it can be
demonstrated. There are, however, in the case of sensitization two dose-response curves, one for induction and one for
elicitation. It is apparent that genetic principles are involved even at the level of the lymphocyte. The surface
antigens on the lymphocyte that determine its specificity to
react with antigen are also associated with separate genetic
loci that determine its ability to respond.

With regard to route of exposure, it should be recognized
that one could choose either topical application or in the
case of the guinea pig, injection, in preference to the
occlusive patch. I have included "Biological properties" of
the chemical because it is well known that certain chemicals
can directly and/or indirectly modify the immune response.
Many cancer chemotherapeutic agents are effective because of
their immunosuppressive properties, while several lymphocyte
mitogens are used experimentally. Finally one must always
remember that animal models are not completely naive immunologically and that dynamically changing their immune status
can have a significant effect on both primary and secondary
responses. This is particularly true with humans who have
considerable environmental contact via the skin to numerous
chemicals. The guinea pig, on the other hand, although
otherwise immunologically active, because of its protective
hair and isolated existence, is naive to skin contact with
most environmental chemicals.

I will now discuss an experimental approach that can be
used for safety assessment. The intent is to detect and
identify the potential to sensitize so that this biological
property of a new ingredient can be assessed along with any
other inherent toxicity that might be present. The guinea
pig test (Fig. 3) that we use is diagrammatically presented.
It is intended to be a screening procedure prior to the human
repeated insult patch test and other subsequent human exposures. The concept is simple. Single occlusive patches
containing solubilized test material are applied to a test
group of guinea pigs at weekly intervals for three weeks.
It is a prerequisite that the chemical penetrate into at
least the upper layers of the skin. Patches are removed
after 6 h exposure. During the fifth week, challenges, with
the highest non-irritating concentration of the same test
material are made on a naive site. An appropriate challenge
control is used. Eighty percent ethanol is generally used
as a vehicle for induction and acetone is generally used for
challenge. At 24 and 48 h after application of the challenge
patch, the sites are graded for degree of erythema and are

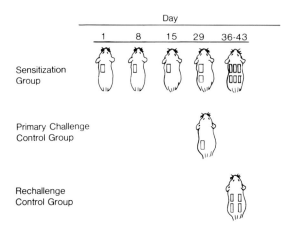

Fig. 3 Buehler topical patch technique.

Table 5 *Primary sensitization*

Experimental group	Response grade					Incidence	Severity
	0	0.5	1	2	3		
Test group (24 h)	6	2	7	4	1	13/20	1.0-0.8
(48 h)	8	2	6	4	0		
Control group (24 h)	7	3	0	0	0	0/10	0.2-0.1
(48 h)	9	1	0	0	0		

assigned numbers of 0 through 3, three being intense erythema.
Illustrative results are presented in Table 5. The severity
score represents the average skin grades of all animals at
24 and 48 h. The incidence is the fraction of animals responding with greater severity than the controls. The 0.5
scores represent barely susceptible irritation and are an
assurance that an adequate concentration has been tested.
The incidence of 13/20 reflects that there was a guinea pig
with a barely discernible, i.e., 0.5, reaction at 24 h that
was stronger, i.e., 1.0, at 48 h. One animal reversed that
sequence. Both animals are considered to be sensitized.
  The guinea pig has six test sites available for patching,
which means there is a certain degree of flexibility with
regard to challenge/re-challenge situations. An important
criterion for re-challenges is that they should be accomplished within a couple of weeks of the primary challenge.

It is often important, therefore, to anticipate follow-up experiments, prior to induction and elicitation. I should also mention that there are occasions when it is important to have a stable of highly reactive guinea pigs available for elicitation. On these occasions we use a procedure that has been presented by Ritz [2], that involves a single injection of the test material in Freund's adjuvant. This process usually provides several highly sensitive guinea pigs even when weak sensitizers are used.

Table 6 *Supplementary information after primary challenge*

---

1. Confirmation of sensitization

   a) Re-challenge at $\geq$ concentration
   b) Dose response — no effect level

2. Cross reactions

   a) Chemically related
   b) Components of mixtures
   c) Fractions or impurities

3. Re-design for comparative toxicology

   a) Dose response
        induction/elicitation
   b) Other variables

Table 6 is a summary outline of the kinds of experiments that can be useful for safety assessment. The most common circumstance will be the need to confirm reactivity in the case of relatively weak sensitizers or to determine the dose response and the no-effect level of stronger sensitizers. The latter information could be important for designing the human repeated insult patch test.

Table 7 *Cross reactivity of chemically similar materials*

Re-challenge test compound*	Animals sensitized
Primary sensitizer	6/7 (2.2 - 2.1)**
Homologue A	6/7 (1.9 - 1.1)
Homologue B	3/7 (0.9 - 0.9)

  * Tested at equimolar concentrations
 ** Number sensitized/number tested

The next most important question usually relates to the
specificity of the reaction and how broadly it might apply to
chemically related materials. In addition, the ingredient
being tested is often a mixture of materials and will always
contain impurities. It is important to establish the actual
sensitizing component in these mixtures. If the individual
chemicals can be identified and synthesized in a relatively
pure state the re-challenge sites can be used appropriately
to identify the causative agent. For example, the experiment
shown in Table 7 was designed to investigate the structure
activity relationship of three chemically similar materials,
taken from unpublished data by Ritz [10]. Homologue A showed
the highest cross-reactivity and molecular modelling confirmed
its three-dimensional similarity. Table 8 shows a hypothetical
situation with re-challenges subsequent to primary challenge,
where only sensitized animals were used. Component A-3 would
clearly be implicated.

Table 8 *Identification of the sensitizing component in a
mixture*

	Incidence	Severity
Primary challenge		
Test substance A	10/20	1.2 - 1.4
Re-challenge		
Component A-1	0/10	0.1 - 0.2
Component A-2	0/10	0.1 - 0.2
Component A-3	7/10	0.9 - 1.1

* No significant response in controls

A specific batch of alkyl ether sulfate designated LES
13-2035, was implicated as a sensitizer during a dermatitis
epidemic in Scandinavia (Table 9) [11]. Animals sensitized
by closed patch to the surfactant reacted not only with a
formulation containing the surfactant, but also to the hexane
extractable fraction. Further extraction and considerable
guinea pig testing extablished that a change in processing
had resulted in low levels of sultones. These sultones were
extremely potent as sensitizers and changing the chemical
process resolved the problem. Table 10 shows the dual dose
response and the quantitative relationship of two of these
synthesized sultones. The C_{16} moiety is apparently less
potent although in this particular case, it is probably due
to its inability to penetrate the skin.

Table 9 *Re-challenge of LES 13-2035 sensitized animals*

		Incidence*	Severity
Dishwashing liquid	20% aqueous	50/91 (55)	0.8 - 0.7
Hexane extract	1% acetone	18/30 (70)	0.9 - 0.7
	0.33% acetone	31/67 (48)	0.7 - 0.5

* Number sensitized/number tested: number in parentheses -
% reacting.
* Average score at 24 and 48 h.

Table 10 *Sensitization with 1-alkenyl-1,3-sultones*

Compound	Induction nmole	Challenge 2	Response 20	Dose, nmole[a]) 200
C_{12}	71	2/15	4/15	9/15
	710	6/15	8/15	13/15
	7100	9/14	10/14	13/14
C_{16}	71	0/14	0/14	0/14
	710	0/15	0/15	1/15
	7100	1/15	1/15	6/15

a) Number sensitized/number tested.

For materials of interest, that have been tested in the
guinea pig without producing delayed hypersensitivity or are
intended to be used at low levels, it is also necessary to
do human testing [12]. In these instances not only ingredients but also the complete formulation will generally be
tested (Table 11). We consider 200 to be an adequate number
of subjects so 2-3 panels of 60-80 subjects will be run at
different times. There are significant differences in the
details of the protocols, as indicated on the Table. These
differences are more or less intentional since both tests
have evolved empirically and both have been modified to
maximize their separate utilities. It is the purpose of each
test to describe the allergenic potential of test materials.
Most of the differences are related to inherent differences
in the test subjects. The most significant is the difference
in vehicles and the numbers and time of exposure. The actual
patch may vary, but is always occlusive. Two challenges are
conducted; one on the original site of application and
another on the opposite arm. The variation in responses

Table 11 *Human repeated insult patch test*

---

1. Occlusive patch

2. Vehicle

     a) Aqueous
     b) Dilute formulation

3. Induction
     3 x /week for 3 weeks

4. Challenge

     a) Original site
     b) Alternate site

5. Scoring

Table 12 *Supplemental human studies*

---

1. Dose response to challenge

2. Identification

     a) Ingredient
     b) Fraction

3. Recycle to guinea pig

4. *ad libitum* use tests

---

requires a complex scoring system to describe the lesion and
to account for uncontrollable events (such as lost patches).
   Interpretation of the human test (Table 12) in many ways is
more difficult than it is with the guinea pig test.   The
variability in the gross appearance of the lesion is one factor.   Another is that the human test can result in cumulative
irritation and very often other reactions are seen that are
attributable to prior exposures, e.g., pre-sensitization.
It is, therefore, imperative that human tests be pre-
programmed for re-challenges.   The only limitations on what
can be done are those imposed by the subjects themselves.
Otherwise, the same types of studies as those described for
the guinea pig can also be done.   Additionally and most
importantly, humans can be used for *ad libitum* or provocative
tests at whatever extent of exposure might be required.   The
ability of a "sensitized individual" to use a formulation
containing a material that has a low potential to sensitize
is substantive data and permits a well informed safety
assessment.   Provocative tests can be used to define the

threshold level of reactivity. In addition, it is often very
useful to utilize the information from the human tests to recycle the problem of the guinea pig. This can be very informative particularly in the cases where vehicle can have significant effects on penetration.

Table 13 *Utility of human testing*

Panelist	Primary challenge* (96 h after removal)	Two month Usage Study Lotion	Soap	Diagnostic (96 h after removal) A	B	C
006	1	0	0	0	1	1
025	0	0	0	0	0	0
045	1	0	0	0	0	0
106	0	0	0	0	0	0
060	0 (1E)**	0	0	1E	1E	1E
065	1E	0	0	2	2	2
076	1E	0	0	2	2	2
082	1 (1E)**	0	0	2	1	1
087	1E	0	0	2	1E	2
088	1E	0	0	2	2	2
091	2E	0	0	2	2	2

* Erythema (1-3).   ** 264 h after removal.
Papules or edema (E).   J. Powers, personal communication.

Table 13 summarizes some data that illustrate the utility of
the proposed approach [13]. Subsequent to the finding in the
guinea pig that an experimental preservative had relatively
weak allergenic potential, a series of human repeated insult
patch tests were initiated and completed in 230 subjects. At
preservative levels in two separate experimental formulations,
there were no positive responders. In another test, however,
at increased concentration in a different vehicle and after
heating to solubilize the material there were 17 out of 99
subjects with reactions that were considered to be typical
for sensitization. Seven of these subjects as well as four
test controls agreed to further studies. Each subject was
exposed for two weeks at a time to gradually increasing exposure levels to two seperate formulations containing differing levels of this preservative. Finally, they were able
to use these products *ad libitum* with no clinical or subject-
ive effect. While this phase of testing was proceeding in
the human, groups of highly sensitized guinea pigs were
challenged with pure materials that were known to be present
as impurities. This established that the reactivity was

most likely due to the preservative itself, rather than to an
impurity present during synthesis or that was formed during
processing. Re-challenging the human subjects with three
separate but typical batches of the preservative would tend
to confirm this observation. Our specific conclusion was that
the choice of vehicles was critical and substantive for its
allergenic potential. More generally, it is also clear that
practical thresholds can be described for potentially useful
sensitizers.

SUMMARY

The guinea pig model can be used to detect and identify the
allergenic properties of low-molecular weight chemicals.
Discovering this biological property of a chemical does not
necessarily predict that this material will induce clinically
relevant dermatitis in the consumer. However, by fully
utilizing the sites available for challenge, it is possible
to quantify this reaction and provide other relevant data
that are important in the design of human studies. In addition, comparison of these quantitative data to similar data
on chemicals with known epidemiology can provide a "risk
factor". Furthermore, *ad libitum* and provocative data in the
human are even more substantive data for safety assessment.
   The final point I would like to make is that the information
from the market place with regard to incidence and severity of
reactions is an essential element, if knowledgeable safety
assessments are to continue to be made. Knowledge of the
presence or absence of adverse reactions during intended use
or accidental misuse are critical for evaluation of safety
assessment.

REFERENCES

1. Buehler, E.V. (1965). *Arch. Dermatol.* **91**, 171-177.
2. Ritz, H.L. and Buehler, E.V. (1980). In "Current Con-
    cepts in Cutaneous Toxicity", pp.25-40. Academic Press.
3. Magnusson, B. and Kligman, A.M. (1969). *J. Inv. Dermatol.*
    52, 268-276.
4. Klecak, G. (1977). In "Dermatotoxicology and Pharmacology"
    (eds. F.H. Marzulli and H.I. Maibach), pp.305-340.
    Halsted Press, N.Y.
5. North American Contact Dermatitis Group (1975). *Contact
    Dermatitis* **1**, 277-280.
6. Mitchel, J.C. (1977). *Contact Dermatitis* **3**, 315-320.
7. Fisher, A.A. (1973). "Contact Dermatitis", pp.1-448.
    Lea & Febiger, Philadelphia.
8. Prystowsky, S.D., Allen, A.M., Smith, R.W., Nonomura,
    J.H., Odom, R.B. and Akers, W.A. (1979). *Arch. Dermatol.*
    115, 959-962.

9. Ben-Efraim, S. and Maurer, P.H. (1966). *J. Immunol.* **97,** 577-587.
10. Ritz, H.L. (1982). Personal Communication.
11. Ritz, H.L., Conner, D.S. and Sauter, E.D. (1975). *Contact Dermatitis* **1,** 349-358.
12. Buehler, E.V. and Griffith, J.F. (1975). In "Animal Models in Dermatology" (ed. H.I. Maibach), pp.56-66. Churchill Livingston, N.Y.
13. Powers, J. (1982). Personal Communication.

ANIMAL MODELS OF SENSITIZATION
VIA THE RESPIRATORY TRACT

J.E. Doe

*Imperial Chemical Industries PLC,
Central Toxicology Laboratory,
Alderley Park, Macclesfield, Cheshire, UK*

INTRODUCTION

Sensitization via the respiratory tract leading to occupational asthma is an important cause of morbidity in industry.
At least thirty non-protein, simple chemicals have been
reported to cause occupational asthma and some are listed in
Table 1. They have been reported to cause three classes of
pulmonary reaction in sensitized individuals; an immediate
reaction which occurs within minutes of exposure to the
allergen, a late reaction which occurs several hours after
exposure, and a dual reaction where an immediate reaction
precedes a late reaction. Despite the efforts of many
investigators to define the process of sensitization and to
devise suitable testing regimes, there are no accepted
experimental methods for identifying those chemicals which
are likely to cause respiratory sensitization. It is the
industrial toxicologist's role to try to predict the effects
of chemicals in man to aid in the development of safe ways of
handling them, by using models which are predictive both
qualitatively and, if possible, quantitatively. In this case
there are two phases involved, the sensitization of the individual and the reaction in sensitized subjects. This paper
describes some of the work which has investigated both of
these phases in experimental animals.

SENSITIZATION VIA THE RESPIRATORY TRACT

The Entry of Chemicals into the Respiratory Tract

In order to be a sensitizer by inhalation, the chemical must
gain entry into the respiratory tract, which means it must be
present as a gas, a vapour, droplets or particles small

Table 1 *Some simple chemicals reported to cause occupational asthma*

Abietic acid (23)	Enflurane (31)	Phthalic anhydride (37)
Aminoethylethanolamine (24)	Ethylenediamine (28)	Platinum salts (38)
6-Aminopenicillanic acid (25)	Formalin (32)	Potassium dichromate (28)
Ammonium thioglycollate (26)	Hexamethylenetetramine (26)	Sodium benzoate (39)
Ampicillin (25)	1,5-Naphthylene diisocyanate (33)	Spiramycin (40)
Amprolium hydrochloride (27)	Monoethanolamine (26)	Sulphathiazole (28)
Benzylpenicillin (25)	Nickel sulphate (34)	Tartrazine (39)
Chloramine-T (28)	Phenylenediamine (28)	Toluene diisocyanate (TDI) (8)
Dimethylmethane diisocyanate (MDI) (30)	Phenylglycine hydrochloride (35)	Triethylenetetramine (23)
	Piperazine hydrochloride (36)	Trimellitic anhydride (41)

( ) = reference number

enough to be inhaled. Inhaled particles may be deposited in the respiratory tract as a result of impaction, sedimentation, Brownian motion, turbulent diffusion and electrostatic forces, the appropriate mechanism involved and the site of deposition are determined by the size, shape and density of the particle and by the air velocity during respiration [1]. Particles can be deposited throughout the respiratory tract from the nose, where most particles larger than 10 μm are deposited, the bronchi where particles of 5 to 10 μm are deposited and the alveolar regions where particles between 0.1 and 5 μm may deposit [2]. Vapours may reach all levels of the respiratory tract and form hapten conjugates if reactive.

The lymphoid tissue in the respiratory tract has been classified into three levels by Nagaishi [3] into: lymph nodes found close to the trachea, the carina and the major bronchi; lymphoid nodules closely related to bronchial walls; and lymphoid infiltrations scattered throughout the respiratory bronchioles and the broncho-alveolar junction. There is evidence that the lung is capable of mounting a purely local immune reaction in response to the presence of antigenic material [4], but a strong stimulus can apparently overcome the "barrier" function of the lung and systemic sensitization may result [5,6]. Mackaness [7] has postulated that the major function of the lymphoid apparatus in the lung is the exclusion of antigenic material, but this obviously fails when sensitization occurs.

Experimental Studies of Sensitization via the Respiratory Tract

Much of the experimental work in this area has centred around the isocyanates, especially toluene diisocyanate (TDI) which has been shown to cause occupational asthma in a proportion of those exposed to it [8]. Scheel *et al.* [9] were able to demonstrate the presence of precipitating antibodies, following the exposure of rabbits to TDI at a concentration of 0.1 ppm for six hours a day for five days a week for five weeks using a conjugate of TDI with ovalbumin as an antigen. More recently, these observations have been followed up by the work of Karol and her associates with TDI and Tolyl-p-isocynate (TMI) [10,11]. Exposure of guinea pigs to 1 ppm TMI on day one for three hours, 2 ppm for one hour on day two, and 1 ppm for one hour per day on days three, four and five resulted in the production of cytophilic antibodies detected with a TMI-bacterial amylase conjugate on day 14. Karol was able to obtain a dose-related response in the production of precipitating and cytophilic antibodies in guinea pigs following exposure to TDI for three hours a day for five days. At

0.25 ppm and 0.5 ppm there were minimal antibody titres as
assayed by passive cutaneous anaphylaxis with a TDI-guinea
pig serum albumin, whereas exposures to 1.0 ppm resulted in
significant titres by day 21 in all animals exposed.

Similar results have been obtained following the intratracheal instillation of simple chemicals. Patterson *et al.*
[12] instilled trimellitic anhydride intratracheally into
rhesus monkeys leading to the finding of specific IgA and IgM
in broncho-alveolar fluid and specific IgG and IgM in serum
using a conjugate of trimellitic anhydride with human serum
albumin (TM-HSA). Reactivity of peripheral lymphocytes to
TM-HSA was also noted. Patterson *et al.* [13] have also instilled diphenylmethane diisocyanate (MDI) intratracheally
into dogs and provoked the production of specific IgA, IgG
and IgM as detected by an MDI dog serum albumin conjugate
(MDI-DSA). The dogs also showed immediate skin reactivity to
MDI-DSA, and there was peripheral lymphocyte reactivity to
MDI-DSA. Stein-Streilein [14] instilled picryl sulphonic
acid intratracheally into hamsters and demonstrated delayed
hypersensitivity reactions on the ears following the application of TNCB on day five.

However, sensitization is not the only response to be seen
following the administration of simple chemicals to the
respiratory tract. Parker and Turk [15] instilled potassium
dichromate or nickel sulphate intratracheally into guinea pigs
nine days before attempting to sensitize them parenterally to
the appropriate hapten. The intratracheal instillation resulted in the inhibition of the sensitization of the guinea
pigs as measured by skin tests. Instillation with potassium
dichromate did not affect the response to nickel sulphate and
vice versa, indicating a state of specific unresponsiveness
or tolerance. Doe *et al.* [16] observed a similar phenomenon
following the exposure of guinea pigs to TDI by inhalation at
1 ppm for five hours. This treatment inhibited subsequent
dermal sensitization for up to seven weeks, but did not affect
the ability of DNCB to sensitize the guinea pigs. Pretreatment with cyclophosphamide before exposure to TDI not
only prevented the induction of tolerance, but also allowed
the TDI inhalation to sensitize the animals shown by positive
skin reaction 21 days later.

The experimental work summarized above indicates that it is
possible to sensitize laboratory animals by the administration
of simple chemicals by inhalation or by intratracheal instillation and to show both humoral and cellular responses. There
are, however, indications that tolerance may also result from
exposure to chemicals via the respiratory tract, and it is
possible to postulate that perhaps this is the normal response
to inhaled antigens as the majority of those exposed occupationally to sensitizing chemicals do not become sensitized [17].

PULMONARY REACTIONS IN SENSITIZED ANIMALS

Immediate Reactions

Guinea pigs sensitized with a protein react to the inhalation
of that protein by going into anaphylactic shock. At lower
concentrations of antigen the guinea pig responds with an increase in respiration rate within minutes which has been used
as an index of response by Karol et al. [10,11]. Using guinea
pigs sensitized by the inhalation of TMI vapour, TMI-ovalbumin
conjugate and TDI vapour, Karol et al. have shown that a conjugated hapten is necessary for the guinea pigs to express its
sensitized state. Guinea pigs sensitized with TMI-ovalbumin
to the inhalation of TMI-ovalbumin aerosol but not to an aerosol of ovalbumin. Guinea pigs sensitized with TMI vapour respond positively to an aerosol of TMI-bovine albumin, but they
do not respond to TMI vapour. This is in marked contrast to
sensitized humans where reactions follow exposure to TDI
vapour [8].

Delayed Reactions

Work in our own laboratories using guinea pigs sensitized with
subcutaneous or footpad injections of antigen or hapten in
Freund's Complete Adjuvant (FCA), has indicated that a similar
state of unreactivity to haptens may exist with delayed reactions. Guinea pigs sensitized by 0.25 mg of ovalbumin in FCA
on days one and 15 and challenged with a 0.5% aerosol of
ovalbumin for one hour on day 24 showed a slow rise in respiration rate and resistance, as measured by a non-invasive
method of rat measuring pulmonary function [18], see Fig. 1.
Roska et al. [19] described a similar reaction in guinea pigs
sensitized with ovalbumin which was attributed to a type III
antibody-mediated reaction. In guinea pigs sensitized with
FCA alone on days one and 15 and challenged with an aerosol
of purified protein derivative of old tuberculin (PPD), an
increased respiration rate and decreased tidal volume were
observed at 24 hours and 48 hours after challenge, but not
one or three hours after challenge (Fig. 2). These results
are similar to those described by Miyamoto et al. [20] using
a similar experimental regime. After 48 hours the guinea
pigs were killed and the free pulmonary cell population was
examined using a lavage technique [21] and showed an increase
in total cells, made up of lymphocytes and macrophages (Fig.
3). In contrast, challenge with the appropriate hapten
failed to show any change in either respiratory parameters or
cells recovered by pulmonary lavage in guinea pigs sensitized
with either dinitrochlorobenzene or potassium dichromate in
FCA which showed reactions on skin test. Guinea pigs

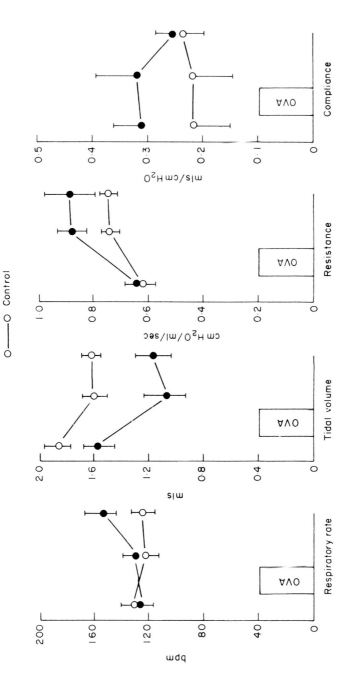

Fig. 1 The effect of exposure to an ovalbumin aerosol on the pulmonary function of guinea pigs sensitized to ovalbumin in FCA.

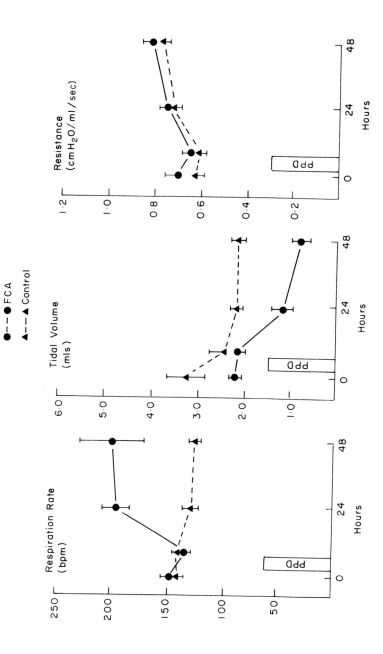

Fig. 2 The effect of PPD aerosol on the lung function of guinea pigs sensitized with FCA.

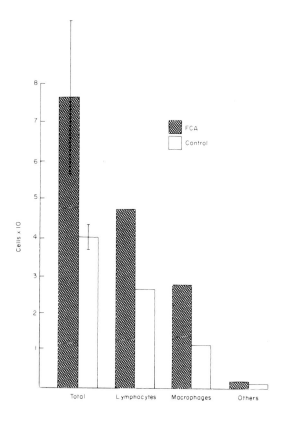

Fig. 3 The effect of PPD aerosol on cells recovered by lung
lavage in guinea pigs sensitized with FCA.

sensitized by TDI in FCA showed skin reactions when challenged
dermally, but exposure to 2 ppm TDI vapour for two hours did
not cause a change in respiratory parameters. There was however, an increase in the total cells recovered from the lungs
by pulmonary lavage consisting of an increase in polymorphonuclear cells (Fig. 4). Thus again there appears to be a
difference between the ability of guinea pigs to respond to
protein and to unconjugated haptens, the reasons for which
represent an interesting area for research. This phenomenon
makes the study of the pulmonary hypersensitivity of simple
chemicals very difficult.

THE PREDICTION OF PULMONARY SENSITIZATION POTENTIAL

As there are no accepted experimental models for pulmonary
sensitization, it is difficult to offer advice on predicting

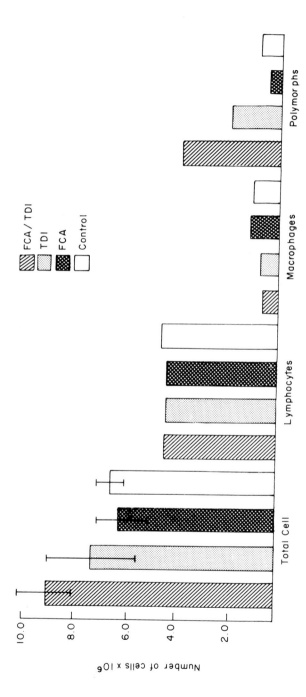

Fig. 4 The effect of exposure to 2 ppm TDI for 2 hours on cells recovered by lung lavage in guinea pigs sensitized with TDI in FCA.

the potential of a new chemical to cause pulmonary sensitization. Obviously, unless a chemical can become airborne either as a vapour or as inhalable droplets or particles it cannot be inhaled and therefore cannot become a pulmonary sensitizer, and any potential problem is avoided. This proviso effectively limits the number of chemicals which need to be considered, and good occupational hygiene and handling precautions for dusty and volatile materials can reduce it even further. There remains however, a possibility that a very potent pulmonary sensitizer would still exert its action at very low exposure levels and there is, unfortunately, little that can be done to predict this type of compound at present. A knowledge of its skin sensitizing ability does not appear to be of great value in this matter, for compounds, such as dicyclohexylmethane diisocyanate, have been shown to cause contact dermatitis but little or no pulmonary sensitization has been reported, although inhalation exposure is thought to have occurred [22]. Development of the guinea pig models where sensitization has been achieved by inhalation exposure should be considered. The major obstacle has been the difficulty in eliciting pulmonary reactions to inhaled simple chemicals. Perhaps this problem should simply be shelved at the moment and the response of guinea pigs to inhaled chemicals be further evaluated in terms of whether the production of a specific cytophilic antibody occurs or sensitized lymphocytes are produced.

There is an outside chance that it would be possible to predict the type of sensitivity that might be produced i.e., immediate, late or dual if such procedures could be investigated with a wide range of chemicals with known properties in humans. Such experimentation would also provide indications of the exposure concentrations at which sensitization is likely to result so that appropriate hygiene standards could be suggested.

ACKNOWLEDGEMENT

I thank Mrs G.M. Milburn and Mr L. Pinto for their experimental assistance.

REFERENCES

1. Hatch, T.F. and Gross, P. (1964). "Pulmonary Deposition and Retention of Inhaled Aerosols" Academic Press, New York.
2. Lipmann, M. (1981). In "Inhalation Toxicology and Technology" (Ed. B.K.J. Leong) pp.107-120, Ann Arbor Science, Ann Arbor.
3. Nagaishi, C. (1972). In "The Lymphatic System" pp.102-179,

Baltimore University, Rank Press, Baltimore.
4. Burrell, R. and Hill, H.O. (1975). *Clin. Exp. Immunol.* **24**, 116-124.
5. Nash, D.R. and Holle, B. (1973). *Clin. Exp. Immunol.* **13**, 573-583.
6. Galindo, B. and Myrvik, Q.D. (1970). *J. Immunol.* **105**, 227-237.
7. Mackaness, G.B. (1971). *Am. Rev. Respir. Dis.* **104**, 813-828.
8. Pepys, J., Pickering, C.A.C., Breslin, A.B.Y. and Terry, D.J. (1972). *Clin. Allergy* **2**, 225-236.
9. Scheel, L.D., Killens, R. and Josephson, A. (1964). *Amer. Ind. Hyg. Assoc. J.* **25**, 179-184.
10. Karol, M.H., Dixon, C., Brady, M. and Alarie, Y. (1980). *Tox. Appl. Pharmac.* **53**, 260-270.
11. Karol, M.H. In "Inhalation Toxicology and Technology" (Ed. B.K.J. Leong) pp.233-246, Ann Arbor Science, Ann Arbor.
12. Patterson, R., Zeiss, R.C., Roberts, M., Pruzansky, J.J., Wolkonsky, P. and Chacon, R. (1978). *J. Clin. Invest.* **62**, 971-978.
13. Patterson, R., Harris, K.E., Pruzansky, J.J. and Zeiss, C.R. (1982). *J. Lab. Clin. Med.* **99**, 615-623.
14. Stein-Streilein, J. (1982). *Amer. Rev. Respir. Dis.* **125**, 58.
15. Parker, D. and Turk, J.L. (1978). *Int. Archs. Allergy Appl. Immunol.* **57**, 289-293.
16. Doe, J.E., Hicks, R. and Milburn, G.M. (1982). *Int. Archs. Allergy Appl. Immunol.* **68**, 275-279.
17. Butcher, B.T., Karr, R.M., O'Neill, C., Davies, R.J. and Salvaggio, J.E. (1978). *J. Allergy Clin. Immunol.* **60**, 138-147.
18. Hiett, D.M. (1974). *Brit. J. Ind. Med.* **31**, 53-58.
19. Roska, A.K.B., Garancis, J.C., Moore, V.L. and Abramoff, P. (1977). *Clin. Immunol. and Immunopath.* **8**, 213-224.
20. Miyamoto, T., Kabe, J., Noda, M., Kobayashi, N. and Miura, K. (1971). *Amer. Rev. Respir. Dis.* **103**, 509-515.
21. Brain, J.D. and Frank, R. (1968). *J. Appl. Physiol.* **25**, 61-69.
22. Emmett, E.A. (1976). *J. Occ. Med.* **18**, 802-804.
23. Fawcett, I.W., Newman-Taylor, A.J. and Pepys, J. (1977). *Clin. Allergy* **7**, 1-14.
24. Pepys, J. and Pickering, C.A.C. (1972). *Clin. Allergy* **2**, 197-204.
25. Davies, R.J., Hendrick, D.J. and Pepys, J. (1974). *Clin. Allergy* **4**, 227-247.
26. Gelfand, H.H. (1963). *J. Allergy* **34**, 374-381.
27. Greene, S.A. and Freedman, S. (1976). *Clin. Allergy* **6**, 105-108.

28. Popa, V., Teculescu, D., Stanescu, D. and Garislescu, N. (1969). *Dis. Chest* **56**, 395-404.

29. Vallieres, M., Cockroft, D.N., Taylor, D.M., Dolorich, J. and Hargreave, F.E. (1977). *Amer. Rev. Resp. Dis.* **115**, 867-887.

30. Tanser, A.R., Bourke, M.P. and Blandford, A.G. (1973). *Thorax* **28**, 596-600.

31. Schwettmann, R.S. and Casterline, J. (1976). *Anaesthesiol.* **44**, 166-199.

32. Hendrick, D.J. and Lane, D.J. (1977). *Brit. J. Ind. Med.* **34**, 11-18.

33. Harries, M.G., Burge, P.S., Jameson, M., Newman-Taylor, A.J. and Pepys, J. (1979). 762-766

34. McConnell, L.II., Fink, J.N., Schleueter, D.P. and Schmidt, M.C. (1973). *Ann. Intern. Med.* **78**, 888-890.

35. Kammermeyer, J.K. and Mathews, K.P. (1973). *J. Allergy Clin. Immunol.* **52**, 73-84.

36. Pepys, J., Pickering, C.A.C. and Loudon, H.W.B. (1972). *Clin. Allergy* **2**, 189-196.

37. Chester, E.H., Schwartz, H.J., Payner, C.B. and Greenstein, S. (1977). *Clin. Allergy* **7**, 15-20.

38. Pepys, J., Pickering, C.A.C. and Hughes, J. (1972). *Clin. Allergy* **2**, 391-396.

39. Freedman, B.J. (1977). *Clin. Allergy* **1**, 407-415.

40. Davies, R.J. and Pepys, J. (1975). *Clin. Allergy* **5**, 99-107.

41. Zeiss, C.R., Patterson, R., Pruzansky, J.J., Miller, M.M., Rosenburg, M., Suszko, I. and Levitz, D. (1977). *J. Allergy Clin. Immunol.* **60**, 96-103.

IMMUNE DRUG-INDUCED BLOOD DYSCRASIAS

E.C. Gordon-Smith

*Royal Postgraduate Medical School,
Du Cane Road, London W12 OHS, U.K.*

INTRODUCTION

Haematology has many advantages over other specialities in
medicine which derive from the ease with which the blood may
be biopsied and studied in the laboratory. It is not surprising, therefore, that the study of human blood has provided
the basis for so many important fields of medicine and science,
from immunology itself to molecular biology, from the physiology of gas exchange to the new speciality of rheology. Nor
is it to be wondered at that a large proportion of the studies
which have led to an understanding of the functions of the
blood and what may go wrong with them has been carried out on
man himself and that animal models have played a relatively
minor role. Nowhere is this more evident than in the investigation of immune disorders of the blood, particularly the
drug-induced disorders.

Immune-mediated Drug-Induced Disorders of the Blood

Drugs may cause blood dyscrasias in a number of ways, through
immune mechanisms, by interfering with the metabolism of the
cells and by direct cytotoxic action. Since the management
and prognosis of the cytopenias produced by these different
actions are different it is essential to work out the pathogenetic mechanisms in each case. The involvement of the
immune system may broadly be classified in two ways, first
through the production of antibodies directed against various
cell types, either directly (autoimmune) or indirectly (drug-
dependent immune cytopenias) or secondly, through less well
characterized mechanisms involving the cellular components of
the immune system. Antibodies tend to cause destruction of
peripheral blood cell lines, usually one at a time, whereas

IMMUNOTOXICOLOGY
ISBN 0-12-282180-7

the cellular disorders seem to be associated with destruction
or malfunction of blood cell precursors in the bone marrow.

Drug-induced Haemolytic Anaemia

There are three ways in which red cell survival may be shor-
tened by the presence of antibodies in the blood, each producing a characteristic clinical picture and spectrum of
laboratory tests. In the first, the immune complex mechanism,
the cell may be considered an innocent victim of a reaction
between the drug, perhaps combined with a plasma protein or
other macromolecule and antibody generated in response to the
drug. Absorption of the complex on to the surface of the red
cells leads to the fixation of the complex on the surface and
intravascular lysis of the red cell. In the second, the drug
binding mechanism, the drug is bound to the membrane of the
cell, perhaps modifying it in some way. Antibodies directed
against the drug are bound to the surface but here complement
is not activated and destruction of red cells takes place
through binding of F_c portions of the antibody by the macrophage system. The most intriguing of the immune haemolytic
anaemias is that where the drug induces antibodies directed,
not against the drug, but against a component of the red cell
membrane producing a true autoimmune haemolytic anaemia. It
is worth examining these three mechanisms in some detail
since they are probably the pathways by which the majority of
blood dyscrasias are produced. Table 1 summarizes the main
features.

Immune Complex Haemolytic Anaemia

That immune complexes may be involved in blood cell destruction was first suggested by the work of Ackroyd in 1949 where
the target cell was the platelet, not the red cell. Subsequent work has been mainly on the red cell, however, mostly
because techniques for identifying antibodies and complexes
and observing their effects are more readily carried out
using that cell. Typically, the haemolysis is acute, intravascular in type with haemoglobinaemia and haemoglobinuria.
Renal failure may occur if hypotension or dehydration are
present. Usually there is a history of prior exposure to the
drug and very small quantities of the drug produce the haemolysis. The list of drugs which have been found to cause this
type of haemolysis is very long but with a few exceptions the
number of cases reported for each drug is small. Reviews may
be found in Petz and Garraty [1] and Worlledge [2,3]. Exceptions include the drug rifampicin which is particularly interesting since intermittent exposure to the drug, two or
three times a week, commonly produces haemolysis (or

Table 1 *Clinical and laboratory features of haemolysis caused by different mechanisms.*

Mechanism	Drug examples	Clinical features	Direct antiglobulin test	Antibody identification
Immune complex	Quinidine Rifampicin	Small dose of drug. Previous exposure. Rapid effect. Intravascular haemolysis.	Usually complement only	Serum acts with RBC in presence of drug. Eluate non-reactive.
Drug absorption	Penicillin Cephalosporins*	Large, prolonged dose of drug. Extravascular haemolysis.	IgG or IgG + c'	Serum and eluate react with drug-treated RBC.
Autoimmune	Methyldopa Levadopa	Delayed onset of haemolysis. Positive DAT without haemolysis common. Dose related.	IgG only	Serum and eluate react with normal RBC. Rh specificity common.

* May also cause positive DAT by non-immunological protein absorption.

thrombocytopenia) whereas continuous daily exposure is much
less likely to do so. The antibody response to the drug is
usually IgM in type and the complexes are loosely bound to
the red cell surface. The direct antiglobulin test is positive with anti-complementary sera but negative with anti-IgM
or anti-IgG sera. The eluate from the red cell surface does
not usually react with normal red cells but the patient's
serum, containing the anti-drug antibody but not the rapidly
metabolized drug, will react with normal red cells only if
the drug (or the antibody producing metabolite) is added *in
vitro*. Once the drug is withdrawn the haemolytic anaemia
resolves rapidly and the direct antiglobulin test becomes
negative within a few days. Whilst therapeutic agents are
the most commonly observed causes of this type of haemolytic
anaemia various industrial/agricultural compounds have also
been implicated. Trimellitic anhydride, a compound used as
a plasticizer and as a curing agent for epoxy resins, is well
known as a cause of bronchospasm possibly through the generation of IgE antibodies but it may also give rise to IgG
antibodies which are associated with haemolytic anaemia and
pulmonary alveolar haemorrhage [4].

Drug Absorption Mechanism

Penicillin is bound to the surface of red cells, the amount
of binding being dependent on the concentration of penicillin
and the concentration of penicillin antigenic determinants on
the red cell. Anti-penicillin antibodies of the IgG type
bind directly to the membrane bound drug and, if the concentration of antibody and its avidity are high, sufficient
binding of antibody occurs to produce destruction of red
cells via F_c binding to macrophages [5]. The haemolysis is
extravascular and subacute, the direct antiglobulin test is
positive with anti-IgG anti-sera and the indirect antiglobulin
test is positive with penicillin coated red cells. Although
the haemolysis is extravascular it may be very marked and
even fatal. Occasionally there is evidence of complement
fixation and it is possible that in these patients with drug-
binding and immune complex mechanisms act at the same time.

Autoimmune Drug-induced Haemolysis

In 1966 Worlledge and her colleagues found that a high proportion of patients taking methyldopa developed a positive
direct antiglobulin test [6] and that some of them had
haemolytic anaemia [7]. The antibody responsible was IgG in
type and the free serum antibody and the eluate from the red
cells reacted with normal red cells in the absence of the
drug. Further work showed that the antibody may have

specificity to the Rh blood group system, the antibody failing
to react with the rare Rh_{null} cells. In many patients a number of different antibodies may be found, some with anti-c or
anti-e specificity and others which react with all cells including Rh_{null} cells. Typically the antibody develops after
several weeks of exposure to methyldopa and the titre and
incidence of positive test is dose-dependent. When the drug
is withdrawn the direct antiglobulin test remains positive
for weeks or months before gradually becoming negative. Re-
introduction of the drug leads to reappearance of the antibody, again with a similar lag period.

Several theories have been propounded to account for the
appearance of autoantibodies. Worlledge et al. [7] suggested
that the methyldopa alters red cell antigens in a subtle
fashion so that they stimulate the production of antibodies
which react with the normal antigen. If the incorporation of
the alteration occurs at an early stage in red cell development and the altered antigen is not presented for antibody
formation until the red cell is destroyed this would account
for the delay in appearance of the antibody [8]. However,
occasionally there is a rapid disappearance of antibody after
the drug is withdrawn which is difficult to explain on such
a basis. Another suggestion has been that methyldopa alters
the nature of immunoglobuulin so that it will bind to red
cells [9] but this does not explain the Rh specificity of so
many of these antibodies. An attractive hypothesis is that
methyldopa alters the cellular immune response so that there
is an increased tendency to produce antibodies against "self"
antigens. Worlledge [2,3] suggested that methyldopa might
alter T-cell regulation of antibody production and, indeed,
subsequent work showed that methyldopa may inhibit T-cell
suppression of IgG production by pokeweed-mitogen stimulated
mononuclear cells [10]. However, the mechanism does not explain the prediliction of methyldopa induced autoantibodies
to react with the Rh antigens of red blood cells.

Drug-induced Agranulocytosis

Drug-induced agranulocytosis is a relatively rare disorder
which may cause catastrophic results. It is recognized that
whilst most cases of agranulocytosis are caused by the presence of antibodies which cause destruction of peripheral
blood granulocytes by immune lysis a number of cases are
caused by inhibition of granulocyte production. Much the
same mechanisms of immune lysis and destruction of granulocytes have been identified as for red cells. Amidopyrine has
been the main culprit in immune complex-mediated granulocyte
destruction which has led to its withdrawal from most

countries in the developed world, though it is still supplied
in some poorer lands. The marked systemic symptoms of drug-
induced agranulocytosis are caused by the sudden release of
granulocyte contents into the blood and include fever, sometimes with rigors, abdominal pain and occasionally hypotension.
In addition to this acute agranulocytosis with apparent lysis
of cells some drugs, again penicillin, may cause neutropenia
by opsonizing neutrophils with antibody directed against membrane bound molecules.

   Amidopyrine (aminophenazone) and its analogue antipyrine
(phenazone) provide an interesting example of the effects of
minor alterations on chemical structure on the ability to
induce toxic antibody. The deaminated phenazone was widely
used as an antipyretic but has not been demonstrated to cause
agranulocytosis whereas the incidence with aminophenazone is
high. Another example is in the H_2 antagonists metiamide and
cimetidine. The former causes an unacceptably high incidence
of neutropenia whereas cimetidine has a low incidence (though
some immune thrombocytopenia may be caused). The substitution
of =N-CN in cimetidine for =S in metiamide in the side chain
of otherwise identical molecules is associated with this
change. In this case agranulocytosis is caused through inhibition of granulocyte precursors in the marrow and the different activity of the compounds may be related to the binding of metiamide but not cimetidine in the marrow rather than
differences in antibody stimulation [11]. It seems that
several drugs owe their myelotoxic activity to selective or
relatively marked uptake by the marrow and it is not clear
whether their adverse reactions are antibody-mediated or
whether they have a direct toxic action. Unlike most immune
reactions, there is dose dependence and recovery may be delayed depending on how long it takes for the drug to be
eliminated from the marrow. Chlorpromazine and possibly gold
salts are in this category.

Drug-induced Thrombocytopenia

Ackroyd's [12] pioneering work on immune mechanisms in drug-
induced cytopenias showed that sedormid induced thrombocytopenia through the absorption of antibody-drug complex by
platelets and then subsequent sequestration in the reticulo-
endothelial system. The mechanism was thought to be similar
to that seen in experimental serum sickness. Drug-induced
thrombocytopenia of this type is usually abrupt and follows
a second or subsequent exposure to a small amount of drug.
Since the bone marrow has not had time to mount a compensatory
hyperplasia of megakaryocytes the thrombocytopenia may be
catastrophic and virtually precludes the *in vivo* challenge

by the drug to prove the association. Certain drugs, again
penicillin and possibly cephalothin and trimethaprin, may be
bound to platelets in sufficient concentration to produce the
same method of destruction as seen in the drug-membrane interaction in red cells [13,14]. Platelet-associated IgG is found
in the latter group of immune thrombocytopenias but, as with
red cells, the immune complexes are loosely bound to the surface and may readily be washed off [15].

Aplastic Anaemia

Aplastic anaemia, that is pancytopenia associated with an
empty bone marrow in the absence of malignant disease or
exposure to cytotoxic drugs or radiation, is the most serious
of the drug-induced cytopenias not only because all cell
lines are affected but because the disease itself does not
get better when the offending drug is removed. Despite a
great deal of study, very little is known about the pathogenesis of aplasia. Certain clinical features have to be
explained by any hypothesis on the pathogenesis. The development of aplasia is rare and idiosyncratic. Aplasia more
commonly follows second or subsequent exposure to a particular drug [16], but may develop during a single prolonged exposure. There is no clear cut relationship between the
structures of drugs which cause aplastic anaemia except that
there is a preponderance of nitroso- or amino-containing ring
compounds (e.g., aminophenazone, the pyrazolones and chloramphenicol). Indeed, it was predicted when chloramphenicol
was first marketed that blood dyscrasias were to be expected
[17] and shortly afterwards the first case of chloramphenicol-
induced aplasia was documented [18] in a patient who received
a prolonged course of the drug. Evidence that chloramphenicol
does cause aplastic anaemia is circumstantial rather than
experimental since no animal model exists and *in vitro* studies
have failed to show the effect of the drug on precursor cells
(with possibly a few exceptions) [19]. One of the problems
is that there is a delay, usually 6 to 12 weeks, between exposure to an agent suspected of causing aplasia and the development of pancytopenia so that studies are only possible
after the presumed damaging event. This delay in expressing
damage also makes it difficult, if not impossible, to monitor
patients for the occurrence of aplasia in a way which will
prevent the disaster.

There is some evidence that at least in a proportion of
cases of aplastic anaemia (perhaps 20-25%) immune mechanisms
may play a part in prolonging the aplasia. For example,
Bacigalupo and colleagues [20] found that in 10 out of 20
patients with severe aplastic anaemia removal of T-cells

from marrow aspirate before *in vitro* culture enhanced the growth of CFU_c and that in six of these patients putting the T-cells back inhibited colony growth again. Torok-Stord *et al.* [21] were also able to identify immune factors which inhibited marrow growth *in vitro* and to distinguish the inhibitors from allosensitization caused by multiple blood transfusions. Even so, in the majority of patients with aplastic anaemia it is not possible to identify specific immunological factors in the disease.

Treatment of asplastic anaemia with antilymphocyte globulin leads to remission in a proportion of cases, though the more severe and prolonged the disease before treatment the less likely is a response [22].

Screening of Drugs for Toxicity in the Cytopenias

The identification of a drug responsible for an immune cytopenia is fairly straightforward if the native drug is responsible for the production of antibodies. In this case the patient's serum which contains anti-drug antibodies will cause changes on the target cell which can be measured. With red cells this is simple with the indirect antiglobulin test, more difficult with platelets where agglutination tests are difficult and the release of platelet factors such as serotonin or platelet factor 3 must be measured, and most difficult with granulocytes. Occasionally, a drug may be found to inhibit granulocyte colony growth *in vitro* in the presence of patient's serum [23] but only in cases of granulocytopenia, not aplastic anaemia. When antibodies develop against a metabolite of the drug it may be much more difficult to identify the offending substance, particularly if there are many metabolites and when the patient has been exposed to several drugs at the same time. Where drugs are essential to the patient's management all should be withdrawn and reintroduced one at a time with very careful monitoring of the blood count. In both agranulocytosis and thrombocytopenia, testing the patient with the putative offending drug should be avoided unless it is absolutely necessary to know. As mentioned before, test doses may cause a very rapid (hours) fall to virtually zero in these cells in susceptible patients and death may result.

In aplastic anaemia implication of the drug can only be based on the evidence that the patient took the drug with a reasonable temporal relationship to the onset of the disease and upon precedent, both from experience and the literature. This emphasizes yet again the need for reporting possible associations as quickly as possible to the confidential records of the Committee of Safety of Medicines.

REFERENCES

1. Petz, L.D. and Garratty, G. (1980). In "Drug Induced Immune Hemolytic Anemia in Acquired Immune Hemolytic Anemias", pp.267-304. Churchill Livingstone, New York.
2. Worlledge, S.M. (1973). In "Immune Drug Induced Haemolytic Anaemias in Blood Disorders Due to Drugs and Other Agents" (ed. R.H. Girdwood), pp.11-26. Excerpta Medica, Amsterdam.
3. Worlledge, S.M. (1973). *Semin. Hematol.* **10**, 327-344.
4. Ahmad, D., Patterson, R., Morgan, W.K.C., Williams, T. and Zeiss, C.R. (1979). *Lancet* **ii**, 328-330.
5. Petz, L.D. and Fudenberg, (1966). *New Engl. J. Med.* **274**, 171-178.
6. Carstairs, K.C., Breckenridge, A., Dollery, C.T. and Worlledge, S.M. (1966). *Lancet* **ii**, 133-135.
7. Worlledge, S.M., Carstairs, K.C. and Dacie, J.V. (1966). *Lancet* **ii**, 135-139.
8. Worlledge, S.M. (1969). *Brit. J. Haematol.* **10**, 5-8.
9. Gottlieb, A. and Wurzel, H.A. (1974). *Brit. J. Haematol.* **43**, 85-97.
10. Kirtland, H.H., Mohler, D.N. and Horwitz, D.A. (1980). *New Engl. J. Med.* **302**, 825-832.
11. Young, G.A.R. and Vincent, P. (1980). *Clinics Haematol.* **9**, 483-504.
12. Ackroyd, J.F. (1949). *Clin. Sci.* **7**, 249-285.
13. Sheiman, L., Spielvogel, A.R. and Horowitz, H.I. (1968). *J. Am. Med. Assoc.* **203**, 601.
14. Claas, R.H.J., van der Meed, J.W.M. and Langerak, J. (1979). *Brit. Med. J.* **ii**, 898.
15. Miescher, P.A. and Graf, J. (1980). *Clinics Haematol.* **8**, 505-519.
16. Williams, D.M., Lynch, R.E. and Cartwright, G.E. (1973). *Semin. Hematol.* **10**, 195.
17. Recinos, A., Ross, S. and Olshaker, T.E. (1949). *New Engl. J. Med.* **241**, 733.
18. Rich, M.L., Ritterhof, R.J. and Hoffman, R.J. (1950). *Ann. Intern. Med.* **33**, 1459.
19. Howell, A., Andrews, T.H. and Watts, R.W.E. (1975). *Lancet* **i**, 65-69.
20. Bacigalupo, A., Podest, M. and Vam Lint, M.T. (1981). *Brit. J. Haematol.* **47**, 423-433.
21. Torok-Stord, B., Sieff, C. and Thomas, E.D. (1980). *Blood* **55**, 211-218.
22. Gluckman, E., Devergie, A., Poros, A. and Degoulet, P. (1982). *Brit. J. Haematol.* **51**, 541-550.
23. Barrett, A.J., Weller, E., Rozengurt, N., Longhurst, P. and Humble, J.G. (1976). *Brit. Med. J.* **ii**, 850-851.

TOXIC AND IMMUNOLOGICAL MECHANISMS
IN HALOTHANE HEPATITIS

M. Davis

Dudley Road Hospital, Birmingham B18 7QH, U.K.

The fact that there is no entirely satisfactory classification of hepatic drug reactions is a reflection of our poor understanding of their pathogenesis. This particularly applies to the so-called "unpredictable" or "idiosyncratic" reactions which arise as rare, but often life-threatening, complications of therapeutic doses of drugs. Because many of these adverse effects are accompanied by clinical and laboratory manifestations of hypersensitivity, it has long been suggested that they might arise as a result of an immunological reaction to the offending agent.

Despite such features, however, attempts to document *in vitro* sensitization to drugs, or artificially-prepared drug-protein hapten conjugates, in typical cases have generally produced equivocal results [1]. This is perhaps not surprising in view of the small molecular weights of most of these compounds, which makes it unlikely that by themselves they could be immunogenic. In an attempt to circumvent this problem, sensitization has also been tested to serum from normal individuals, taken after exposure to the offending agent. The rationale behind this approach was that the serum might contain the parent drug or its metabolite in a form more readily recognized by the immune system. Using this technique, Berg and colleagues have been able to demonstrate lymphocyte sensitization to such "metabolite containing sera" in a number of allergic drug reactions, including some which involved the liver [2].

However, the interpretation of all such studies is difficult; demonstration that patients have circulating antibodies to drugs or their metabolites, or lymphocytes which are sensitized to them, indicates only that immunological recognition has occurred to the compounds in question, and does not necessarily imply a role in pathogenesis of liver damage.

IMMUNOTOXICOLOGY
ISBN 0-12-282180-7

An alternative possibility is that sensitization is directed specifically towards liver cell components which in some way have become altered by the drug or its metabolites. An important advance in this direction stems from experimental observations that a number of chemicals and drugs produce tumours or necrosis of the liver via chemically highly-reactive metabolites, which bind covalently to, and denature, liver cell macromolecules [3]. Such a sequence of events is now well documented for the "predictable" dose-related hepatotoxicity from carbon tetrachloride [4] and paracetamol (acetaminophen) [5]. Recently, however, similar events have been described in experimental hepatic injury from a variety of drugs, including isoniazid [6], methyldopa [7] and halothane [8], where there is no clear relationship between dose and the appearance of hepatic damage in man.

Although experimental hepatic necrosis from such drugs appears to arise as a direct toxic effect of the covalently-bound metabolite, it is possible that liver cells could in addition become more subtly altered, and provide the antigenic stimulus for an immune attack.

In order to produce hepatic damage from "idiosyncratic" hepatotoxins in experimental animals, it has generally been necessary to administer the compounds under very precise conditions, in order to favour a particular route of metabolism which gives rise to chemically-reactive derivatives [6,8]. There is a small but growing body of evidence that in man individual variations in drug metabolism via hepatotoxic derivatives are important in determining susceptibility to hepatic damage [1]. This is likely to be the case whether the reaction is mediated by direct toxicity or via an immunological attack directed against drug-metabolite altered liver cell components. Any consideration of immune mechanisms in pathogenesis of drug-induced liver injury must therefore take into account possible variations in drug metabolism which ultimately lead to the development of sensitization.

The hepatocellular necrosis associated with the anaesthetic agent halothane provides an example of how such metabolic and immunological processes might co-operate in the production of liver cell damage.

Two patterns of hepatic damage are encountered in patients exposed to halothane. Controlled clinical trials have shown that up to 20% of patients repeatedly anaesthetized with the drug develop minor elevations in serum transaminases accompanied by focal hepatocellular necrosis [9]. In contrast, severe hepatitis is so uncommon that accurate estimates of its frequency cannot be made; the incidence probably lies between 1 in 22,000 and 1 in 35,000 halothane anaesthetics [10].

The minor changes are not associated with features of hypersensitivity, but several features of the severe reaction
point indirectly to a possible immunological basis [11].
These include the association with multiple exposures, suggesting the need for an earlier sensitizing dose, while some
affected patients have a history of allergy and others have
organ-specific antibodies, especially antithyroid, which persist after recovery from the illness. This suggests a predisposition to autoimmune reactions. About 25% have antibodies direct against guinea pig liver and kidney microsomes
(LKM antibodies), which are not seen in acute hepatitis from
other causes.

However, despite these suggestive findings, early attempts
to document sensitization to halothane or its metabolites in
typical cases were largely unrewarding [11]. This led to a
proliferation of experimental studies to investigate the
direct hepatotoxic potential of the drug.

Halothane is metabolized via at least two pathways, oxidative and reductive, depending on the ambient oxygen concentration [8], and both can generate chemically reactive metabolites which bind to liver cell macromolecules. It appears
that the compound produced by the oxidative pathway is an
intermediate of the main halothane metabolite, trifluoroacetic
acid, while the reductive pathway appears to involve removal
of one of the halogen atoms from the parent compound to form
a reactive metabolite [8].

The relevance of such reactive metabolites in the pathogenesis of liver injury has been demonstrated by the development of an experimental animal model of direct hepatotoxicity
from halothane [8]. This involves the administration of
anaesthetic doses of the agent, under hypoxic conditions, to
phenobarbitone-pretreated rats. The extent of covalent binding of reactive halothane metabolites paralleled the degree
of liver damage, which was dose-related. The specific
involvement of metabolites produced via the reductive pathway could be documented by the failure of the drug to produce hepatic necrosis when given under high oxygen tensions,
and by the progressive increase in severity of liver damage
as the degree of hypoxia was increased.

The environmental manipulations needed to produce this
effect were more extreme than those likely to be encountered
during halothane anaesthesia in patients. Nevertheless,
halothane is known to undergo reductive metabolism in man
[12], albeit to a small degree, when the drug is given under
normal oxygen tensions. Individual variations in metabolism
via this pathway could at least partially govern susceptibility to hepatic damage in man.

Apart from any direct hepatoxic potential of reactive

halothane metabolites, it seemed possible that they could
also lead to alterations in liver cell antigens, with the
triggering of a cell-damaging immune response. If immune
mechanisms were involved in the pathogenesis of the hepatic
damage, it should be possible to detect sensitization *in
vitro* to halothane-altered liver cell antigens.

A major problem in testing such a hypothesis is the preparation of appropriate antigenic material. The approach we
have used is to prepare it *in vivo* [13] in the rabbit whose
hepatocyte membranes have been shown to share some antigenic
determinants in common with human liver cells. Animals were
anaesthetized with halothane for 45 minutes, then allowed to
recover, and killed 12 to 18 hours later. This was to allow
metabolism of the drug, with any attendant antigenic alterations to proceed *in vivo*. The livers were removed and
hepatocyte components used as antigens in *in vitro* tests for
sensitization.

In early studies, using the leucocyte migration test,
lymphocytes from 8 or 12 patients with severe halothane
hepatitis were shown to be sensitized to a liver homogenate
prepared from halothane pretreated rabbits [14]. Further
studies demonstrated that lymphocytes from such patients were
strongly cytotoxic *in vitro* to halothane-pretreated rabbit
hepatocytes [15]. Sensitization could not be blocked by
incubation of lymphocytes with a purified preparation of a
normal liver membrane lipiprotein (liver specific protein
(LSP)). This indicated that the immunological reaction was
directed towards a different, possibly halothane-altered
antigen not normally expressed on the hepatocyte. Having
obtained this preliminary evidence for cellular sensitization,
subsequent studies were carried out using indirect immunofluorescence to investigate the presence of circulating antibodies directed against hepatocytes isolated from halothane-
pretreated rabbits [13]. Sera were tested from 13 patients
with severe, unexplained hepatocellular necrosis arising
within 28 days of a second or subsequent halothane anaesthetic.
All cases were negative for markers of Hepatitis B virus
infection and recent infection with the Hepatitis A virus,
and in no patient was there a history of excess alcohol ingestion or recent exposure to known hepatotoxic drugs. As controls, apart from normal individuals, sera were tested from
patients who had recently undergone a second or subsequent
halothane anaesthetic, with no abnormalities in liver function
tests, and from patients with acute viral, alcohol-, or drug-
induced hepatitis.

Initial studies in which sera from patients with severe
halothane hepatitis were incubated with "halothane hepatocytes" revealed a linear pattern of immunofluorescence.

However, this was a non-specific finding, being seen in 30%
of sera from patients with other liver diseases. This linear
pattern of immunofluorescence could be abolished by pre-
incubating sera with control hepatocytes, indicating that the
antibody absorbed was directed against normal hepatocyte membrane components.

Using such absorbed sera from patients with severe halothane-
associated hepatitis, a distinct granular pattern of immunofluorescence was observed, indicating the presence of other
antibodies. On further incubation, the granules coalesced to
form a cap over one pole of the cell. This phenomenon of
capping indicates that the antibody, and thus the relevant
antigenic determinants, are localized on the cell surface
membrane [16]. Such granular fluorescence on halothane-
pretreated hepatocytes was seen using sera from 9 of 13
patients, while results were uniformly negative with absorbed
sera from all the control groups.

The localization of the altered antigen on the cell surface
suggests that it could be relevant in the pathogenesis of the
liver lesion, because it would be accessible to immunological
attack *in vivo*. This could occur either via complement-
mediated cytolysis, or through co-operation with cellular
components of the immune system, and to investigate the
latter mechanisms, studies were carried out using an induced
cytotoxicity assay [13].

The rationale for this technique lies in the fact that a
proportion of the normal lymphocyte subpopulation is made up
of killer (K) lymphocytes, which themselves have no antigenic
specificity, but which are capable of lysing antibody-coated
cells [17]. Their target is thus determined by the specificity of the antibody. Thus, if the halothane-related antibody were able to induce K cell cytolysis, it should be
possible, by coating halothane-pretreated hepatocytes with
the antibody, to render them susceptible to cytotoxicity by
normal lymphocytes. Apart from demonstrating the existence
of co-operation between humoral and cellular components of
the immune system, the induced cytotoxicity assay is a
valuable tool for demonstrating the presence of circulating
antibody, being many times more sensitive than immunofluorescence techniques [13].

For the induced cytotoxicity assay [13], hepatocytes were
isolated from halothane-pretreated or control rabbits, and
established in microculture test wells. Heat inactivated
serum, absorbed with normal hepatocytes, was then added to
the wells and incubated for two hours to allow any antibody
present to react with the cell membrane and coat the hepatocytes. After washing, lymphocytes from normal healthy individuals were added. After a further 36 h incubation, the

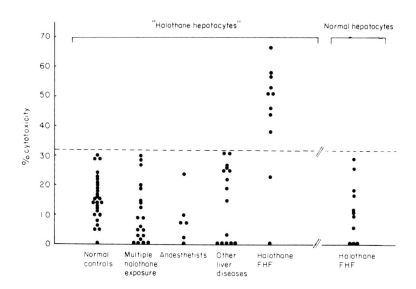

Fig. 1 Percentage cytotoxicity of normal lymphocytes towards
isolated hepatocytes from halothane pretreated and control
rabbits after pre-incubation with absorbed serum. The dotted
line represents the upper limit of normal.

remaining hepatocytes were counted, and a percentage cytotoxicity calculated by reference to control wells to which
lymphocytes had not been added.
   Of the 16 patients with severe halothane-associated hepatitis studied, absorbed sera from all but two induced signi-
cant cytotoxicity (Fig. 1). Positive results were obtained
with all serum samples producing granular immunofluorescence,
and three of the immunofluorescence negative sera also induced cytotoxicity, reflecting the greater sensitivity of the
cytotoxicity assay. Using this technique, it was also possible to demonstrate the presence of the halothane-related
antibody in sera from two surgeons, with histories of recurrent episodes of hepatitis coinciding with occupational exposure to halothane. Negative results were obtained using
hepatocytes from non-anaesthetized or ether-anaesthetized
rabbits as targets.
   We were also able to study sera from patients who developed
only minor elevations in transaminases after repeated exposures to halothane [9]. In marked contrast to the severe
group, results in these cases were uniformly negative, indicating absence of the "halothane antibody" [18].
   The specificity of these findings to severe halothane-

associated hepatitis was demonstrated by uniformly negative
results using absorbed sera from all the control groups studied. Thus, the presence of the halothane-related antibody
could not be explained solely as a result of halothane anaesthesia, and the failure to demonstrate a similar phenomenon
after minor halothane-related liver damage makes it unlikely
that it arose secondary to a direct hepatotoxic effect of the
drug.

These results therefore show that patients with severe
halothane-associated hepatitis have a circulating antibody
reacting specifically with a halothane-altered liver membrane
antigen, and that this antibody renders liver cells from
halothane-pretreated rabbits susceptible to cytotoxicity by
normal lymphocytes.

The experimental findings of Sipes and colleagues had shown
that direct hepatotoxicity from halothane was mediated via
the reductive pathway of metabolism [8]. Studies were therefore carried out to investigate the relative importance of
oxidative and reductive metabolism of halothane in the expression of the altered hepatocyte antigen [19].

The halothane-altered antigen was detected by a modification
of the induced cytotoxicity assay. Sera from patients known
to contain the antibody reacting with the altered membrane
determinants were incubated with hepatocytes isolated from
rabbits anaesthetized with halothane under different oxygen
tensions. In the presence of the altered antigen, the antibody will bind to the cell, and render it susceptible to
cytotoxicity *in vitro* by normal K lymphocytes, as discussed
earlier.

In marked contrast to the findings in relation to the direct
toxicity of halothane, the altered antigen could only be detected after anaesthesia under higher oxygen concentrations
(Table 1) indicating the exclusive involvement of the oxidative pathway of metabolism [19]. The demonstration in the
patients of circulating antibodies directed against the
rabbit liver antigen indicates that similar, if not identical
antigenic determinants were generated in their own livers,
also via the oxidative route.

Demonstration of an immunological event *in vitro* is not
proof of a pathogenetic process *in vivo*. Nevertheless, based
on these experimental observations, it can be hypothesized
that the relatively common minor hepatic damage, where there
is no evidence for involvement of immune mechanisms [18], is
due to a direct hepatotoxic effect of the drug, and that
susceptibility may be determined by individual variations in
metabolism via the reductive pathway. Accentuation of this
pathway by genetic or environmental factors could lead to the
development of a more severe lesion. However, because the

Table 1 *Expression of altered hepatocyte antigen following preferential stimulation of oxidative or reductive halothane metabolism.*

Metabolic route stimulated	O_2 tension	Pretreatment	Expression of altered antigen
Oxidative	99%	nil	7/7
	99%	BNF	7/7
	14%	BNF	7/7
Reductive	14%	nil	0/7
	99%	PB	0/7
	14%	PB	0/7

BNF — β-naphthoflavone.   PB — phenobarbitone.

majority of patients thus affected had evidence of sensitization to halothane-altered hepatocyte antigens [13] it is tempting to postulate the involvement of an additional immune process in these cases. Susceptibility to such an immune component is unlikely to be due to individual differences in the metabolism of halothane because the altered antigen is expressed via the oxidative pathway, which is the major route for the biotransformation of the drug in man. A more likely basis for its development is an abnormal immune system, and in keeping with this is the high frequency of organ specific autoantibodies in patients with the condition [20].

The relative contributions of direct hepatotoxicity and immune mechanisms in pathogenesis of the severe lesion in man is not known, but both may be involved. Hepatic histology from such cases often shows co-existence of centrilobular necrosis, suggesting direct toxicity, and periportal lymphocyte infiltration, suggesting immunological events, in the same specimen [21].

CONCLUSION

There is increasing evidence that hepatotoxicity from many drugs and chemicals arises as a result of overproduction of reactive hepatotoxic metabolites. In some instances, as in severe halothane hepatitis, immune reactions directed against drug or metabolite-altered liver antigens may also be involved.

A clearer understanding of these mechanisms and their interactions is needed to enable the development of diagnostic tests, the screening of patients at risk, and the evolution of safer drugs.

REFERENCES

1. Zimmerman, H.J. (1979). In "Hepatotoxicity", pp.91-121. Appleton Century Crofts, New York.
2. Berg, P. and Brattig, N. (1981). In "Drug Reactions and the Liver" (eds. M. Davis, J.M. Tredger and R. Williams), pp.105-110. Pitman Medical, Tunbridge Wells.
3. Mitchell, J.R. and Jollow, D.J. (1975). *Gasteroenterol.* **68**, 392-410.
4. Slater, T.F. (1972). In "Free Radical Mechanisms in Tissue Damage". pp.118-120. J.W. Arrowsmith Ltd., Bristol.
5. Jollow, D.J., Mitchell, J.R., Potter, W.Z., Davis, D.C., Gillette, J.R. and Brodie, B.B. (1973). *J. Pharmacol. Exp. Ther.* **187**, 195-202.
6. Nelson, S.D., Mitchell, J.R., Timbrell, J.A., Snodgrass, W.R. and Corcoran, G.B. (1976). *Science* **193**, 901-902.
7. Dybing, E., Nelson, S.D., Mitchell, J.R., Sasame, H. and Gillette, J.R. (1976). *Molc. Pharmac.* **12**, 911-914.
8. Sipes, I.G. (1981). In "Drug Reactions and the Liver" (eds. M. Davis, J.M. Tredger and R. Williams), pp.157-171. Pitman Medical, Tunbridge Wells.
9. Wright, R., Eade, O.E., Chisholm, O.M., Lloyd, B., Edwards, J.C., Moles, T.M. and Gardner, M.J. (1975). *Lancet* **i**, 821-823.
10. Strunin, L. (1977). In "The Liver and Anaesthesia" pp.166-167. W.B. Saunders Co., London.
11. Davis, M., Vergani, D., Eddleston, A.L.W.F. and Williams, R. (1979). In "Immune Reactions in Liver Disease" (eds. A.L.W.F. Eddleston, J.C.P. Weber and R. Williams), pp. 235-246. Pitman Medical, Tunbridge Wells.
12. Cohen, E.N., Trudell, J.R., Edmunds, H.N. and Watson, E. (1975). *Anaesthesiol.* **43**, 392-396.
13. Vergani, D., Mieli-Vergani, G., Alberti, A., Neuberger, J.M., Eddleston, A.L.W.F., Davis, M. and Williams, R. (1980). *N. Engl. J. Med.* **303**, 66-71.
14. Vergani, D., Tsantuolas, D., Eddleston, A.L.W.F., Davis, M. and Williams, R. (1979). *Lancet* **2**, 801-803.
15. Miele-Vergani, G., Vergani, D., Tredger, J.M., Eddleston, A.L.W.F., Davis, M. and Williams, R. (1980). *J. Clin. Lab. Immunol.* **4**, 49-57.
16. Schreiner, G.F. and Unanue, G.R. (1977). *J. Immunol.* **119**, 1549-1552.
17. Cochrane, A.M.G., Moussouros, A., Thomson, A.D. and Williams, R. (1976). *Lancet* **i**, 441-443.
18. Davis, M., Vergani, D., Miele-Vergani, G., Eddleston, A.L.W.F., Neuberger, J.M. and Williams, R. (1981). In "Drug Reactions and the Liver" (eds. M. Davis, J.M.

Tredger and R. Williams), pp.237-244. Pitman Medical,
Tunbridge Wells.

19. Neuberger, J., Mieli-Vergani, G., Tredger, J.M., Davis, M.
and Williams, R. (1981). *Gut* **22**, 669-672.

20. Walton, B., Simpson, R.R., Strunin, L., Doniach, D.,
Perrin, J. and Appleyard, A. (1976). *Brit. Med. J.* **i**,
1171-1173.

21. Zimmerman, H.J. (1979). In "Hetapotoxicity. The Adverse
Effects of Drugs and Other Chemicals on the Liver"
pp.370-394. Appleton Century Crofts, New York.

ALTERED IMMUNE FUNCTION
IN MICHIGAN RESIDENTS
EXPOSED TO POLYBROMINATED BIPHENYLS

J.G. Bekesi*, J.P. Roboz*, S. Solomon*,
A. Fischbein** and I.J. Selikoff**

*Department of Neoplastic Diseases,
**Environmental Sciences Laboratory,
Mount Sinai School of Medicine,
New York, New York 10029, U.S.A.

INTRODUCTION

A commercial preparation of polybrominated biphenyls (PBB) was inadvertently used in place of magnesium oxide in the preparation of a feed supplement for lactating cows [1,2]. The contaminating chemical preparation, consisting of 2-penta-, 4-hexa-, 4-hepta-, and 2-octabromobiphenyls was used as a flame retardant (called Firemaster FF-1) and manufactured by the Michigan Chemical Company.

Toxic effects exhibited by animals that consumed PBB-contaminated feed included reduced milk production, joint swelling, hyperkeratosis, persistent mastitis, cutaneous and subcutaneous infections, and abscess formation on back, legs and udder. Moreover, wasting and death occurred between 6 to 24 months following PBB exposure for a group of 400 cows and in 10 to 14 young heifers and bulls [3-5]. Some of the young bulls had atrophied testicles and abnormal semen that showed no spermatozoal motility with numerous headless and tail-less spermatozoa [3].

Identification of PBB as a toxic agent in the feed did not occur until 9 months after the initial accident. Feed containing PBB was used by dairy farmers throughout Michigan during 1973 and for most of 1974. The meat and dairy products containing PBB as a bioconcentrate were widely distributed within the state before the nature and magnitude of the problem was recognized [1-5]. Even though, in accordance with state regulations that set a ceiling on acceptable PBB

COURSE OF POLYBROMINATED BIPHENYLS (PBB) CONTAMINATION IN STATE OF MICHIGAN

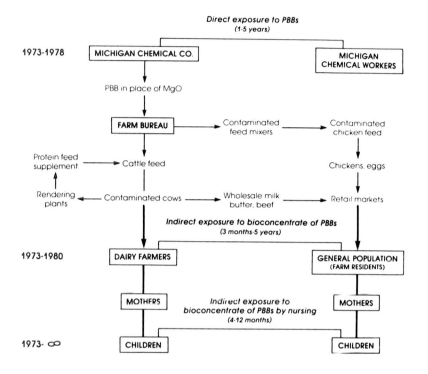

content, about 500 farms were quarantined and approximately 32,000 cattle, 1.6 million chickens, and 5 million eggs were destroyed, the potential still existed for large-scale human contamination with these halogenated hydrocarbons until 1978 when it was banned. This concern, however, was not limited to the dairy farm residents alone, inasmuch as there was extensive dissemination of PBB contaminated produce (beef, poultry, eggs, milk, cheese, butter etc) to the general population of Michigan as well (Table 1). Indeed, subsequent indepth investigation of Michigan farm residents and consumers conducted in both 1976 and 1978 revealed that most of the subjects examined had detectable serum and fat PBB levels [7-9]. Follow-up studies of the same individuals in 1977 and 1980, respectively, confirmed that both serum and adipose PBB levels remained essentially unchanged [4,6-10].

Clinical symptoms included fatigue, a striking decrease in the capacity for physical and intellectual work, and an unusual increase in the requirements for sleep. Some of those examined also showed slow reactivity in answering questions, reduced energy of expression and movement, and poor memory which suggests a diffuse cortical involvement [14]. In addition to arthritis-like changes in a significant portion of the PBB-exposed farm residents, symptoms of joint pain, swelling of joints, and deformity were also observed. The knees and ankles seemed to be most often affected, but the small joints of the fingers and hands were frequently involved. Tendonitis, with swelling, pain and crepitations present, in some cases with joint involvement more often affected the tendons of the extensor and flexor muscles of the hands [11]. It was concluded, therefore, that a "toxic PBB syndrome" existed in humans and it was primarily characterized by deleterious effects to the hepatic, neurological and musculoskeletal systems [11].

Experimental data to date have indicated that polybrominated biphenyls, similar in chemical structure to polychlorinated biphenyls, are fat soluble and stored in the thymus, liver, brain and adipose tissues; and suggest that they persist in those tissues for prolonged periods. Because of such factors as toxicity, tumour promoting activity, and a lack of active PBB metabolism, there is major concern regarding the acute as well as the chronic consequences to the health of Michigan residents [4,6,9-13]. In fact, several routine tests of liver function are frequently abnormal in these subjects as compared with either a comparable group of Wisconsin dairy farmers or a group of apparently healthy New York City residents who were not exposed to PBB contaminated produce [11].

IMMUNOLOGICAL DYSFUNCTION DETECTED AMONG THE PBB-EXPOSED MICHIGAN DAIRY FARM RESIDENTS

In 1976, our studies of the manifestations of the "toxic PBB syndrome" in humans were extended to include the assessment of immunological dysfunctions of 45 adult Michigan dairy farm residents who consumed PBB contaminated food products for periods ranging from three months to three years [10,12]. Test comparisons were made with a group of 46 dairy farm residents in central Wisconsin who had not been exposed to PBB contaminated food and to a group of 76 healthy subjects from the New York Metropolitan area. Marked changes in various immunological parameters were noted among the Michigan dairy farm residents compared with both the Wisconsin and New York control populations [10,12,13]. The peripheral blood lymphocytes (PBL) of only 27 of the 45 Michigan subjects exhibited a normal response to the T-cell mitogens phytohaemagglutinin (PHA) and concanavalin A (ConA), to the alloantigens in the MLC reaction, and to the B-cell mitogen (pokeweed mitogen). In the remaining 18 subjects, the

Table 2 *Comparison of T-lymphocyte subpopulation and function in the PBL of Wisconsin residents vs the PBB-exposed Michigan dairy farm residents.*

Subjects	T-lymphocytes [1] [2] Absolute number	Mitogens for T-cells [2] PHA Maximum stimulation (c.p.m.)	CONA Maximum stimulation (c.p.m.)	Proliferative T-cell response [2] Maximum stimulation (c.p.m.)
New York City (Control) N = 76	1,986 ± 251	102,226 ± 8,720	98,151 ± 5,600	40,952 ± 960
Wisconsin dairy farm residents N = 46	1,473 ± 63	97,662 ± 2,693	96,662 ± 3,151	38,172 ± 1,209
PBB-exposed Michigan dairy farm residents a) with normal T-cell function N = 27	1,341 ± 79	92,272 ± 2,231	94,634 ± 4,502	28,248 ± 2,072
b) with decreased T-cell function N = 18	917* ± 119	28,457* ± 3,406	36,117* ± 2,694	10,147* ± 317

(1) Spontaneous E-rosette-forming PBLs at 4°C with sheep red blood cells.

(2) Data are means ± standard deviation.

* Statistical significance (Student's T-test) between maximum lymphoblastogenesis of Wisconsin farm residents and that of Michigan dairy farm residents, p < 0.001.

Table 3 B-lymphocyte subpopulation and function in the PBL of Wisconsin residents vs the PBB-exposed dairy farm residents.

Subjects	Total number of mononuclear cells per mm³ [1]	B-lymphocytes Absolute number [1]	B-lymphocyte response PWM Maximum stimulation [1] (c.p.m.)
New York City (Control) N = 76	2,589 ± 380	521 ± 52	95,130 ± 6,369
Wisconsin dairy farm residents N = 46	2,103 ± 149	487 ± 29	90,636 ± 3,406
PBB-exposed Michigan fairy farm residents:			
a) with normal T-cell function N = 27	2,214 ± 162	467 ± 34	93,199 ± 7,412
b) with decreased T-cell function N = 18	2,098	331 ± 32	39,159 ± 3,537*

(1) Data are means ± Standard deviation. P < 0.001

lymphocytes showed an impaired functional response to all
mitogens and alloantigens (Table 2). It is important to note
that the lymphocytes of all PBB-exposed study subjects showed
a reduced proliferative T-cell response in mixed leukocyte
cultures. In fact, the group of 18 individuals had values
measuring one-third to one-fourth of those obtained from the
normal controls (Table 2,3). The number of viable cells in
the various sub-populations of peripheral blood lymphocytes
were measured by their ability to form stable rosettes with
sheep erythrocytes for the T-cells and the B-lymphocytes were
quantified by either direct immunofluorescence or by sheep
erythrocytes sensitized with antibody and complement (EAC).
The 27 Michigan farm residents with normal lymphocyte functions also exhibited the normal distribution of T and B-
lymphocytes. Eighteen of the 45 subjects with lymphocyte
dysfunction showed significantly reduced population of T-cells
(Table 2,3). Despite the marked changes in the characteristic cell surface markers detected in the peripheral blood
lymphocytes of the PBB-exposed Michigan farm residents, the
marker for monocytes, determined by peroxidase staining or
latex digestion, were not different when compared to either
control group. The most significant deviation, therefore,
from the control samples was in marked increase in lymphocytes without detectable surface markers (Figs. 1 and 2).

PERSISTENT IMMUNE DYSFUNCTION IN MICHIGAN DAIRY FARM RESI-DENTS EXPOSED TO POLYBROMINATED BIPHENYLS.

In 1981, we were able to re-examine 40 of the original
Michigan farm residents tested in 1976 and 41 of the Wisconsin
farmers and this provided the opportunity to study the persistence of the immunological abnormalities [10,12,13,15].
Comparing the Wisconsin control data of 1976 to 1981, it was
found that 1) the mean total number of mononuclear cells was
2,106 vs 2,097 per mm^3; 2) 71.0% vs 69.8% E-rosette forming
PBLs with 1,473 vs 1,464 in the absolute numbers of T-lymphocytes; and 3) 23.1% vs 22.5% EAC-rosette forming PBLs with
487 vs 472 in the absolute numbers of B-lymphocytes. Seven-
teen of the 40 Michigan farmers examined in 1976 and again
in 1981 showed a consistent deviation from the normal range
in both percent and absolute number of T-lymphocytes (Fig. 1).
Significant group differences were found with respect to the
percent and total number of T-lymphocytes both in 1976 and
in 1981. In terms of the B-lymphocytes, the Michigan farmers
fell within the normal range on both occasions.
    A second important feature of the PBL of PBB-exposed
Michigan farmers was a marked prevalence of lymphocytes without detectable membrane markers (null (N) cells). While the

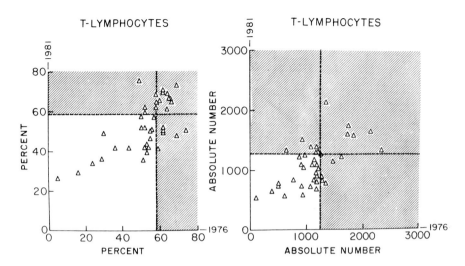

Fig. 1 Scatter plots of the percents and absolute numbers
of the T-lymphocyte subpopulation obtained from PBB-exposed
Michigan dairy farm residents (N = 40) during 1976 and then
again in 1981. The shaded areas represent regions which contain the upper 95% of a matched control group of Wisconsin
dairy farmers (N = 41) determined concurrently on respective
measures. (r = 0.57, p < 0.01).

aetiology of this result is not clear, it is possibly due to
either a defect in the maturation of the cells and/or a
selective binding of PBB to the surface membrane of the T-
lymphocytes (Fig. 2).

The functional integrity of the PBL was assessed through
lymphoblastogenesis with selected mitogens, i.e., phytohaemagglutinin (PHA) for T-cells and pokeweed mitogen (PWM)
for B-cells [10]. The Wisconsin mean maximum stimulation
values for 1976 and 1981 were 97.6 x 10^3 c.p.m. vs 101.2 x 10^3
c.p.m. and 87.2 x 10^3 c.p.m. vs 90.9 x 10^3 c.p.m. for PHA
and PWM, respectively. Group differences were significant
(p < 0.0001) in 1976 and in 1981 for both parameters; with 15
of the 39 Michigan farmers exhibiting persistently lower PHA
values. The constancy of this deficit is further reflected
in the rather high correlations computed between the two
surveys for the T-cell function (r = 0.87, p < 0.01) and the
B-cell function (r = 0.85, p < 0.01). In general, a decreased
response to the T-cell mitogen was accompanied by a corresponding decrease in the number of T-lymphocytes (Fig. 3). In
a few Michigan subjects, however, an abnormally low T-lymphocyte function occurred in the presence of a normal number of

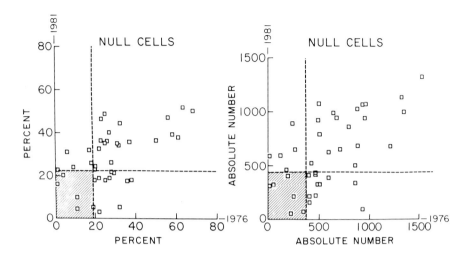

Fig. 2   Scatter plots of the percents and absolute numbers
of the "Null-cell" subpopulation obtained from PBB-exposed
Michigan dairy farm residents (N = 40) during 1976 and then
again in 1981.   The shaded areas represent regions which contain the upper 95% of a matched control group of Wisconsin
dairy farmers (N = 41) with concurrent determinations on the
respective measures.

T-cells.   The implications of this observation are at present
under investigation.

While the B-lymphocytes of PBB-exposed individuals are, for
the most part, within normal limits, there is a functional
anomaly reflected by the decreased response to the B-cell
mitogen.   This result may represent either a defect in the
B-cells per se and/or some alteration in the ratio of helper
T-cell to suppressor T-cell sub-populations.

In conclusion, the lower numbers and impaired function of
the T-lymphocytes observed approximately eight years after
onset of PBB exposure in a small group of Michigan dairy farm
residents is indicative of a persistent PBB-induced immune
suppression that is likely to be characteristic of the larger
segment of the subjects studied.

FAMILY CLUSTERS AND IMMUNE DYSFUNCTIONS

The immunological abnormalities were examined with respect to
family units in order to address the issue of a genetic predisposition to the "toxic PBB syndrome".   Eight families were
tested that consisted of 27 adults ranging in age from 19 to

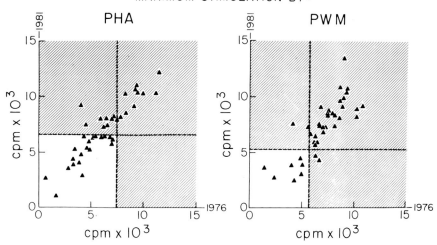

Fig. 3 Scatter plots of the T- and B-lymphocyte functions obtained from 41 PBB-exposed Michigan farm residents back in 1976 and again in 1981. The shaded areas represent regions which contain the upper 95% of a matched control group of 40 Wisconsin dairy farmers with concurrent determinations on the respective measures.

76 years [12]. Data derived from this study indicate that the numerical and functional changes in the T- and N-cells affected the PBB-exposed Michigan family as an integral unit and the values were relatively independent of age and sex [12]. These findings do not indicate genetic predisposition as an important factor in explaining the impaired lymphocyte function. It is important to note that similar intra-family clusterings were observed for the serum and adipose PBB levels of quarantined and non-quarantined families which emphasizes the crucial role of a common dietary source [7,8, 10,12,13].

IDENTIFICATION AND QUANTIFICATION OF BLOOD COMPARTMENTS

The presence of PBB in the plasma, red and white cells, and the β-lipoprotein fractions of plasma was established by positive chemical ionization mass spectrometry in samples from Michigan subjects, but not for the controls [13,15]. A highly sensitive technique, based on negative chemical ioniz-ation, was developed for trace quantification of PBB [16,17]. The distribution of PBB in blood compartments was: red blood cells: white blood cells: plasma proteins: β-lipoproteins

= 1 : 85.5 : 14.9 : 334.4, respectively. In our initial report, no correlation was found between immune dysfunction and plasma PBB levels. The β-lipoprotein fraction appears to be the major protein carrier in the plasma. There is a strong suggestion that a correlation exists between the high PBB content in the white blood cells as well as in the β-lipoprotein fraction and the decreased immunological function found in the PBL of the PBB-exposed subjects [15].

CONCLUSIONS

In 1973, a commercial preparation of polybrominated biphenyls (PBB), Firemaster FF-1, was inadvertently substituted as a supplement to cattle feed and was distributed to farms throughout the State of Michigan. Dairy products from contaminated animals (beef, poultry, eggs, milk, cheese, butter) were widely consumed in that State until 1978. The presence of PBB has been confirmed in the blood, fat and breast milk in nearly every Michigan resident tested. In a significant portion of the PBB-exposed dairy farm residents a "toxic PBB syndrome" was recognized, which was primarily characterized by abnormalities in the hepatic, neurological and musculoskeletal systems. Our original study in 1976 identified the existence of immunological dysfunctions associated with PBB exposure. More recently, in 1981, we re-examined the same individuals and the data strongly suggest the presence of persistent immunotoxicological effect. This syndrome consists of a decrease in the percent and absolute number of T-lymphocytes, with a concomitant increase in the occurrence of lymphocytes without detectable membrane surface markers; and, in 30% of the subjects retested, there was a reduction in the T-cell function. The immunological dysfunction detected among PBB-exposed subjects tended to affect families as a unit and was independent of age or sex. The possibility of genetic predisposition was excluded based on data from non-related co-consumers.

ACKNOWLEDGEMENTS

We gratefully acknowledge the excellent technical help of Patricia Mason, Khanitha Tangnavarad and Sophie Kurdziel and the secretarial assistance of Diane Andujar. This research was supported by NIEHS contract NO1-ES-9-0004.

REFERENCES

1. Carter, L. (1976). Science 192, 240-243.
2. Dunckel, A.E. (1975). J. Am. Vet. Med. Assoc. 167, 838-841.

3. Jackson, T.F. and Halbert, F.L. (1974). *J. Am. Vet. Med. Assoc.* **165**, 437-439.
4. Humphrey, H.E.B. and Hayner, N.S. (1974). In "Polybrominated Biphenyls; an Agricultural Incident and its Consequences. An Epidemiological Investigation of Human Exposure". Michigan Department of Health, Lansing, Michigan.
5. Kay, K. (1977). *Envir. Res.* **13**, 74-93.
6. Meester, W.D. (1979). *Vet. Hum. Toxicol.* **21**, 231-235.
7. Wolff, M.S., Aubrey, B., Camer, F. and Haymes, N. (1978). *Environ. Health Perspect.* **23**, 177-181.
8. Wolff, M.A., Haymes, N., Anderson, H.A. and Selikoff, I.J. (1978). *Environ. Health Perspect.* **23**, 315-319.
9. Wolff, M.S., Anderson, H.A. and Selikoff, I.J. (1982). *JAMA* **247**, 2112-2116.
10. Bekesi, J.G., Holland, J.F., Anderson, H.A., Fischbein, A.S., Rom, W., Wolff, M.S. and Selikoff, I.J. (1978). *Science* 1207-1211.
11. Anderson, H.A., Lillis, R. and Selikoff, I.J. (1978). *Environ. Health Perspect.* **23**, 217-223.
12. Bekesi, J.G., Anderson, H.A., Roboz, J.P., Roboz, J., Fischbein, A.S., Selikoff, I.J. and Holland, J.F. (1979). *N.Y. Acad. Sci.* **320**, 717-728.
13. Bekesi, J.G., Roboz, J., Anderson, H.A., Roboz, J.P., Fischbein, A.S., Selikoff, I.J. and Holland, J.F. (1979). *Drug and Chem. Toxicol.* **2**, 179-191.
14. Valcuikas, J.A., Lillis, R., Wolff, M.S. and Anderson, H.A. (1978). *Environ. Perspect.* **23**, 199-210.
15. Roboz, J., Suzuki, R.K., Bekesi, J.G., Holland, J.F. and Selikoff, I.J. (1980). *J. Env. Path. Toxicol.* **3**, 363-378.
16. Roboz, J., Greaves, J., Holland, J.F. and Bekesi, J.G. (1982). *Anal. Chem.* **54**, 1104-1108.

VARIOUS MECHANISMS IN CHEMICALLY-INDUCED THYMIC INJURY

K. Miller

Immunotoxicology Department,
British Industrial Biological Research Association,
Woodmansterne Road, Carshalton, Surrey, U.K.

Before discussing the biological effects of compounds known to produce thymic injury it might be well to briefly consider the nature and function of the thymus. It is less than 20 years ago that the thymus was characterized as a lympho-epithelial organ with immunological activity. Since then an extraordinary number of investigations dealing with the function of the organ itself as well as with its cellular products, the so-called thymus-derived lymphocytes (T-cells) have been performed. It is now well established that T-cells are implicated in most aspects of immunity, either as direct effector cells (cytotoxicity phenomena, secretion of various mediators of delayed hypersensitivity) or as regulatory, helper or suppressor cells in humoral and cell-mediated responses.

Haematopoietic stem cells originating from embryonic tissues such as liver or from adult bone marrow migrate to the thymus where they are induced to proliferate and differentiate. This differentiation is marked by morphological alterations and the expression of characteristic T-cell surface antigens. The extensive intra-thymic lymphopoiesis that takes place can be considered as a mechanism to generate random genetic variation which would provide the lymphoid cells with different immune reactivity patterns, while the large amount of intra-thymic cell death that occurs could be concerned with elimination of self-reactive or non-concordant clones [1]. Intra-thymic death appears to be a constant and normal aspect of thymic function and approximately 60% of newly formed thymocytes die within the thymus [2]. The extent of intra-thymic cell death compared to emigration and the magnitude of export at different ages is still an unresolved question. Cells emigrate from the thymus to the spleen, lymph nodes and

IMMUNOTOXICOLOGY
ISBN 0-12-282180-7

thoracic duct in a unidirectional fashion and several studies
have identified two classes of thymus-derived cells, one
short-lived and the other long-lived, which interact with
each other to regulate B-lymphocyte antibody responses [3].
   The respective role of direct contact of the precursor cells
with the thymic epithelial microenvironment and of the humoral
substances (or hormones) produced by the thymus is not yet
clearly established, although both actions, cellular and
humoral, represent necessary steps in T-cell maturation. The
requirement for appropriate major histocompatibility complex
(MHC) matching for cellular cooperation in the immune response
is acquired by thymocytes from MHC antigens present on the
epithelial cells [4]. The presence of humoral factors in the
thymus has been demonstrated by a number of investigators,
who have extracted and purified a number of different thymic
peptides, as well as demonstrating that these extracts have
numerous and often specific biological effects on the differentiation and functional activity of the lymphocytes. The
reticular epithelial cells, known to have secretory activity,
are generally considered to be the source of thymic hormones
and a strict relationship exists between the morphological
state of thymic epithelial cells and the production of thymic
humoral factors [5]. Thus the basic processes for T-cell
differentiation in the thymus involve selection of the T-cell
repertoire as well as specialization into different functional
subsets of T-cells.
   Similarly to other endocrine glands, the thymus is involved
in various endocrine feedback mechanisms. After thymectomy,
the gonads of experimental animals begin to mature but ultimately degenerate unless treated with a thymic hormone extract,
whereas adrenal cortical secretions affect lymphatic structure
and function. In the tiny amounts that circulate normally
from day to day, glucocorticoids chronically suppress the
growth and development of thymocytes. This physiological
suppression may be abolished by removing the adrenal glands
which causes the size and cellularity of the thymus to increase. Conversely, when increased amounts of steroids are
secreted by the adrenals during periods of stress, great numbers of thymus cells are destroyed. Apart from this function,
steroids play another important regulatory role. Oestradiol,
testosterone and corticosterone have been demonstrated, at
physiological levels, to modify the synthesis of thymic factors by epithelial cells [6]. That there is some common
immunoendocrine control is borne out by studies with compounds
such as theobromine where both thymic and testicular atrophy
have been shown to occur in the rat [7]. Preliminary studies
in our laboratories have also demonstrated that in the rat,
loss of thymic weight occurs after exposure to theobromine

Table 1   *Theobromine administration: effect on relative weight of thymus and gonads.*

	Organ weight (g) after:	
	2 week gavage	4 week gavage
Thymus		
Control	0.400 ± 0.063	0.407 ± 0.059
250 mg/kg/day	0.261 ± 0.035[b]	0.225 ± 0.045[c]
500 mg/kg/day	0.147 ± 0.027[c]	0.157 ± 0.069[c]
Testes		
Control	0.941 ± 0.017	0.950 ± 0.073
250 mg/kg/day	0.907 ± 0.192	1.025 ± 0.037
500 mg/kg/day	1.044 ± 0.030[a]	0.978 ± 0.108
Prostate		
Control	0.073 ± 0.006	0.080 ± 0.018
250 mg/kg/day	0.071 ± 0.025	0.080 ± 0.025
500 mg/kg/day	0.061 ± 0.017	0.052 ± 0.021[a]
Seminal vesicles		
Control	0.059 ± 0.010	0.130 ± 0.050
250 mg/kg/day	0.040 ± 0.017[z]	0.100 ± 0.027[b]
500 mg/kg/day	0.037 ± 0.004[b]	0.051 ± 0.025[b]

[a] $p > 0.05$ [b] $p > 0.005$ [c] $p > 0.001$.

at concentrations which do not produce testicular effects (Table 1). Thus whilst the thymus is involved in the hypophyso-cortico-adrenal and hypophyso-testicular axes via the intermediary of thymic humoral factors [8], it may also be the most sensitive indicator of toxic effects associated with endocrine regulation.

Various industrial and environmental chemicals have also been shown to have a profound effect on thymus and on thymus-dependent functions. The ability of the pesticide contaminant 2,3,7,8-tetrachlorodibenzo-p-dioxin (TCDD) to impair immune mechanisms is well documented. TCDD causes thymic atrophy in all mammalian species studied [9,10] and mouse pups from mothers fed low levels of TCDD have been shown to develop thymic atrophy and certain types of immunosuppression at exposure levels that were insufficient to produce overt symptoms of toxicity [11]. The mode of action of TCDD is not caused by endocrine regulatory factors, or by a direct

cytotoxic effect on lymphocytes. The possibility that TCDD
has an effect on bone marrow stem cells has been raised as an
alternative hypothesis [12]. As with many other substances,
controlled studies to evaluate the functional effects of TCDD
on the lymphoid system are clearly needed.

Recently, particular attention has been paid to the selective effect on the thymus by the dioctyltin compounds which
are used as heat and light stabilizers in PVC food packaging
material. In 1976 Seinen and Willems reported that dioctyltin
dichloride (DOTC) caused severe reduction of thymic weight in
weanling rats after exposure to diets dontaining 50 or 150 ppm
of this compound [13]. Subsequent publications by this group
have been concerned with the effect of DOTC as an immuno-

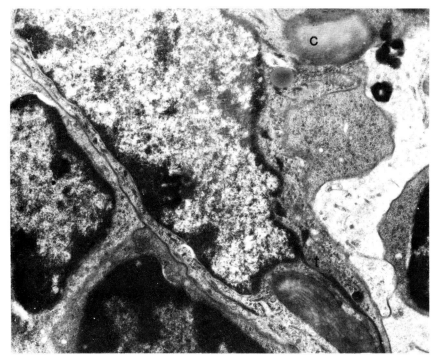

Fig. 1 Thymic reticular epithelial cells from untreated rat,
showing cytoplasmic tonofilaments (t) and bundle of collagen
fibrils.

suppressive agent. Histologically, the observed thymic changes
were described as severe depletion of cortical thymocytes and
the loss of cortical medullary boundaries. The effect seemed
limited to thymocytes and neither bone marrow cells nor mature
lymphocytes appeared to be affected [14]. As no indication of
direct thymocyte destruction *in vivo* had been observed [15],
we decided to investigate the ultrastructure of the rat thymus
during DOTC-induced involution and during return to normal
diets.

Inbred PVG rats were exposed to standard laboratory diets
containing 150 ppm DOTC over 2 or 4 weeks respectively, followed by 1,2,3 or 4 weeks on normal diets. When the thymuses
from animals were examined, a number of reticular epithelial
cells were observed with extensive vacuolation after 2 weeks

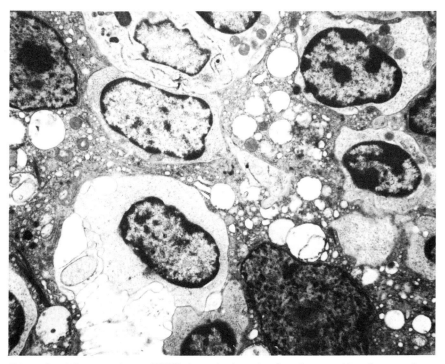

Fig. 2   Thymus from DOTC-treated rat showing reticular epithelial cells with extensive cytoplasmic vacuolation (x 3000).

on the DOTC-containing diet, whilst examination of thymuses
of control rats showed the normal ultrastructure of the organ,
with epithelial cells characterized by the presence of tonofilaments and small flocculent deposits (Fig. 1). The number
of reticular epithelial cells observed with vacuolation in
the thymuses of treated animals increased with the time of
exposure to DOTC. After four weeks many vacuolated epithelial
cells were easily observed because of the severe thymocyte
depletion, and a low number of macrophages were also present
(Fig. 2). Circulating levels of corticosteroids did not
appear to play a part in the action of DOTC as thymic involution was as marked in adrenalectomised as in intact rats
following DOTC exposure, and the ultrastructural changes were
of the same order. After three weeks on DOTC-diets an increased number of secreting granules in the distal cytoplasm
of normal-appearing reticular epithelial cells was also
apparent possibly due to inhibition of secretory activity of
the cells [16] or alternatively, by decreased secretion from
the cells. It thus appears that DOTC acts selectively on the
thymus in such a way that the humoral function of the organ
may be affected.

After return to the normal diet, thymuses were examined
weekly and even though there was considerable repopulation of
the thymuses, some areas remained depopulated and vacuolated
epithelial cells were still present. Thymic weight remained
significantly reduced, although to what extent the damaged
reticular epithelial cells may account for the incomplete
recovery of the thymus in these experiments is not clear.
The question arose, however, as to when reversibility of
thymic involution caused by DOTC would occur as well as to how
exposure to DOTC might effect the physiological involution of
the thymus related to age. Longer recovery experiments
demonstrated that a progressive decrease of the relative size
of the thymus with age occurred in both control and treated
animals, but as the thymuses of treated animals never fully
recovered in terms of weight, age-dependent decay of the
thymuses was completed earlier in this group (Fig. 3). The
functional significance of such involution needs further
study.

In other studies in our laboratories the effect of DOTC-
induced thymic atrophy on immunological competence was investigated by exposing animals to diets containing 75 ppm DOTC
for either eight or twelve weeks. At this concentration
neither food intake nor growth-rate was decreased compared
with animals on a normal diet. A marked decrease in circulating lymphocytes was found and the ability of the circulating mononuclear cells to respond to mitogen-induced
blastogenesis was reduced at the three dose levels of

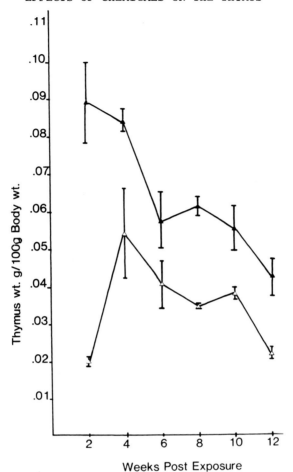

Fig. 3 Age-related decrease in thymic weight in rats fed 150 ppm DOTC for 4 wk after return to normal diet (△——△) compared to untreated rats (▲ —— ▲).

phytohaemagglutinen (PHA) used. When these results were plotted as graphs it was evident that the response of the lymphocytes to PHA was similar over the concentrations used, and that the effect therefore was likely to be due to a dilution in responding cells rather than a qualitative effect (Fig. 4). In the *in vitro* culture assay, no account is taken of the reduction of the total lymphocytes obtained from the treated animals so the actual loss of PHA-responsive cells in the host may well be greater. Animals were also investigated as to their ability to respond to a heterologous T-cell dependent antigen, e.g. sheep red blood cells (SRBC) after five and nine weeks on the DOTC-containing diet. The haemagglutinin assays did not reveal any differences in the

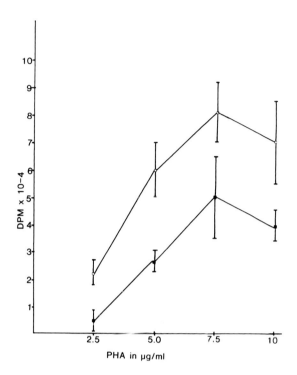

Fig. 4 Uptake of ^{3}H-Thymidine (mean ± s.e.) in response to
PHA stimulation of 2 x 10[5]/well blood mononuclear cells from
rats fed 75 ppm DOTC for 12 wk (■———■) compared to untreated rats (□———□).

ability of the treated animals to mount specific antibody
responses against SRBC as compared to control animals (Fig.
5). These results correlate with the lack of any significant
alteration in spleen weight or splenic lymphocyte populations
indicating that there is little release of splenic lymphocytes for a considerable time after "chemical" thymectomy.
   Thus the investigations in our laboratories all indicate
that DOTC does not include the characteristic and dramatic
alterations of the immune system associated with immunosuppressive drugs, but rather a slow decline in immunocompetence due to loss of regulatory T lymphocytes similar
to the changes reported after adult thymectomy [17]. It is
also possible that damage to reticular epithelial cells produced by DOTC leads to some thymocytes entering alternate
pathways of differentiation which generate non-functional
T lymphocytes [18].
   Various environmental chemicals are also known to act

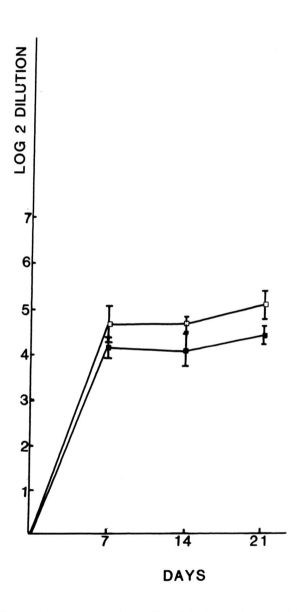

Fig. 5 Humoral response to a T-cell dependent antigen (SRBC) immunised after 9 wk DOTC feeding (75 ppm) during the follow-ing 3 wk on DOTC-diets (■———■) compared to untreated rats (□———□).

preferentially on the immune system, in particular a number
of metabolites synthesized by different species of fungi.
The best known metabolite is undoubtedly Cyclosporin A which
selectively inhibits T-cell responses to antigens and mitogens
and has minimal effects on B lymphocytes [19]. Virtually
nothing is known of its mode of action except that it prevents
lymphocyte activation and appears to act early in the cell
cycle. The trichothecene group of Fusarium mycotoxins are
also known to be potent immunosuppressants producing thymic
atrophy in experimental animal models [20]. The tricothecenes
have been implicated in both human and animal outbreaks of
mycotoxicosis. They are known to inhibit protein synthesis
specifically [1] but whether this condition is the precise
mechanism of action leading to its toxic effects is unknown.
There appears to be a preferential cytotoxicity for lymphoid
cells, and depression of PHA responses and atrophy of the
thymus has been shown to occur as an early response in mice
[21]. The thymus appears sufficiently sensitive to these
toxins to be impaired at doses too low to provoke cellular
lesions or perceptible signs of toxicity.

The different compounds described here all have an effect
on the thymus, but many act at several different levels,
directly on the intrathymic rapidly dividing cells, directly
on the reticular epithelial cells of the thymic stroma, or
indirectly through changes in endocrine control. Discernment
of the mechanisms by which a compound acts will greatly aid
in understanding how toxicological effects may be influenced
by alteration in immune regulation.

ACKNOWLEDGEMENTS

Dr J. Forster and Miss M.P. Scott participated in the studies
carried out at the BIBRA laboratories. These studies form
part of a research project funded by the U.K. Ministry of
Agriculture, Fisheries and Food. The results of this research
are Crown Copyright.

REFERENCES

1. Stutman, B. (1978). *Immunological Rev.* **42**, 139-184.
2. Joel, D.D., Chanana, A.D., Coltier, H., Cronkite, G.P.
    and Laissue, J.A. (1979). *Cell Tissue Kinet.* **10**, 57-63.
3. Zimmerman, B. and Tsui, F. (1980). *Thymus* **1**, 293-304.
4. Jenkinson, E.J., Ewijk, W. and Owen, J.J.T. (1981).
    J. Exp. Med. **153**, 280-292.
5. Garaci, E., Pecci, G., Rinaldi Garacia, C., del Gobbo, V.
    and Tonietti, G. (1978). *Clin. Imm. Immunopathol.* **11**,
    157-167.
6. Stimson, W.H. and Grilly, P.J. (1981). *Immunology* **44**,
    401-407.

7. Tarka, S.M., Zoumas, B.L. and Gans, J.H. (1979). *Toxicol. Appl. Pharmac.* **49**, 127-149.
8. Deschaux, P., Massengo, B. and Fontanges, R. (1979). *Thymus* **1**, 95-108.
9. Vos. J., Moore, J. and Zinkel, J. (1973). *Environ. Health Perspect.* **5**, 149-162.
10. Faith, R.E., Luster, M.I. and Vos, J.G. (1980). In "Reviews in Biochemical Toxicology" (eds. E. Hodgson, J.R. Bud and R.H. Philpot), Vol.2, pp.173-211, Elsevier, Oxford.
11. Thomas, P.T. and Hinsdill, R.D. (1979). *Drug and Chemical Toxicol.* **2**, 77-98.
12. Vos, J.G. (1977). *CRC Crit. Rev. Toxicol.* **5**, 67-101.
13. Seinen, W. and Willems, M.I. (1976). *Tox. Appl. Pharmacol.* **35**, 63-75.
14. Penninks, A.H. and Seinen, W. (1980). *Tox. Appl. Pharmacol.* **56**, 221-231.
15. Seinen, W., Vos, J.G., Van Spanje, I., Snoele, H., Brands, R. and Hooykaas, H. (1977). *Tox. Appl. Pharmacol.* **42**, 197-212.
16. Shoham, J., Ben David, E. and Sandbank, V. (1982). *Immunology* **45**, 31-38.
17. Stutman, O. and Hood, R.A. (1974). *Ser. Haemat.* **7**, 505-523.
18. Cantor, H., McVay-Boudreau, L., Hugenberger, F., Naidorf, K., Shen, F.W. and Gershon, R.K. (1978). *J. Exp. Med.* **147**, 1116-1125.
19. Klaus, G.G.B. (1981). *Immunology Today* **2**, 88-97.
20. LaFarge-Frayssinet, C., Lespinats, G., Lafont, P., Loisillier, F., Mousset, S., Rosenstein, Y. and Frayssinet, C. (1979). *Proc. Soc. Exp. Biol. Med.* **160**, 302-311.
21. Cardliffe, E. and Davies, J. (1977). *Antimicrob. Agents Chemother.* **11**, 491-499.

APPROACHES AND METHODOLOGY FOR EXAMINING THE IMMUNOLOGICAL EFFECTS OF XENOBIOTICS

J.H. Dean, M.I. Luster,[*] M.J. Murray and L.D. Lauer

[*] *Chemical Industry Institute of Toxicology*
and National Institute of Environmental Health Sciences,
Research Triangle Park, North Carolina 27709, U.S.A.

INTRODUCTION

Traditional toxicological methods have implicated the immune system as a potential target for toxic insult. In many studies, morphologic and gravimetric alterations in lymphoid organs, as well as quantitative changes in peripheral leukocyte counts or bone marrow cellularity were reported in animals exposed to xenobiotics at dose levels where other manifestations of toxicity were not apparent. Cellular injury and functional impairment of immunoresponsive cells can now be quantitated using sensitive and reproducible *in vitro* and *in vivo* assays of immune function and host resistance following chemical or drug exposure.

The sensitivity of the immune system in assessing toxic injury results from innate biological characteristics of immune cell function and response. Biological amplification, a key concept in the immune response requires interactions between multiple cell types within a highly organized and precisely regulated network. Minor perturbations in this network, perceived as changes in one or more components of immunity, are detectable by well-defined *in vivo* and *in vitro* assays evaluating immune function. Not every alteration, however, leads to significant acute or chronic immune impairment *in vivo*. There appears to be a certain resiliency and reserve within the immune response. On the other hand, concomitant changes in host resistance and immune function following chemical exposure in laboratory animals might indicate potentially significant health effects to be considered in human risk assessment of chemicals and drugs.

The primary strategies among immunologists working in the

toxicology and safety assessment arena are to select or de-
develop, validate and apply a tiered panel of methods (e.g.,
Dean et al. [1]) that can reproducibly characterize immune
alterations occurring following in vivo exposure to chemicals
of concern. Although many of these methods are widely used
in clinical medicine, validation of these methodologies in
rodent models appears necessary. The selection and validation
of these immunological methods for toxicological studies have
addressed several issues. These include the following: 1)
does the method yield results that are consistent and reproducible within and between laboratories?; 2) does the method
have sufficient sensitivity to detect biologically significant
changes (e.g. alterations in host susceptibility to infectious
agents or neoplastic cell growth); 3) does the method predict
immunotoxic potential in humans?

Presently under development or validation in rodents, are
methods for assessing delayed-hypersensitivity to novel antigens such as keyhole limpet haemocyanin or bovine gamma globulin; lymphoproliferative responses to T- and B-cell mitogens
and alloantigens in one-way mixed leukocyte culture (MLC);
quantitation of B- and T-cell subpopulations using monoclonal
antibodies to cell surface markers; in vitro lymphocyte cytotoxicity and macrophage cytostatis against specific tumour
target cells; quantification of antibody plaque forming cells
and specific immunoglobulin levels in serum; macrophage effector function with and without activation; bone marrow cellularity and progenitor cell colony-forming units; and models
of host resistance to bacteria, viruses, parasites or trans-
plantable tumour cell challenge. These assays can be subsequently employed to evaluate the integrity of the immune
system following chemical exposure and the resulting data
used as a base for predicting no effect levels and potential
human health risk.

In this respect acute and chronic exposure to toxic chemicals and drugs have been shown to produce immune dysfunction
and in some cases, alter host susceptibility to bacteria,
viruses, tumours and parasites [2,3,4]. Experimental animals
exposed to polychlorinated or polybrominated biphenyls or
2,3,7,8-tetrachlorodibenzo-p-dioxin (TCDD) for example have
been shown to exhibit alterations in immune function and host
resistance [5,6] similar to those observed in humans acci-
dentally exposed to these same chemicals [7,8].

A second strategy is to demonstrate the utility of the
immune system for studying injury at a cellular and functional
level i.e., as a sensitive indicator of toxicity. Routine
parameters measured in toxicology studies, such as blood or
tissue cellularity are often considerably less sensitive
indicators of toxicity than immune function tests. The

lymphocyte, in particular, possesses a number of characteristics that make it an appropriate model for examining the effects of various agents on cell growth, differentiation and function [9,10]. Among these are its capacity to undergo blastogenesis and division *in vitro* in response to mitogens or alloantigens; expression of gene products on its surface that can be utilized as markers of differentiation; and its potential to undergo terminal differentiation resulting in production of soluble mediators (e.g. lymphokines or antibody) or providing effector function (e.g. tumour target cell killing).

Because cellular differentiation and proliferation are closely linked processes, disruption of normal differentiation can alter proliferation or some measurable function associated with differentiation. Most leukaemias and lymphomas, for example, represent proliferating populations of cells arrested at a single point in differentiation. A variety of chemicals of environmental concern, including benzene, halogenated hydrocarbons, polycyclic aromatic hydrocarbons, and several chemicals with tumour promoting potential (e.g. TCDD and 12-0-tetradecanoylphorbol-13-acetate, TPA) produce toxicity to the immune system that appears to alter this orderly process of differentiation and maturation.

RESULTS AND DISCUSSION

Three prototype chemicals were studied using our multifaceted Tier 1 assay panel [11] to assess chemical and drug-induced effects on the immune system and host resistance. Representative chemicals included a polycyclic hydrocarbon carcinogen (benzo(a)pyrene), a potent tumour promoter (12-0-tetradecanoyl phorbol 13-acetate (TPA)) and a synthetic environmental estrogenic drug (diethylstilbestrol (DES)). These results, in part, summarize data and methodology previously published in detail by the authors [12-16].

Benzo(a)pyrene (BAP) represents a large and ubiquitous class of chemicals collectively known as polycyclic aromatic hydrocarbons (PAHs). PAHs are found in coal tar, soot and other fossil fuel combustion products. Most, including benzo(a)pyrene are potent carcinogens, and have been shown to modulate immunity [17]. In contrast, TPA, a phorbol diester derived from croton oil, is a potent promoter of multiple tumours in the skin tumour promotion model [18]. *In vitro*, TPA has been shown to enhance transformation of fibroblasts following exposure to carcinogens such as PAH [19,20] and can also modulate function in certain immunoresponsive cells [11,21-24].

Diethylstilbestrol, a human carcinogen, has been associated

with a rare, latent, clear cell vaginal carcinoma of young
women exposed to DES *in utero* [25]. A non-steroidal synthetic
compound with potent estrogenic activity, DES is widely utilized as a growth promoting agent in livestock and for numerous
therapeutic purposes in humans. DES exposure in rodents has
been shown to produce multiple immune alterations [12-14,26].

In the studies described here, adult, female B6C3F1 mice
received subcutaneous injections of BAP, TPA, or DES dissolved
in corn oil over a 14 day period (BAP or TPA) or a 5 day
period (DES). Control groups received corn oil injections on
an identical schedule. Total dosages were 50, 200, or 400 mg
BAP/kg body weight; 2, 20, or 40 mg TPA/kg body weight; and
0.2, 2, or 8 mg DES/kg body weight. Assays were performed
2-5 days following administration of the final dose.

Administration of these three agents at the dosages described
above did not result in lethality or overt signs of toxicity
during the exposure period. Significant loss of body weight,
a traditional indicator of generalized toxicity, did not occur,
although there was a dose-related decrease in body weights of
BAP-exposed mice (Table 1). In contrast, mice treated with
DES exhibited a slight, though insignificant increase in body
weight, consistent with the growth promoting effects of this
drug.

Lymphoid organ weights, which can serve as indicators of
potential immunotoxicity of an agent, are presented in Table 1.
Thymic atrophy, for example, is often coincident with quantitative changes in T-lymphocyte numbers, characteristics and
functions. In the experiments summarized here, both DES and
TPA induced a dose-related thymic atrophy. In the case of
DES this decrease was significant at all dosage levels and
ranged from 56% at 0.2 mg/kg to 75% at 8.0 mg/kg. In contrast,
a significant dose-dependent hypertrophy occurred in the
spleens of DES and TPA-treated animals, while BAP did not influence either splenic or thymic weights.

Peripheral leukocytosis (Table 1) occurred in all DES-
exposed groups and following high dose (40 mg/kg) exposure
to TPA. A relative increase in lymphocytes appeared to be at
least partially responsible for the increase following DES
treatment.

Quantitative changes in lymphoid organ weights and peripheral blood composition is suggestive of possible immunological
effects, but may occur in the presence of normal immune function [27] ; and thus, functional parameters must be examined.
Assays quantitating lymphoproliferation in response to mitogens or alloantigens allow quantitative assessments of co-
operation and function between cellular components responsible
for both cell-mediated and humoral immunity. Of the three
agents tested, DES most consistently and dramatically

Table 1 *Effects of chemical exposure on body weights, lymphoid organ weights and leukocyte counts*[a].

Chemical (dosage μg/g)	Body weight (g)	Thymus (mg)	Spleen (mg)	Leukocytes x 10^3/mm^3	Lymphocytes x 10^3/mm^3
DES 0	20.8 ± 0.4	49.2 ± 1.6[b]	118 ± 27	3.8 ± 0.3	2.9 ± 0.2
DES 0.2	21.6 ± 0.6	21.8 ± 1.1[b]	140 ± 80	5.7 ± 0.6[c]	4.4 ± 0.4[c]
DES 2.0	22.8 ± 1.0	14.5 ± 1.1[b]	161 ± 9[c]	8.4 ± 1.5[b]	7.2 ± 1.3[b]
DES 8.0	22.1 ± 0.5	12.1 ± 0.7[b]	205 ± 8[b]	11.0 ± 1.0[b]	9.1 ± 0.8[b]
Dose response	NS[d]	< 0.01	< 0.01	< 0.01	< 0.01
BAP 0	21.2 ± 0.5	63.3 ± 5.2	97 ± 4	6.8 ± 0.4	5.8 ± 0.3
BAP 50	20.9 ± 0.8	59.4 ± 4.6	97 ± 3	8.8 ± 1.4	7.1 ± 1.1
BAP 200	20.2 ± 0.2	57.0 ± 3.6	92 ± 4	8.1 ± 0.7	6.5 ± 0.7
BAP 400	19.8 ± 0.5	48.4 ± 6.9	100 ± 7	7.9 ± 0.6	5.5 ± 0.5
Dose response	< 0.05	< 0.05	NS	NS	NS
TPA 0	20.5 ± 0.5	49.5 ± 3.4	110 ± 7	5.8 ± 0.5	4.6 ± 0.4
TPA 2.0	21.0 ± 0.5	44.8 ± 3.2	110 ± 9	7.5 ± 0.6	5.8 ± 0.4
TPA 20.0	20.6 ± 0.5	33.0 ± 1.3[b]	192 ± 14[b]	7.6 ± 0.9[b]	3.8 ± 0.4
TPA 40.0	20.9 ± 0.6	36.7 ± 2.4[c]	245 ± 18[b]	10.0 ± 0.7[b]	3.9 ± 0.4
Dose response	NS	< 0.01	< 0.01	< 0.001	< 0.05

[a]Mean value ± SEM of 6–8 mice per group

[b]Significantly different from control, p < 0.01

[c]Significantly different from control, p < 0.05

[d]Not significant

Table 2 Lymphocyte function following exposure to BAP, TPA and DES

Chemical (dosage µg/g)	Proliferative response in CPM x 10³[a] ^{3}H-TdR ± SEM (% change)				Effector function	Surface markers[a]	
	PHA	Con A	LPS	MLC	% Spontaneous cytolysis of YAC-1	% T cells	% B cells
BAP 0	77.7±2.7	82.0±8.4	15.9±0.9	10.0±0.05	19.6	28.0±1.0	37.4±2.1
BAP 50	71.3±5.0 (8% ↓)	87.3±6.7 (6% ↑)	22.4±2.1[b] (32% ↑)	9.3±0.03 (7% ↓)	ND[c]	ND	ND
BAP 200	52.8±4.5 (32% ↓)	54.7±9.2 (33% ↓)	16.8±2.5 (0%)	10.5±0.04 (5% ↑)	ND	ND	ND
BAP 400	31.3±2.7[d] (60% ↓)	37.9±4.8 (54% ↓)	7.7±1.2[d] (54% ↓)	10.7±0.02 (7% ↑)	18.1	28.6±0.9	39.2±1.0
Dose response	< 0.01	< 0.01	< 0.05	NS[e]	ND	ND	ND
TPA 0	41.5±2.7	66.3±2.8	10.7±0.8	14.0±1.2	20.3	50.3±4.0	44.0±2.6
TPA 2.0	47.4±2.9 (14% ↑)	69.0±6.1 (4% ↑)	11.3±1.4 (5% ↑)	15.4±2.0 (10% ↑)	4.4[b]	ND	ND
TPA 20.0	36.3±3.4 (13% ↓)	54.1±7.2 (20% ↓)	9.3±0.9 (13% ↓)	15.0±1.0 (7% ↑)	3.3[b]	ND	ND
TPA 40.0	26.6±3.8[b] (36% ↓)	32.5±3.2[b] (51% ↓)	5.9±0.5[b] (45% ↓)	9.6±1.2[b] (31% ↓)	2.7[b]	20.5±2.9[d] (59% ↓)	36.0±2.1[b] (18% ↓)
Dose response	< 0.005	< 0.01	< 0.01	< 0.05	ND	ND	ND

Table 2 (cont'd)

DES 0	27.5±3.6	23.4±2.8	8.2±0.8	4.0±0.3	19.5	38.0±0.8	34.2±4.1
DES 0.2	17.3±1.5[b] (37% ↓)	16.1±3.1 (31% ↓)	13.6±1.0[d] (65% ↑)	3.9±0.4 (2% ↓)	ND	ND	ND
DES 2.0	12.2±1.5[d] (56% ↓)	12.1±1.7[d] (48% ↓)	10.0±0.9 (22% ↑)	2.8±0.2[d] (30% ↓)	ND	ND	ND
DES 8.0	4.8±0.7[d] (82% ↓)	8.3±0.8[d] (64% ↓)	5.8±1.2 (29% ↓)	3.0±0.2[d] (25% ↓)	18.8	28.5±2.3[d]	37.6±3.4
Dose response	< 0.01	< 0.01	< 0.01	< 0.01	ND	ND	ND

[a] Mean value ± SEM of 6–8 mice per group

[b] Significantly different from control, $p < 0.05$

[c] Not determined

[d] Significantly different from control, $p < 0.01$

[e] Not significant

suppressed T-cell proliferative responses (Table 2). Similarly mixed leukocyte cultures (MLC), measuring alloantigenic stimulation of responder splenocytes were significantly affected in the 2 and 8 mg DES/kg dosage groups where a decrease in proliferation was observed. Relative percentages of splenic lymphocytes bearing T-cell surface markers were also decreased in the high-dose DES group while percentages of splenocytes with B-cell markers remained unchanged. This suggests a direct toxic effect of DES on T-cells, or effects upon T-cell differentiation and/or maturation. Lymphoproliferative responses to phytohaemagglutinin (PHA) and Concanavalin A (Con A) stimulation following BAP and TPA exposure were also reduced in a dose-related manner. While percentages of splenocytes with B- and T-cell markers were not altered following BAP exposure, both populations decreased in TPA-exposed mice compared to controls. Thus, TPA may also disrupt normal differentiation, maturation or surface marker expression in splenocytes. Lipopolysaccharide (LPS)-induced B-cell proliferation was significantly decreased only in the high dose BAP and TPA groups, and not altered in the DES groups except at 0.2 mg/kg, where the response was elevated.

An additional in vitro assay of cell-mediated immune function examined spontaneous cytolysis of tumour targets by natural killer (NK) cells. NK-mediated cytolysis of TAC-1 targets was not changed in BAP or DES-treated mice, but was dramatically suppressed in all TPA-treated groups (Table 2). Since spontaneous cytolysis of tumour cells in vivo may represent a mechanism of natural tumour resistance, suppression of NK activity may be expected to influence tumour resistance. Spontaneous tumour incidence in mice with genetically deficient or enhanced NK activity has correlated with modulation of natural resistance to tumours [28].

Antibody-mediated parameters (Table 3) were evaluated in mice exposed to the three test agents by quantitating plaque-forming cells (PFC) to sheep red blood cell (SRBC) antigens, a T-cell dependent response, and to LPS, a T-cell independent response. With DES, serum antibody titres to LPS rather than PFC were determined. PFC response to SRBC decreased in a dose-related manner in both DES and BAP-exposed mice. In the BAP-treated groups the suppression ranged from 40% to 89%, while suppression in the high-dose (8 mg/kg) DES-treated group was 43% of control values. In general, PAHs have been shown to be immunosuppressive for B-cells and humoral immunity [17].

Suppression of PFC response to LPS of approximately the same magnitude as seen with PFC responses to SRBC were observed in BAP-treated mice. More recent studies have shown that BAP appears to selectively affect either B2 cells directly, or their terminal maturation to plasma calls [15].

Table 3 *Antibody mediated parameters following BAP, TPA or DES exposures*

Chemical (dosage μg/g)	SRBC PFC/spleen ± SEM x 10^{-4} (% change)[a]	LPS PFC/spleen ± SEM x 10^{-4} or HA titre (Log_2) (% change)[a]
BAP 0	30.9 ± 5.4	13.4 ± 1.2
BAP 50	18.6 ± 4.0 (30% ↓)	6.3 ± 1.0[b] (53% ↓)
BAP 200	7.5 ± 0.7[b] (76% ↓)	4.7 ± 0.5[b] (65% ↓)
BAP 400	3.3 ± 0.4[b] (89.3% ↓)	2.0 ± 0.4[b] (82% ↓)
Dose response	< 0.01	< 0.01
TPA 0	29.8 ± 8.1	83.3 ± 13.0
TPA 2.0	19.2 ± 3.5 (36% ↓)	ND[c]
TPA 20.0	25.3 ± 3.5 (15% ↓)	70.5 ± 12.0 (15% ↓)
TPA 40.0	28.3 ± 8.2 (5% ↓)	57.9 ± 6.1 (30% ↓)
Dose response	NS[d]	NS[d]
DES 0	16.0 ± 1.9	6.67 ± 0.21
DES 0.2	13.0 ± 1.0 (19% ↓)	6.00 ± 0.26 (10% ↓)
DES 2.0	8.7 ± 0.9[b] (46% ↓)	5.67 ± 0.21 (15% ↓)
DES 8.0	9.1 ± 0.7[e] (43% ↓)	3.67 ± 0.49[b] (45% ↓)
Dose response	< 0.01	< 0.01

[a] Mean value of 6-8 mice per group

[b] Significantly different from control, $p < 0.01$

[c] Not determined

[d] Not significant

[e] Significantly different from control, $p < 0.05$

Following DES exposure, antibody titres to LPS were reduced
up to 45%. In contrast, no significant alterations were observed in PFC responses to either SRBC or LPS in TPA-treated
mice.

Although BAP, TPA and DES were shown to alter various immunologic parameters, demonstration of the biological relevance of
such changes is essential in the immunotoxicological assessment of a chemical. Measurement of host resistance, in infectivity models provides a means for correlating immune dysfunction with a significant biological effect *in vivo*. Host
resistance in mice challenged with the bacterium *Listeria*
monocytogenes was affected differently by exposure to each of
the three agents tested (Table 4). BAP did not significantly
influence mortality at any dosage. This result might be expected since pathogenesis of this agent is controlled by
T-cells and macrophages [29]. After exposure to DES, however,
there was a dramatic increase in *Listeria*-associated deaths.
A possible T-cell defect implicated by altered T-cell functional assays, severe thymic atrophy, and the concurrent loss
of splenocytes bearing T-cell markers may, in part, explain
the increased susceptibility to *Listeria* observed in DES-
exposed mice. Alternatively the macrophages alterations previously reported [11] may also help to define host resistance
mechanisms to *Listeria*. Related studies using Swiss mice
challenged with *Pneumococcus* Type 1 and *Pasturella septica*
have shown that DES stimulates phagocytosis and prolongs animal survival [30]. The apparent discrepancy between these
studies and our own may, in part, involve a mechanism of host
resistance to *Pneumococcus*, believed to be T-cell independent.
In contrast to DES exposure, after an initial LD_{20} challenge
dose, in which no deaths occurred in TPA-treated animals, an
LD_{80} challenge dose was employed (Table 4). No deaths
occurred at the two higher doses of TPA, compared to 89%
mortality observed in controls. Although the basis for this
increased resistance is not clear, we have recently observed
enhanced H_2O_2 generation and macrophage-mediated cytostasis
of tumour cells by macrophages from TPA-exposed mice (Dean
et al, unpublished observation).

Host resistance to challenge with cells from two syngeneic
tumour lines, PYB6 and B16F10, was examined in chemically
treated animals (Table 4). In BAP-exposed mice, the percentage of successful transplants was not significantly altered
between groups, consistent with observations that BAP-exposure
results primarily in B-cell and not macrophage or T-cell
dysfunction. Following DES or TPA exposure, however, successful PYB6 tumour transplants increased significantly in the
medium and high dosage groups. The mechanisms of allograft
and tumour resistance is believed to require both macrophages

Table 4 *Alterations in host resistance parameters following BAP, TPA or DES exposure*

Chemical (dosage µg/g)	Listeria challenge		PYB6 Challenge		B16F10 Challenge[a]	
	Mortality per no. challenged	% Mortality	No. tumours per no. challenged	% tumour takes	No. of lung modules per mouse	CPM ^{125}I-IudR incorporation per lung
BAP 0	0/10	0%	0/10	0%	ND	ND
BAP 50	1/10	10%	1/10	10%	ND	ND
BAP 200	1/10	10%	0/10	0%	ND	ND
BAP 400	0/10	0%	2/10	20%	ND	ND
TPA 0	17/19	89%	8/35	23%	15 ± 2	1509 ± 296
TPA 2.0	6/10	60%	11/30	37%	41 ± 5[b]	2673 ± 392[c]
TPA 20.0	0/10[c]	0%	17/30[b]	57%	68 ± 4[b]	9805 ± 1803[b]
TPA 40.0	0/6[c]	0%	17/28[b]	61%	81 ± 7[b]	9355 ± 1530[b]
DES 0	2/10	20%	2/10	20%	ND	ND
DES 0.2	10/10	100%	3/10	30%	ND	ND
DES 2.0	10/10	100%	8/10	80%	ND	ND
DES 8.0	8/8	100%	9/10	90%	ND	ND

[a]Mean value ± SEM of 6–8 mice per group

[b]Significantly different from control, $p < 0.01$

[c]Significantly different from control, $p < 0.05$

and immunocompetent T-lymphocytes [31]. Our results indicate
a T-cell dysfunction in DES and TPA exposed mice which provides
an immune environment more favourable to tumour development.
In the case of DES, they also correlate previous studies indicating decreased tumour latency and increased mortality in
DES-treated, B6C3F1 mice challenged with Lewis lung carcinoma,
[14] and also with dose-related increases of spontaneous
mammary tumours in C3H mice exposed to DES [32].

TPA exposure also coincided with increased numbers of PYB6
tumour takes and B16F10 melanoma lung nodules in mice sacri-
ficed three weeks following challenge (Table 4). In addition,
pulmonary radioisotope incorporation correlated well with
total pulmonary tumour burden. Radioactivity increased from
1509 cpm per lung in controls to 9355 cpm per lung in the high
dose TPA group. These data suggest impaired host resistance
in TPA-treated mice and are consistent with impaired T-cell
function, decreased numbers of splenocytes bearing T-cell
markers, reduced thymic weights, and loss of NK activity, also
observed in these animals. In addition, recently demonstrated
cell surface receptors on murine lymphocytes capable of binding TPA could provide a rationale for the apparent specific
lymphoid toxicity observed in our assays [33] and may suggest
a role for immunoalteration in TPA-induced tumour promotion.

SUMMARY

Drug and chemical-induced toxicity can be assessed in assays
quantitating immune function and host resistance. These
assays can be utilized to demonstrate potentially important
functional alterations in immunoresponsive cells in the
absence of overt in vivo toxicity. Three prototype chemicals,
BAP, TPA and DES were evaluated using a comprehensive panel
of immune function and host resistance assays. This approach
allows for the determination of immunologic alteration following chemical or drug exposure, and for the assessment of the
biological relevance of these effects upon host resistance.
Furthermore, it serves to elucidate mechanisms of toxicity at
cellular and subcellular levels. For example, BAP, a potent
initiator of carcinogenesis, had no effect upon our host
resistance models, a result not unexpected since PAHs have
previously been shown to primarily modulate humoral immunity.
In contrast, the tumour promoter, TPA, had little effect upon
antibody-mediated plaque formation, but significantly altered
lymphoproliferation, NK-mediated tumouricidal activity, and
host resistance to tumours. Similarly, DES exposure predominantly affected T-cell function, which correlated with
decreased host resistance to bacterial and tumour challenge.
Thus, there appears to be evidence that alterations in T-cell

numbers and function may predict potential changes in host
resistance to tumour and bacterial challenges. This would
agree with current concepts implicating T-cells as important
mediators of host resistance although macrophage alterations
cannot be ruled out. In contrast, TPA-induced *in vivo* protection against *Listeria* challenge probably results from
activation of bactericidal systems following TPA-exposure.
These data demonstrate the importance of multifaceted panels
in assessing potential immunotoxicity. Infectivity and tumour
challenge models allow for the correlation of immunological
effects with other biologically relevant endpoints that can
provide potentially important information in the safety assessment of chemicals and drugs.

REFERENCES

1. Dean, J.H., Padarathsingh, M.L. and Jerrels, T.R. (1979).
    Drug and Chem. Toxicol. **2**, 5-17.
2. Vos, J.G. (1977). *CRC Crit. Rev. Toxicol.* **5**, 67-101.
3. Faith, R.E., Luster, M.I. and Vos, J.G. (1980). In
    "Reviews in Biochemical Toxicology" (eds. E. Hodgson,
    J.R. Bend and R.M. Philpot), Vol.2, pp.172-212. Elsevier,
    New York.
4. Dean, J.H., Luster, M.I. and Boorman, G.A. (1982). In
    "Immunopharmacology - Research Monographs in Immunology"
    (eds. M. Rola-Plezczynski and P. Sirois). Elsevier/North
    Holland Biomedical Press, Amsterdam, (In press).
5. Luster, M.I., Boorman, G.A., Harris, M.W. and Moore, J.A.
    (1979). *Int. J. Immunopharmacology* **2**, 69-80.
6. Luster, M.I., Boorman, G.A., Dean, J.H., Harris, M.W.,
    Luebke, A.W., Pardarathsingh, M.L. and Moore, J.A. (1980).
    Int. J. Immunopharmac. **2**, 301-310.
7. Bekesi, J.G., Holland, J.F., Anderson, H.A., Fischbein,
    A.S., Rom, W., Wolff, M.S. and Selikoff, I.J. (1978).
    Science **199**, 1207.
8. Chang, K.-J., Hseih, K.-H., Lee, T.-P., Tang, S.-Y. and
    Tung, T.-C. (1981). *Toxicol. Appl. Pharmacol.* **61**, 58.
9. Katz, D.H. (1977). In "Lymphocyte Differentiation,
    Recognition and Regulation" (ed. D. Katz). Academic Press,
    New York.
10. Pfeifer, R.W. and Irons, R.D. (1982). *J. Reticulo-
    endothelial Soc.* **31**, 155-170.
11. Dean, J.H., Luster, M.I., Boorman, G.A. and Lauer, L.D.
    (1982). *Pharmacol. Rev.* **34**, 137-148.
12. Luster, M.I., Boorman, G.A., Dean, J.H., Luebke, R.W.
    and Lawson, L.D. (1980). *J. Reticuloendothelial. Soc.*
    28, 561.
13. Boorman, G.A., Luster, M.I., Dean, J.H. and Wilson, R.E.

(1980). *J. Reticuloendothelial. Soc*. **28**, 547.

14. Dean, J.H., Luster, M.I., Boorman, G.A., Luebke, R.W., Lauer, L.D. (1980). *J. Reticuloendothelial Soc*. **28**, 571-583.

15. Dean, J.H., Luster, M.I., Boorman, G.A., Lauer, L.D., Luebke, R.W. and Lawson, L. (1982). *Clin. Exptl. Immunol*. (In press).

16. Luster, M.I., Dean, J.H. and Moore, J.A. (1982). In "Principles and Methods in Toxicology" (ed. W. Hayes), pp.561-586. Raven Press, New York.

17. Ball, J.K. (1970). *J. Natl. Cancer Inst*. **44**, 1.

18. Berenblum, I. (1975). In "Cancer" (ed. Becker), Vol.1, pp.323-344. Plenum Press, New York.

19. Lasne, C., Gentile, A. and Chouroulinkov, I. (1974). *Nature* **247**, 490-491.

20. Fisher, P.B., Weinstein, B., Eisenberg, D. and Ginsberg, H.S. (1978). *Proc. Nat. Acad. Sci*. (Wash.) **75**, 2311.

21. Touraine, J.L., Hadden, J.W., Touraine, F., Hadden, E.M., Estensen, R. and Good, R.A. (1977). *J. Exp. Med*. **145**, 460.

22. Kwong, C.H. and Mueller, G.C. (1982). *Cancer Res*. **42**, 2115.

23. Keller, R. (1979). *Nature* (Lond.) **282**, 729-731.

24. Laskin, D.L., Laskin, J.D., Kessler, J. (1982). Weinstein, I.B. and Carchman, R.A. (1981). *Cancer Res*. **41**, 4523-4528.

25. Herbst, A.L., Ulfelderand, H. and Poskanzer, D.C. (1971). *New Eng. J. Med*. **284**, 878.

26. Kalland, T., Strand, O. and Forsberg, J. (1980). *J. Natl. Cancer Inst*. **63**, 413-421.

27. Vos, J.G., Krajns, E.I., Beckhof, P.K. and Van Logten, M.J. (1982). In "Proceedings of the 4th Congress of Pesticide Chemistry". Kyoto, Japan.

28. Herberman, R.B. and Holden, H.T. (1978). *Adv. Cancer Res*. **27**, 305-372.

29. Tripathy, S.P. and Mackaness, G.B. (1969). *J. Exp. Med*. **130**, 1-16.

30. Nicol, T., Cordingley, J., Charles, L., McKelvie, P. and Bailey, D. (1963). In "Roledu System Reticulo-Endothelial dans L'Immunite. Antibacterionne et Antitumorale" pp.165-175, Paris Colloques International du C.N.R.S. 115.

31. Klein, G. (1966). *Ann. Rev. Microbiol*. **20**, 223-252.

32. Norvell, M.J. and Shellenberger, T.E. (1977). *Proc. 16th. Annual Meeting Soc. Toxicol*. Abstract 115, p.12.

33. Sando, J.J., Hilfiker, M.L., Salomon, D.S. and Farrar, J.J. (1981). *Proc. Natl. Acad. Sci*. **78**, 1189-1193.

TOXICITY OF HEXACHLOROBENZENE IN THE RAT FOLLOWING COMBINED PRE- AND POST-NATAL EXPOSURE: COMPARISON OF EFFECTS ON IMMUNE SYSTEM, LIVER AND LUNG

J.G. Vos, G.M.J. Brouwer, F.X.R. van Leeuwen and Sj. Wagenaar

*National Institute of Public Health,
P.O. Box 1, 3720 BA Bilthoven, The Netherlands.*

INTRODUCTION

In a previous study it was shown that exposure of rats to hexachlorobenzene (HCB) causes (in addition to liver changes) marked effects on the immune system, suggesting immuno-stimulation [1]. Upon functional assessment of the immune system, the main effect was an enhanced antibody response to the thymus-dependent antigen tetanus toxoid [1]. As HCB can cross the placenta [2], and a high excretion occurs in the milk [3], the immune effects of HCB were also studied follow-ing combined pre- and post-natal exposure (dietary levels of 50 and 150 mg/kg). The main effects in this study [4] were again stimulation of the humoral immunity, lymph node and lung pathology which occurred at the 50 mg/kg level, whereas liver effects were only noted in the 150 mg/kg group.

In the present study, we further investigated the compound HCB following combined pre- and post-natal exposure to dietary levels of 4, 20 and 100 mg/kg. Besides histo-pathological examination of the lymphoid system, liver and lung, function studies were undertaken in both the immune system and the liver.

MATERIALS AND METHODS

Chemical and diet. Hexachlorobenzene (BDH Chemicals Ltd., Poole, England; purity > 99.5%) was mixed in a semi-synthetic diet (Trouw Ltd., Putten, The Netherlands) at concentrations of 4, 20 and 100 mg/kg. Dietary concentrations of HCB in the various batches were checked by gas-chromatographic analysis. Mean values (and range) in the 4, 20 and 100 mg/kg diets were

IMMUNOTOXICOLOGY
ISBN 0-12-282180-7

3.6 (3.1 - 4.3), 17.9 (17.0 - 20.3) and 100.1 (88.2 - 107.0),
respectively. The control diet contained less than 0.001 mg
HCB/kg. Thus, the calculated dose levels corresponded reasonably well with the intended ones.

Rats. Virgin female randomly bred Wistar rats, RIV:TOX[M]
were mated overnight. Detection of a vaginal plug indicated
day 0 of pregnancy. Rats that became pregnant in a three-day
period were divided randomly into four groups and were kept
under conventional conditions. Starting at day 1-3 of pregnancy they received diets containing 0, 4, 20 or 100 mg HCB/
kg. Diet and water were provided *ad libitum*. At birth the
number of neonates per litter was standardized to eight.
Animals were weaned after three weeks and continued on the
same HCB exposure regimen as their mothers. At this time
male and female rats were allocated randomly to the various
groups.

**Organ weights, histopathology, haematology and serum IgM and
IgG levels.** Rats were anaesthetized with ether and exsanguin-
ation was done from the aorta. Groups of rats aged five weeks
and seven months were used for the determination of organ
weights and for histopathological examination. For the latter
purpose, tissues were fixed in formalin and embedded in Paraplast. For the study of Peyer's patches in the jejunum, so-
called Swiss rolls were prepared prior to fixation [5].
Sections were stained with haematoxylin and eosin. Lung
tissue was also stained for the detection of collagen
(elastica-van Gieson), mast cells (toluidin blue) and retic-
ulin. In addition, lung tissue was embedded in glyco-
methacrylate for the preparation of 1 μm sections (Giemsa
stain). Finally, cryostat sections of the liver of five-
week-old animals were examined by fluorescence microscopy in
order to detect excessive quantities of porphyrins. Slides
of lymph nodes, jejunum and lung were read under code to
avoid bias in the observations. Of the young age groups,
total leukocyte and differential leukocyte counts were also
carried out, and sera were stored at -20°C for total IgM and
IgG analysis by the enzyme-linked immunosorbent assay (ELISA)
[6,7]. Results (mean value of triplicate analyses) were expressed as percentage of the IgM and IgG level in the pooled
control group.

Resistance to *Trichinella spiralis* infection. Five-week-old
rats were infected orally with 1,000 *T. spiralis* larvae
(8-10 animals per group). Six weeks after infection IgM and
IgG antibodies against *T. spiralis* were determined with ELISA
[8]. IgE analyses were performed by passive cutaneous

anaphylaxy (PCA) reactions. At the same time, the number of
larvae in the tongue were determined using the conventional
method [9].

IgM and IgG response to tetanus toxoid. At an age of 11
weeks, female rats were immunized intravenously with 5 Lf
tetanus toxoid plain (prepared in the Institute) with a ten-
day interval. Blood was drawn from the orbital plexus on
day 10 (prior to the booster injection) and day 21 after the
first immunization. Primary and secondary IgM and IgG titres
to tetanus toxoid were determined by ELISA [6].

**IgM and IgG response and delayed-type hypersensitivity to
ovalbumin.** As described elsewhere [10], the ovalbumin model
offers the advantage that both humoral and cellular immunity
can be studied simultaneously in the same animal. At an age
of five weeks, male rats were immunized in the hind footpads
with 100 µg ovalbumin (crystallized 5 times Serva Fein-
biochemika, Heidelberg, West Germany) dissolved in 0.05 ml
phosphate-buffered saline (PBS) and emulsified in 0.05 ml of
complete H37Ra adjuvant (Difco Laboratories, Detroit, USA).
Rats were challenged on day 18 after immunization by an
intracutaneous injection of 5 µg ovalbumin in 20 µl PBS in
the central pinna of the right ear. The left ear was injected with 20 µl PBS. Skin reactions were measured 24, 48
and 72 hours after challenge using a semi-electronic device
[11]. Delayed-type reactions were expressed as the difference in reaction between the challenged and control ear. IgM
and IgG titres were determined by ELISA in sera obtained at
day 14 and 21 after immunization.

Cytotoxicity assay. The natural cytotoxic activity of spleen
cells against tumour cells was measured in a ^{51}Cr-release
test with murine YAC lymphoma target tumour cells. Details
of the *in vitro* assay are given elsewhere [12]. Results of
this experiment, in which a total spleen population of eight-
week-old male animals was studied, were calculated as the
percentage specific release (experimental release minus
spontaneous release).

Microsomal enzyme assay. Liver tissue of five-week-old and
seven-month-old female rats was minced in ice-cold KCl (11.5
g/l) at a ratio of 1 g tissue to 4 ml and homogenized in a
Potter-Elvejhem homogenizer. The 15,000 g supernatant was
centrifuged by 105,000 g for 1 h. The pellet was re-
suspended in 0.1 M phosphate buffer pH 7.4 and stored at
-90 C. Protein was measured by the method of Lowry *et al.*
[13]. Aminopyrine demethylase activity was determined by

measuring the formation of formaldehyde by combining the
methods of Gram *et al*. [14] and Cochin and Axelrod [15].
Aniline hydroxylase activity was determined by measuring the
formation of p-aminophenol according to Gilbert and Goldberg
[16]. Ethoxyresorufin-0-deethylase activity was determined
by the fluorimetric assay of Burke and Mayer [17].

Statistical analysis. Differences in group means were estimated by the Student-t test (two-sided). In case of insufficient homogeneity of variances, the Welch correction with
respect to the degrees of freedom was applied.

RESULTS

Offspring mortality. HCB exposure of female rats during
pregnancy did not affect the number of litters whelped per
number of pregnant females. However, suckling pups appeared
particularly sensitive as mortality occurred in the 100 mg/kg
group during the lactation period but not after weaning. The
day 5 mortality was 7, 7, 6 and 37% in offspring of dams fed
0, 4, 20 and 100 mg HCB/kg, respectively; the day 21 mortality
in these groups was 15, 15, 8 and 67% respectively. Because
of the high mortality in the 100 mg/kg group, some experiments were only carried out with animals from the 0, 4 and
20 mg/kg groups.

Body and organ weights. As shown in Table 1, the body weight
of five-week-old female rats following combined pre- and
post-natal HCB exposure was unaltered. But, a significantly
increased body weight was recorded in the seven-month-old
animals of the 100 mg/kg group. In both age groups, the
relative liver weight was significantly increased in the 20
and 100 mg/kg groups. In these same dose groups, the relative
weight of the popliteal lymph node of the three-week-old
animals was also significantly higher. In the seven-month-
old rats, marked increases were also recorded for the relative weight of spleen, mesenteric and popliteal lymph nodes
in the 100 mg/kg group. Finally, the relative lung weight
was significantly higher in the 20 and 100 mg/kg groups.

Haematology, serum IgM and IgG levels. Changes in the concentration of white blood cells in the 100 mg/kg group were
confined to the number of basophils: an increase from zero
in the control group to $25 \times 10^6/1$ in the high dose group
(P < 0.01). At the same dose level, the serum IgM level was
also significantly increased (P < 0.01). When expressed
as percentage value in the pooled control serum, the value
rose from 102 ± 33 to 160 ± 28. IgG levels did not differ
significantly from the control value.

Table 1 Body and organ weights of female rats following combined pre- and post-natal HCB exposure.

	Dietary concentration (mg/kg)			
	0	4	20	100
5-week-old				
Body (g)	75 ± 12	78 ± 8	81 ± 9	73 ± 3
Liver (g)	3.19 ± 0.48	3.44 ± 0.39	3.64 ± 0.40[b]	3.88 ± 0.23[c]
Thymus (mg)	396 ± 72	435 ± 64	425 ± 77	336 ± 39
Spleen (mg)	242 ± 34	239 ± 22	267 ± 43	261 ± 24
Mesenteric lymph node (mg)	49 ± 14	60 ± 18	57 ± 17	51 ± 12
Popliteal lymph node (mg)	2.6 ± 1.5	3.9 ± 1.4	4.3 ± 1.3[b]	4.3 ± 1.4[b]
Lung (mg)	526 ± 55	544 ± 26	577 ± 67	557 ± 21
Adrenals (mg)	22 ± 4	23 ± 4	23 ± 3	25 ± 5
7-month-old				
Body (g)	213 ± 15	220 ± 11	223 ± 13	241 ± 13[c]
Liver (g)	5.61 ± 1.12	6.12 ± 0.50	6.55 ± 0.32[b]	8.00 ± 0.96[c]
Spleen (mg)	373 ± 47	389 ± 55	383 ± 61	526 ± 44[d]
Mesenteric lymph node (mg)	74 ± 22	87 ± 14	75 ± 13	111 ± 28[b]
Popliteal lymph node (mg)	6 ± 2	5.2 ± 1.4	7.4 ± 3.4	12.8 ± 3.9[c]
Lung (mg)	1045 ± 77	1105 ± 77	1145 ± 56[c]	1297 ± 57[d]

Mean values ± SD of 10 female animals per group are given, except for animals used in the 100 mg/kg group of 5-week-old animals, and 8 and 6 animals in the 0 and 100 mg/kg group of 7-month-old rats.

[b] $P < 0.05$ [c] $P < 0.01$ [d] $P < 0.001$

Table 2 *Incidence of histopathological changes in female rats following combined pre- and post-natal HCB exposure.*

Dietary concentration (mg/kg)	5-week-old*				7-month-old			
	0	4	20	100	0	4	20	100
Liver examined	10	10	10	6	8	10	10	6
centrilobular cell hypertrophy				2				3
cytoplasmic hyalinization hepatocytes								2
single cell necrosis								2
nuclear enlargement								1
inflammatory infiltrate								1
Spleen examined	10	10	10	6	8	10	10	6
increased extramedullary haemopoiesis	3	3	3	5	1	1	2	1
enlarged white pulp								2
Mesenteric lymph node examined†	10	10	10	6	8	10	10	6
proliferation high-endothelial venules			7	4	2	1	4	5
Popliteal lymph node examined†	8	8	9	5	8	10	10	6
proliferation high-endothelial venules	1		5	3	2	3	4	5
Peyer's patches examined†	3	7	7	5				
proliferation high-endothelial venules			3	4				
Lung examined†					8	10	10	6
slight accumulation alveolar macrophages					1	3	4	
strong accumulation alveolar macrophages						1	5	6
proliferation endothelium capillaries							3	6
proliferation endothelium venules								5
cholesterol crystals in alveoli								3

* No changes were observed in thymus and adrenals
† Slides read under code

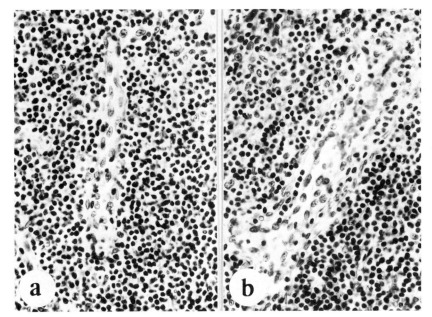

Fig. 1 Mesenteric lymph node of 5-week-old rat of control
(a) and 20 mg HCB/kg group showing proliferation of a high-
endothelial venule in the paracortex (b). Paraplast section,
H.E., x 300.

Histopathology. The results of the histopathological examination are summarized in Table 2. Liver lesions were confined
to the 100 mg/kg group, and were more severe in the older
animals. The most prominent alteration was centrilobular
cell hypertrophy. At the same dose level, increased extra-
medullary haemopoiesis was noted in the spleen of five-week-
old animals, while an enlarged white pulp occurred in low
incidence in seven-month-old rats. A consistent finding in
both age groups was proliferation of high endothelial venules
in mesenteric and popliteal lymph nodes (Fig. 1), which was
observed at high incidence in the 100 mg/kg group and with
lower incidence in the 20 mg/kg group. Proliferation of the
endothelium of the postcapillary venules was also observed
in the Peyer's patches at the same dose levels. Lung tissue
was examined only in the seven-month-old rats. A prominent
finding was a dose-related focal accumulation of macrophages
in the alveoli, which was observed in all HCB groups.
Localization in the 4 mg/kg group was peri-bronchially, and
extended to the periphery of the parenchyma in the higher
dose levels (Fig. 2a). Structural alterations were also
noticed in the blood vessels. The changes consisted of

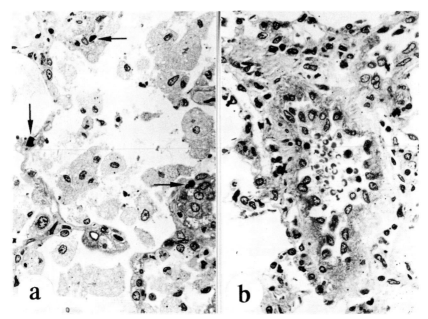

Fig. 2 Lung of 7-month-old rat of the 100 mg HCB/kg group
with intra-alveolar accumulation of macrophages and presence
of mast cells (arrows) in the inter-alveolar septa (a); and
hypertrophy of the lining endothelial cells of venule with
perivascular infiltrate of lymphocytes (b). Glycomethacryl-
ate section, Giemsa, x 300.

hypertrophy and proliferation of the lining of endothelial
cells of capillaries in the 20 and 100 mg/kg group and of
venules in the high dose group only (Fig. 2b and 3). At the
site of the endothelium, macrophage accumulation was observed.
In addition, an increase in mast cells and lymphocytes was
found in these areas (Fig. 2). Finally, intra-alveolar
cholesterol crystals were present in three of the 100 mg/kg
group.

Resistance to *Trichinella spiralis* infection. No significant
differences were found in the number of muscle larvae, nor in
serum IgM, IgG and IgE titres as determined six weeks after
infection, between the control and the 4 and 20 mg/kg groups
(the 100 mg/kg level was not included in this experiment).

IgM and IgG response to tetanus toxoid. As shown in Fig. 4,
both the primary and secondary IgM and IgG responses were
significantly increased in the 4 and 20 mg/kg groups (the
100 mg/kg level was not tested). The largest increase was

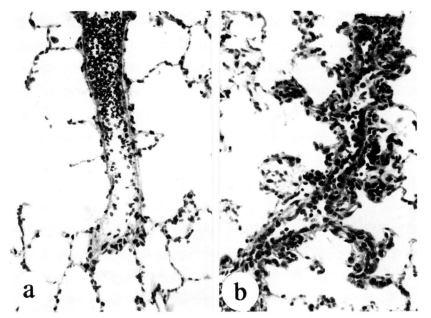

Fig. 3 Lung of 7-month-old rat of control (a) and 100 mg
HCB/kg group (b),   showing hypertrophy and proliferation of
the endothelium of capillaries and venule.   Paraplast section,
H.E., x 190.

found for the secondary IgG titre in the 20 mg/kg group
(approximately 16-fold higher than the titre in the control
group).

**IgM and IgG response and delayed-type hypersensitivity to
ovalbumin.**   In contrast to the marked enhanced antibody response to tetanus toxoid, no significant increase was found
in the day 14 and day 21 IgM and IgG titres against ovalbumin
in rats fed 4, 20 or 100 mg HCB/kg.   However, delayed-type
hypersensitivity reactions against ovalbumin were strongly
enhanced.   As presented in Fig. 5, the 24, 48 and 72 h reactions were significantly increased in the 100 mg/kg group.
The delayed-type reactions were also markedly increased in
the 100 mg/kg group.   The delayed-type reactions were also
markedly increased in the 4 and 20 mg/kg groups, although the
difference with the control group was only statistically
significant for the 48 h reaction in the 4 mg/kg group.

Cytotoxicity assay.   The cytotoxic activity of a total spleen
population of non-tumour bearing rats against murine YAC
lymphoma cells was the same for the 0, 4 and 20 mg/kg group

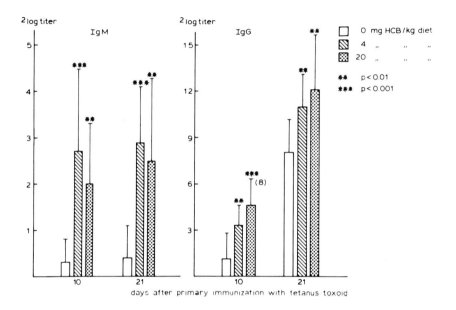

Fig. 4 Primary and secondary IgM and IgG response to tetanus
toxoid in HCB exposed rats immunized intravenously with
tetanus toxoid at an age of 11 weeks and 10 days later.
Values represent means ± SD of 10 rats per group.

(the 100 mg/kg group was not investigated). Effector to
target cell ratios assessed in this experiment were 100, 50
and 10.

Microsomal enzyme assays. Combined pre- and post-natal HCB
exposure to a dietary level of 100 mg/kg significantly
increased the concentration of liver protein, aniline hydroxylase activity and aminopyrine demethylase activity (Fig. 6).
A dose-related and statistically significant increase was
measured in the ERR-O-D activity of all HCB groups at an age
of five weeks as well as seven months. The activity in the
100 mg/kg group of the young animals was six-fold higher than
in the older animals exposed to the same dietary level.

DISCUSSION

Following combined pre- and post-natal HCB exposure, offspring
mortality in the 4 and 20 mg/kg groups was similar to the
control level, while the day 21 mortality in the 100 mg/kg
group was 67%, a value somewhat higher than reported for the

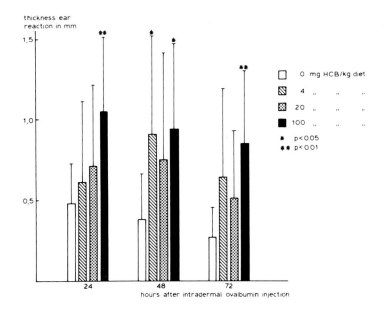

Fig. 5 Delayed-type hypersensitivity reaction in HBC-exposed rats. Animals were immunized at an age of 5 weeks with a mixture of ovalbumin and H37Ra adjuvant and challenged intradermally in the ear 18 days later. Skin reactions were determined 24, 48 and 72 h after challenge. Values represent means ± SD of 7-11 animals.

Sprague-Dawley rat [3,18]. These results confirm the sensitivity of the suckling pup, particularly as after weaning no deaths occurred despite continued dietary HCB exposure.

In the present study, no effect was found on the resistance to a *Trichinella spiralis* infection (yield of muscle larvae, and serum IgM, IgG and IgE titres) following exposure to dietary levels of 4 and 20 mg/kg. These results are in accordance with a previous study [4] in which no effect was found on the IgM and IgG response following combined pre- and post-natal exposure to 50 mg HCB/kg; only the IgG response was significantly increased in the 150 mg HCB/kg group. Also, in the present study no effect was found on the IgM and IgG response to ovalbumin in rats exposed to dietary HCB levels of 4, 20 and 100 mg/kg. In contrast, the primary and secondary IgM and IgG response to tetanus toxoid was significantly enhanced in the 4 and 20 mg HCB/kg group (the 100 mg/kg group was not investigated). These data confirm and extend previous results: enhanced response to tetanus toxoid in

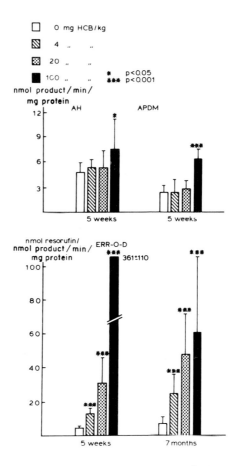

Fig. 6 Activity of aniline hydroxylase (AH), aminopyrine
demethylase (APDM) and ethoxyresorufin-O-deethylase (ERR-O-D)
in liver microsomes of HCB-exposed rats. Means ± SD of the
number of animals as indicated in Table 1.

HCB-exposed young-adult rats [1], and in rats following pre-
and post-natal exposure to dietary HCB levels of 50 and 100
mg/kg [4]. The discrepancy between the present results with
tetanus toxoid on the one hand and ovalbumin and *T. spiralis*
on the other are as yet unexplained; the antibody response
to all three antigens being dependent on the presence of
T-cells [19,20]. Perhaps, the different route of exposure
to these antigens plays an important part.

Delayed-type hypersensitivity to ovalbumin, as a parameter
of the cell-mediated immunity, was significantly increased,
even at the 4 mg HCB/kg level. In an earlier study in which
weaned rats were exposed to a relatively high dietary level

of 1,000 mg HCB/kg, no effect was found on this parameter [1].

The stimulating effect of HCB on immune responses correlates with the observed histological changes in spleen (enlarged white pulp), mesenteric and popliteal lymph nodes and Peyer's patches (proliferation of high-endothelial venules), and the increased serum IgM level. Proliferation of the high-endothelial venules was also observed in previous studies in the rat [1,4], and has been reported to occur following antigenic stimulation of lymph nodes [21]. Recent studies indicate that the high-endothelial venules play an important role in the selective binding and entry of B- and T-lymphocytes from the blood into lymph nodes and Peyer's patches [22]. Humoral factors can be important in the selective binding to high-endothelial venules, as described for a factor in thoracic duct lymph [23]. The effect of HCB on endothelial cells was not limited to lymphoid organs, as proliferation of the lining endothelial cells was observed in lung capillaries and venules. The changes in lung venules have been described earlier [18,24]. As the endothelial hypertrophy and proliferation in lung vessels was accompanied by a peri-vascular infiltrate of lymphocytes, it is tempting to speculate on the relationship with the proliferated high-endothelial venules in lymphoid organs. The altered pulmonary endothelial cells are possibly functionally similar to the high endothelial venules in lymph nodes, resulting in the entry of lymphocytes in the perivascular lung tissue. With respect to the proliferative changes of the endothelium it is of interest to mention the results of a carcinogenicity study in hamsters [25]. In this study dietary HCB exposure induced, besides hepatomas and thyroid adenomas, a relatively high incidence of haemangioendotheliomas in liver and spleen. Thus, the proliferation of the endothelium may also be an expression of an early stage of the development into endotheliomas.

Histologically, the most sensitive parameter in HCB-exposed rats was the intra-alveolar accumulation of macrophages. This effect was dose-related and occurred even at the 4 mg/kg level. Also in earlier studies, this effect was reported albeit at higher dose levels of HCB [4,24,26]. Also, increased peripheral monocyte counts have been recorded [1]. These data indicate that HCB in some way affects the mononuclear phagocyte system of the rat, although in function tests (clearance of intravenously injected colloidal carbon and *L. monocytogenes*) no effect was found [4]. On the other hand, there are experimental data showing that HCB inhibits the Fc receptor activity of alveolar macrophages from rat lung [27].

Besides the pulmonary endothelial changes, the large

increase in intra-alveolar macrophages and the peri-vascular
infiltrate of lymphocytes, and an increase in the number of
mast cells were also observed. These cells were located in the
inter-alveolar septa, often in the foci of pulmonary alteration. In this context, the increase in number of peripheral
basophilic granulocytes as found in the present and previous
studies [1,4] is of interest, as mast cells and basophils play
a prominent part in anaphylactic reactions in the lung [28].
Regarding the pulmonary changes, no interstitial fibrosis was
observed in the present study, as has been reported in
toxicity studies with HCB in the Sherman strain rat [26].
In the latter study, hyperplasia of the adrenal cortex also
occurred, which was not found in the present one with Wistar
rats, and may reflect strain differences.

Combined pre- and post-natal exposure to dietary HCB concentrations of 20 and 100 mg/kg, resulted in a significant
increase of the liver weight. Morphological alterations were
observed only in the high dose group, in particular in the
seven-month-old animals. The main effect was centrilobular
cell hypertrophy which correlates with a modest but statistically significant increased activity of the microsomal enzymes aniline hydroxylase and aminopyrine demethylase. Induction of the latter enzyme has been reported earlier [24].
A remarkable finding was the strong and dose-related increase
in the ethoxyresorufin O-deethylase activity in both five-
week-old and seven-month-old rats, even at the 4 mg/kg level.
The activity in the older animals exposed to 100 mg HCB/kg
was, however, less than in the five-week-old rats, which may
reflect liver damage in the seven-month-old rats, as observed
microscopically. Similar strong increases in the ethoxyresorufin O-deethylase activity have been reported for HCB in
rats [29] and PCB in cockerels [30]. Examination of cryostat
sections of liver of five-week-old rats under the fluorescence
microscope, did not reveal red fluorescence. This indicates
the absence of excessive quantities of hepatic porphyrins.
In comparison, dietary exposure of Charles River CD rats to
100 mg/kg for four months did produce hepatic porphyria which
could be detected macroscopically [24].

From the present study, it may be concluded that HCB stimulates the humoral and cell-mediated immunity in the rat,
which correlates with the effects observed on the lymphoid
organs. Hyperplasia of lymphoid itssue has also been described for HCB-exposed dogs [31]. However, marked species
differences exist in the immune effects of HCB, as this compound is reported to suppress (in mice) serum IgM, IgG and IgA
levels, to reduce antibody forming plaque cell response to
sheep red blood cells and to increase sensitivity to the
lethal effects of a *Plasmodium berghei* infection [32,33].

Reduced resistance to an infectious agent has also been described for invertebrates: clams (*Mercenaria mercenaria*)
exposed to HCB showed an impaired bacterial clearance (*Flavo-
bacterium* sp.) [34]. Species differences may also account
for the effect of HCB on the natural cytotoxic activity to
tumour cells: in mice, HCB exposure reduced the cytotoxic
activity of spleen cells, in particular the adherent fraction
[35], while in the present study no effect was found. Despite
the species differences in the effects of HCB it can be concluded that the compound HCB has immunotoxic properties, in
particular for the developing immune system. The explicit
toxicity for the immune system may be related to the relatively high exposure of lymphoid tissue, as absorption and
transport of orally administered HCB is mainly by lymph
towards the lymph nodes, with only minor involvement of the
portal venous system [36]. The transport of HCB by lymph
will result in relatively high HCB concentrations in the
pulmonary circulation, which may explain the occurrence of
vascular changes in the lung.

ACKNOWLEDGEMENTS

The authors gratefully acknowledge Dr P.A. Greve for the HCB
analyses of the diets, Dr W.H. de Jong for help with the
cytotoxicity assay, and Mr P. Beekhof, Mr K. de Jong, Mr W.
Kruizinga, Mr J. van Sooligen and Mr H. Strootman for excellent technical assistance.

SUMMARY

The effect of hexachlorobenzene (HCB) on the immune system,
liver and lung was studied after combined pre- and post-natal
exposure. Pregnant rats received diets containing 0, 4, 20
and 100 mg HCB/kg. Dosing was continued during lactation and
after weaning. No effect was found on the resistance to a
T. spiralis infection (yield of muscle larvae, and IgM, IgG
and IgE response) on the IgM and IgG response to ovalbumin,
nor on the natural cytotoxic activity of spleen cells against
murine YAC lymphoma cells. In contrast, the primary and
secondary IgM and IgG response to tetanus toxoid, as well as
the delayed-type hypersensitivity to ovalbumin was significantly increased, even at the 4 mg/kg level. Histologically,
proliferation of high-endothelial venules in the paracortex
of mesenteric and popliteal lymph nodes was observed in the
20 and 100 mg/kg groups. In the same dose groups, proliferation of the endothelium of lung vessels and increased numbers
of lymphocytes and mast cells was noted, while intra-
alveolar macrophage accumulation occurred in a dose-related
manner in all three test groups. Morphological changes in

the liver and increased activities of the microsomal enzymes, aniline hydroxylase and aminopyrine demethylase, were observed only in the 100 mg/kg group. However, in all three test groups, a dose-related and significant increase was found in the activity of ethoxyresorufin-O-deethylase. From the results it is concluded that combined pre- and post-natal exposure of rats to a dietary HCB level as low as 4 mg/kg enhanced the humoral and the cell-mediated immunity and caused intra-alveolar macrophage accumulation, while conventional parameters for hepatotoxicity were unaltered. Thus, the developing immune system of the rat seems very sensitive to HCB exposure. Finally, the possible immunopathological relationship between the lung vessel changes and the proliferation of high-endothelial venules in lymph nodes was discussed.

REFERENCES

1. Vos, J.G., van Logten, M.J., Kreeftenberg, J.G. and Kruizinga, W. (1979). *Ann. N.Y. Acad. Sci.* **320**, 535-550.
2. Villeneuve, D.C. and Hierlihy, S.L. (1975). *Bull. Environ. Contam. Toxicol.* **13**, 489-491.
3. Grant, D.L., Phillips, W.E. and Hatina, G.V. (1977). *Arch. Environ. Contam. Toxicol.* **5**, 207-216.
4. Vos, J.G., van Logten, M.J., Kreeftenberg, J.G., Steerenberg, P.A. and Kruizinga, W. (1979). *Drug Chem. Toxicol.* **2**, 61-76.
5. Moolenbeek, C. and Ruitenberg, E.J. (1981). *Lab. Animals* **15**, 57-59.
6. Vos, J.G., Buys, J., Beekhof, P. and Hagenaars, A.M. (1979). *Ann. N.Y. Acad. Sci.* **320**, 518-534.
7. Vos, J.G., Krajnc, E.I. and Beekhof, P. (1982). *Environ. Health Perspect.* **43**, 115-121.
8. Ruitenberg, E.J., Steerenberg, P.A. and Brosi, B.J.M. (1975). *Medikon Nederland* **4**, 30-31.
9. Köhler, G. and Ruitenberg, E.J. (1974). *Bull. Wld. Hlth. Org.* **50**, 413-419.
10. Vos, J.G., Boerkamp, J., Buys, J. and Steerenberg, P.A. (1980). *Scand. J. Immunol.* **12**, 289-296.
11. van Dijk, H., Versteeg, H. and Hennink, H.J. (1976). *J. Immunol. Methods* **12**, 261-265.
12. de Jong, W.H., Steerenberg, P.A., Ursem, P.S., Osterhaus, A.D.M.E., Vos, J.G. and Ruitenberg, E.J. (1980). *Clin. Immunol. Immunopathol.* **17**, 163-172.
13. Lowry, O.H., Rosebrough, A.L., Farr, A.L. and Randall, R.J. (1951). *J. Biol. Chem.* **193**, 265-275.
14. Gram, T.E., Wilson, J.T. and Fouts, J.R. (1968). *J. Pharm. Exp. Ther.* **159**, 172-181.

15. Cochin, J. and Axelrod, J. (1959). *J. Pharm. Exp. Ther.* **125**, 105-110.
16. Gilbert, D. and Goldberg, L. (1965). *Food Cosmet. Toxicol.* **3**, 417-432.
17. Burke, M.D. and Mayer, R.T. (1974). *Drug Metab. Dispos.* **2**, 583-588.
18. Kitchin, K.T., Linder, R.E., Scotti, T.M., Walsh, D., Durley, A.D. and Svendsgaard, D. (1982). *Toxicology* **23**, 33-39.
19. Ruitenberg, E.J., Elgersma, A., Kruizinga, W. and Leenstra, F. (1977). *Immunology* **33**, 581-587.
20. Vos, J.G., Kreeftenberg, J.G., Kruijt, B.C., Kruizinga, W. and Steerenberg, P.A. (1980). *Clin. Immunol. Immunopathol.* **15**, 229-237.
21. Anderson, N.D., Anderson, O.A. and Wyllie, R.G. (1975). *Am. J. Pathol.* **81**, 235-245.
22. Stevens, S.K., Weissman, I.L. and Butcher, E.C. (1982). *J. Immunol.* **128**, 844-851.
23. Carey, G.D., Chin, Y.H. and Woodruff, J.J. (1981). *J. Immunol.* **127**, 976-979.
24. Goldstein, J.A., Friesen, M., Scotti, T.M., Hickman, P., Haas, J.R. and Bergman, H. (1978). *Toxicol. Appl. Pharmacol.* **46**, 633-649.
25. Cabral, J.R.P., Shubik, P., Mollner, T. and Raitano, F. (1977). *Nature* **269**, 510-511.
26. Kimbrough, R.D. and Linder, R.E. (1974). *Res. Comm. Chem. Path. Pathol.* **8**, 653-664.
27. Ziprin, R.L. and Fowler, Z.F. (1977). *Toxicol. Appl. Pharmacol.* **39**, 105-109.
28. Newball, H.H. and Lichtenstein, L.M. (1981). *Thorax* **36**, 721-725.
29. Debets, F.M.H., Strik, J.J.T.W.A. and Olie, K. (1980). *Toxicology* **15**, 181-195.
30. Hansen, L.G., Strik, J.J.T.W.A., Koeman, J.H. and Kan, C.A. (1981). *Toxicology* **21**, 203-212.
31. Gralla, E.J., Fleischman, R.W., Luthra, Y.K., Hagopian, M., Baker, J.R., Esber, H. and Marcus, W. (1977). *Toxicol. Appl. Pharmacol.* **40**, 227-239.
32. Loose, L.D., Pittman, K.A., Benitz, K.F. and Silkworth, J.B. (1977). *J. Reticuloendoth. Soc.* **22**, 253-271.
33. Loose, L.D., Silkworth, J.B., Pittman, K.A., Benitz, K.F. and Mueller, W. (1978). *Infection and Immunity* **20**, 30-35.
34. Anderson, R.S., Giam, C.S., Ray, L.E. and Tripp, M.R. (1981). *Aquatic Toxicology* **1**, 187-195.
35. Loose, L.D., Silkworth, J.B., Charbonneau, T. and Blumenstock, F. (1981). *Environm. Health Perspect.* **39**, 79-91.
36. Iatropoulos, M.J., Milling, A. Müller, W.F., Nohynek, G., Rozman, K., Coulston, F. and Korte, F. (1975). *Environ. Res.* **10**, 384-389.

EVALUATING IMMUNOPATHOLOGICAL EFFECTS
OF NEW DRUGS

E.D. Wachsmuth

*Research Department, Pharmaceuticals Division,
CIBA-GEIGY Ltd., 4002 Basel, Switzerland*

Some drugs have been specifically designed to affect the
immune apparatus and alter immunological reactivity, e.g.,
immunosuppressants administered to inhibit the rejection of
tissue transplants, or immunostimulants used as vaccines
against infection. Other drugs, however, intended for completely different therapeutic applications, have also been
found to cause disorders of the immune response, e.g.,
corticosteroids. Thus the risk of adverse immunological
effects has to be weighed against the benefit expected from
a new drug. In this context, toxicological investigations in
animals are performed to determine undesirable effects of a
compound *in vivo* on different organs and cells, and also on
the lymphatic system, the main component of the immune
apparatus, and thereby to eventually provide the basis for a
risk benefit analysis. Toxicity tests must therefore afford
a qualitative assessment of the effects of a new drug in different species and quantify its toxic or undesirable effects.
The emphasis must be placed upon predicting their possible
occurrence in man and then, in subsequent studies, upon
furthering our understanding of the mechanisms leading to undesirable effects. The initial test systems should consequently be simple, non-selective and reproducible. More
selective tests may be applied later if, in the first instance
some adverse effects have been observed, or if the particular
drug investigated belongs to a group of compounds known to
cause undesirable immunological effects.

Like routine toxicology tests, tests for immunotoxicity may
be hampered, e.g., by species differences in responsiveness;
a compound may cause cumulative effects; the animals may
adapt to the toxic dose, or even develop tolerance. Moreover,
maturing animals may respond differently from adult or old

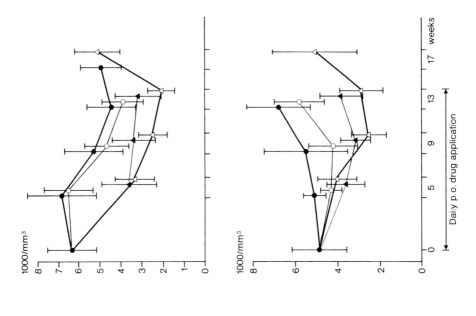

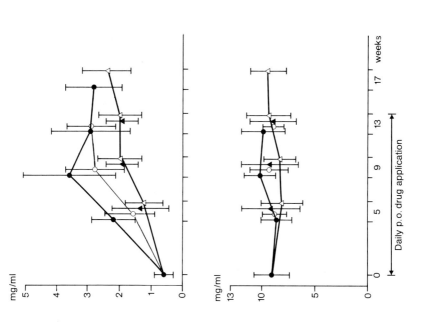

Fig. 1 See legend opposite

animals [1]. The present paper is concerned with how much we
may learn about undesirable immunological effects from the
results of standard toxicity tests of drugs known to affect
the immune system, and whether supplementary investigations
are helpful in recognizing the problem. Some results of our
own previous studies will be discussed in an attempt to
answer these questions.*

TOXICOLOGICAL APPROACH TO THE ASSESSMENT OF IMMUNOSUPPRESSION

The effect of an experimental corticosteroid was investigated
in a 3 month toxicity test in dogs and rats. A dose dependent and reversible effect on blood lymphocytes and γ-globulin
(mostly immunoglobulin) was found in both species (Fig. 1).
The effect on γ-globulin levels was statistically non-
significant in dogs. To obtain significant data, the absolute
counts of lymphocytes and the concentration of γ-globulin
(from total serum protein and the electrophoresis pattern)
have to be calculated. Thymus weights in both species and
spleen weights in rats, but not dogs, decreased parallel to
the findings in blood. It should be noted that the globulin
levels in rats increased during the test period, owing to the
maturation of the initially 6-week-old animals. This decrease
in γ-globulin level and lymphocyte count was obviously biologically relevant, i.e., a sign of immunosuppression, as was
apparent at autopsy of the dogs in the group treated with the
highest dose. Histopathology one month after three months
administration revealed an extensive inflammatory reaction to
parasites in the lung, whereas in the dogs killed immediately
after the administration period, no signs of inflammation
were visible.

Legend to Fig. 1 Rats (top) and dogs (bottom) received oral
doses of 0 μg/kg (●), 10 μg/kg (O), 30 μg/kg (▲) and 100
μg/kg (Δ) of an experimental cortisocteroid once daily for
3 months. Serum γ-globulin concentration (left), blood
lymphocyte counts (right), 1 month recovery group (R).

---

* Experimental drugs: the corticosteroid clobetasolpro-
prionate; the immunostimulators N-acetyl-muramyl-L-alanyl-
-D-iso-glutamine (MDP) and N-acetyl-nor-muramyl-L-alanyl-D-
-iso-glutamine (nor-MDP); the beta-blocker 4-(3-tert-butyl-
amino-2-hydroxypropoxy)-benzimidazole-2-one hydrochloride.

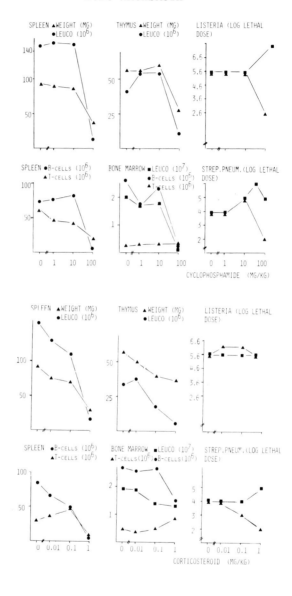

Fig. 2 Dose responses to cyclophosphamide (top) and an experimental corticosteroid (bottom) in mice (female BALB/c x MIW) injected once daily s.c. for 5 days. Morphological analyses were made on day 6 (left and middle) and lethal doses calculated from the surviving mice 10 days after administration of live bacteria (right) to determine inherent resistance (Schedule 1, ▲) and resistance after pretreatment with killed bacteria (Schedule 2, ■).

When the same corticosteroid was administered once-daily to
rats for five days only, the same dose-dependent reductions
in thymus and spleen weights and blood lymphocyte counts were
demonstrable, but the immunoglobulin levels were not affected.
Under these circumstances, there was a clear correlation
between the organ weights and the lymphocyte content of the
organs (correlation coefficients for leucocyte counts with
thymus and spleen weights were r = 0.98 and r = 0.95 respectively). Thus lymphatic organ weights in the rat are a
readily available index of effects on the leucocyte counts
[2].

After daily s.c. injection of the corticosteroid for five
days into mice the results were similar to those found in
rats (Fig. 2). However, whereas the leucocyte counts correlated well with spleen weights, the correlation with the
thymus weights was poor (Table 1). The pattern of correlation
for spleen and thymus after treatment with the corticosteroid
was similar to those obtained with the immunosuppressant
cyclophosphamide and the two presumptive immunostimulating
agents levamisol and nor-MDP (Table 1). Owing to the difficulty of preparing the thymus, the variation in thymus weights
is large and thus more mice have to be used than rats to
arrive at statistically meaningful analyses.

The effect of the two immunosuppressants, cyclophosphamide
and the corticosteroid, and the two presumptive immunostimulants, levamisol and nor-MDP, was further investigated
after daily s.c. injection for five days into mice. The
shape of the dose response curves was specific for each test
compound and alike for one compound with respect to leucocyte
counts in blood and bone marrow, the weights and leucocyte
counts of thymus and spleen, and B-cell counts in spleen and
bone marrow. They decreased in response to increasing doses
of the immunosuppressant agents (Fig. 2) and increased in
response to the immunostimulants. The T-cell counts were
affected less and at higher doses than the B-cell counts, and
the bone marrow was less affected by the corticosteroid than
by cyclophosphamide. Moreover, the counts of granulocyte and
monocyte progenitor cells in the bone marrow (CFU-C) were
decreased more after cyclophosphamide than after corticosteroid treatment.

The weights of secondary tissues of the immune apparatus,
i.e., popliteal and axillary lymph nodes, have proved to be
valuable indices in rats and dogs. Additional information is
obtained by histological analysis of lymphatic tissue. Such
analyses are hardly quantitative and as a rule only extensive
changes become apparent. They can be improved if semi-thin
sections are cut in a standardized plane, preferably trans-
versely through the hilus of lymph nodes and spleen (the

Table 1 *Correlation of organ weights of mice with leucocyte counts in the respective organ. About 10 mice (BALB/c x MIW) per dose-group (4 doses) received s.c. injections daily for 5 days, and organs were analysed on day 6.*

Compound	No.	Thymus Correlation coefficient	Level of significance	No.	Spleen Correlation coefficient	Level of significance
Cyclophosphamide (0, 1–100 mg/kg)	39	0.555	0.0001	39	0.894	0.0001
Corticosteroid (0, 0.01–1 mg/kg)	38	0.575	0.0002	38	0.912	0.0001
Levamisol (0, 0.3–30 mg/kg)	37	0.445	0.0058	38	0.753	0.0001
nor-MDP (0, 1–1000 mg/kg)	36	0.232	0.174	38	0.869	0.0001

spleen of dogs is most difficult to assess with respect to immunocompetent cells) and longitudinally through the thymus [2].

   Although quantitative assessments can be made of dose responses in the lymphatic system, whether such assessments reflect the function of the immune apparatus remains an open question.

RELATION BETWEEN MORPHOLOGICAL FEATURES AND RESISTANCE TO INFECTION

A large number of tests for investigating the function of the immune apparatus have been suggested [3,4]. As its prime function is to defend the body against invasion by foreign matter, including parasites, bacteria, and viruses, the most relevant test is the evaluation of resistance to infection [5,6]. We accordingly administer test compounds once daily s.c. for five days to mice, then infect the mice and determine the lethality. Different doses of bacteria are injected i.p. either after five days' administration of the compound (Schedule 1, Fig. 2) or fifteen days after i.p. injection of 10 heat killed bacteria on day 2 (Schedule 2, Fig. 2). The inherent or natural resistance against infection is tested in Schedule 1, and the potential capacity of the test compound to change resistance after exposure to an immunogen in Schedule 2.

   Cyclophosphamide decreased inherent resistance to infection by *Listeria monocytogenes* and *Streptococcus pneumonia*, whereas the corticosteroid decreased only resistance to the latter (Fig. 2). The shapes of the dose response curves for diminished resistance were very similar to those for changes in morphological features. Low counts of leucocytes and CFU-C in bone marrow and B-cells and T-cells after high doses of cyclophosphamide are therefore consistent with the decreased resistance to both bacteria. Altered resistance to infection with *Listeria* after administration of the corticosteroid is consistent with decreased B-cell counts. Unchanged resistance to infection with *Streptococcus* is consistent with the relatively slight effect on leucocyte and CFU-C counts in the bone marrow, and thus possibly due to remaining functional competence of macrophages, even when T-cell counts are reduced. Whether these changes are attributable to reduced numbers of competent cells for inherent resistance, or to reduction of suppressor cell activity or to altered antigen processing of macrophages for resistance after exposure to immunogen, or whatever else the reason may be, the effect of the two immunosuppressive agents on the resistance to infection appears to be predictable from the morphological features of the lymphatic system. No effect of the two immunostimulants could be

established, i.e. the increase in B-cells was not reflected
in increased resistance to either of the two bacteria.

   These data indicate an approach to the assessment of immunotoxicity, by determining first the dose-dependency of an
effect on the lymphatic system by reference to morphological
features (for which purpose only a very small number of animals
is needed, e.g., 3 to 5 mice or rats per dose group), possibly
followed by a test for resistance to infection (using one
tolerated high dose of the test compound and say, four different bacterial inocula in groups of 5 to 10 mice or rats
each). The relevance of the infectious agent to immunotoxicity
still has to be further evaluated.

TOXICOLOGICAL APPROACH TO THE ASSESSMENT OF IMMUNOSTIMULATION

Therapeutic immunostimulation with vaccines is a well known
and well established practice. Only recently, drugs have
been developed that may prove to be useful immunostimulants,
e.g., levamisol and muramyl peptides [7].

   A 3-month toxicity study in which up to 1000 mg/kg of nor-
MDP was given daily by s.c. injection was performed in BALB/c
mice. To test for a potential autoimmune disease induction,
groups of mice were kept for a further three months without
dosing [8]. No pathological changes were apparent in the
mice. In dogs given i.v. or s.c. injections of MDP, however,
acute-phase proteins in plasma (e.g., fibrinogen, complement-
C3, α3-globulin) increased, as also did alkaline phosphatase
in the liver (demonstrated by histochemistry and tissue
homogenate analyses), indicating drug-induced changes in
liver metabolism. Moreover, the number of monocyte-
granulocyte precursor cells in the bone marrow increased,
leading to an increase in the counts of monocytes and granulocytes in the blood as well as in spleen and liver (Table 2).
Monocytes also became more numerous in secondary lymph nodes
as seen in sinus catarrh and lymph adenitis. These lymph
node monocytes possessed increased numbers of lysosomes (with
immuno-reactive complement-C3 and fibrinogen deposits, but no
immunoglobulin and reduced acid phosphatase activity). They
were homogeneously dense in the electron microscope. So far,
these phenomena resemble a pattern of events to be expected
after administration of a strong adjuvant. However, in
addition to this inflammation, we observed activation of the
mesothelial cells of the epicardium and pericardium, leading
to percarditis and consequently to myocarditis, as well as to
activation of the mesothelial cells of the peritoneum and of
the synovial lining cells in knee joints. The latter effects
are certainly not desirable. As they are dose dependent, the
question arises whether they can be dissociated from the
desired effects by suitable adjustment of the dosage, or

Table 2 *Effect of MDP on the monocytic cell line in dogs (i.v. administration for 10 days).*

Monocytic cells	Control		MDP (5 mg/kg) daily	
	Male	Female	Male	Female
Progenitor cells (10^3/femur)	33 ± 6	9.3 ± 1.6	293 ± 43	285 ± 28
Blood (10^9/1)	0.20	0.25	1.34	0.65
Liver *	5.2 ± 1.0	6.8 ± 1.0	16.1 ± 1.6	21.1 ± 1.0
Spleen *	11.0 ± 1.1	15.5 ± 1.0	15.0 ± 1.0	12.5 ± 1.5
Renal cortex and outer medulla *	0.25 ± 0.01	0.27 ± 0.03	1.04 ± 0.14	1.54 ± 0.36

* Per cent tissue area with endogenous peroxidase-positive cells in 6 μm frozen tissue sections measured by television analysis (TAS-Leitz).

choice of the route of administration, or both. Thus, results of standard toxicity studies complemented by enzyme-histochemical and immunochemical investigations may serve as a basis for a benefit/risk assessment.

HYPERSENSITIVITY REACTIONS IN TOXICITY STUDIES

Special tests for hypersensitivity reactions have been discussed by others at this symposium [9]. The question arises whether such effects of experimental drugs can also be detected in standard toxicity tests. Since any compound may, in principle, act as an immunogen, which could cause hypersensitivity reactions, though the likelihood of such an occurrence (depending on many different factors) is relatively small, and is thus difficult to predict. Hypersensitivity reactions may manifest themselves in anaemia, thrombocytopenia, vasculitis and immune complex deposition. Further evidence of hypersensitivity may be obtained during the course of the toxicity study, e.g., immunoglobulin and complement-C3 levels; occurrence of positive Coomb's tests on red cells and platelets demonstrable with anti-immunoglobulin or anti-complement-C3 or both; occurrence of positive indirect Coomb's tests; presence of circulating immune complexes in plasma and serum; deposition of immune complexes in the kidney. Anaemia and a fall in complement-C3 levels within hours of

administration are pointers towards the diagnosis of allergic
disease. Further evidence may be obtained by means of
special enzyme-histochemical and immunofluorescence techniques.

After administration of an antibiotic to dogs for 3 months,
immune complexes were demonstrated by means of immunofluorescence in some dogs, concomitantly with raised immunoglobulin and complement-C3 levels and immune complexes on red
cells. In frozen spleen sections stained for alkaline phosphatase and peroxidase, the reticular network was seen to be
highly activated, and the monocyte counts increased (Figs. 3
and 4). Moreover, macrophage and Kupffer-cell counts as well
as counts of bile-duct cross-sections were also increased.
Both immuno-chemical analyses and special histochemistry indicated an immune-complex disease in some dogs, the severity of
which increased with increasing doses. The two technical
approaches were complementary (Table 3). Such findings,
however, do not help to distinguish between allergic reactions
to the test compound itself and reactions to other substances
formed as a result of the pharmacological action of the test
compound, e.g., microbial products. Awareness of the dose-

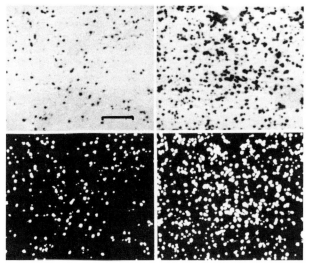

Fig. 3 Morphometry of frozen dog-liver sections by television
analysis. Sections were stained for endogenous-peroxidase
activity in monocytes. Video image in transmitted light (top)
and its digitated television image (bottom). Analysis was
performed with a TAS-Leitz. Control dog (left, stained area
3.2% of total area, 203 counts/mm^2) treated with 5 mg/kg/d MDP
for 10 days (right, stained area 12.2%, 445 counts/mm^2).
Bar: 200 μm.

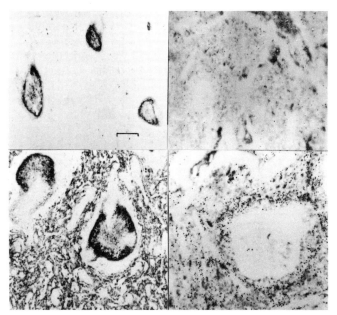

Fig. 4 Frozen spleen sections from 2 dogs, stained for
alkaline phosphatase (left) and endogenous peroxidase (right).
Control (top), after 3 months of administration of an antibiotic causing immune-haemolytic anaemia (bottom). Size of
follicles and contents of enzymic reaction product in the
reticular network (left) and counts of monocytes (right) are
increased in the treated dog. Bar: 200 μm.

and time-dependency of allergic phenomena will be helpful in
the further development of the compound.

AUTOIMMUNE DISEASE

Compounds potentially capable of provoking immunosuppression
or immunostimulation, or even allergy, can be used under
controllable conditions. However, if a generalized autoimmune
disease is caused by a test compound this may not be the case.
Induction of autoimmune disease may occur also in animals as
exemplified in a three month toxicity study in dogs with an
experimental beta-blocker (Table 4). Such occurrences in a
toxicity study preclude the further development in view of
the severe irreversible side-effects in man following treatment with another beta-blocker, practolol [10]. The practolol syndrome resembles an autoimmune disease, though its
mechanism in man is not understood and unfortunately has not
been observed in animals. Moreover, as very little is known

Table 3 *Effect of an experimental antibiotic on dogs in a 3-month toxicity study.*

Dose (mg/kg)	Immunological assays (serum, erythrocytes)		Histochemical assays (kidney, spleen, liver)	
	positive dogs	score	positive dogs	score
0	0/6	0	0/6	0
20	2/6	0.4	3/6	1.5
60	3/6	0.6	3/6	0.6
200	3/6	2.0	6/6	3.1
200R	4/6	1.4	4/6	2.9

R = 4 weeks recovery, score maximum = 10.

about induction of autoimmune diseases (whether due to poly-clonal activation, loss of T-cell suppression, production of non-specific helper factors, or cross-reacting antigens), it cannot reasonably be assumed that the potential risk may be diminished by lowering the dose. Once triggered off, the disease may progress indefinitely.

A lupus erythematosus-like disease may be induced in man e.g., by procainamide or hydralazine, but it is reversible if administration is discontinued [11,12]. We have not been able to induce such a syndrome with hydralazine in rats, dogs or even baboons [2]. However, judging from findings made in a study with procainamide in dogs, it appears that a pre-requisite for the induction of such a syndrome may be long-term administration to dogs older than four years of age [13]. Failing sufficient experience of toxicity studies in old animals, it is not yet possible to estimate the useful-ness of testing drugs for induction of autoimmune diseases under such conditions.

CONCLUSIONS

The few examples cited illustrate that indications of immuno-toxic effects of test compounds can be obtained by intelligent analysis of data from standard toxicity tests. If the data are supplemented by more refined immunochemical plasma or serum analyses, by enzyme- and immuno-histochemistry, they appear to provide sufficient information for the diagnosis of the immunopathology caused by drugs. Thereby, the potential capacity of a test compound to provoke immunosuppression, immunostimulation, allergy or autoimmune disease may be determined, with a view to making benefit/risk assessment.

Table 4 *Summary of immunopathological findings in dogs after 3 months' daily p.o. administration of an experimental beta-blocker.*

	After 3 months' administration	1 month after 3 months' administration
Serum analysis		
Anti-nuclear antibody	2/4	2/5
Anti-lacrimal-gland antibody	1/4	4/5
Increase in immunoglobulin-G	4/4	5/5
" in complement-C3	1/4	2/5
Tissue analysis		
Lymphatic nodules in lacrimal gland (negative for immuno-globulin)	4/4	3/5
Immune complexes (demonstrated with anti-IgG and anti-C3)		
in parotid gland	4/4	5/5
in lacrimal gland	4/4	2/5
in renal glomeruli	2/4	2/5
Increase in the degree of capillarization		
pancreas	1/4	2/5
submandibular gland	3/4	5/5
parotid gland	3/4	4/5

* Frequency of occurrence is given for dogs in the highest dose group. Note that the increased degree of capillarization may be due to an inflammatory response.

However, as knowledge of the relationship between the morphology and function of the immune system is still limited, in particular with respect to toxicology, an open minded and critical approach to the evaluation of immunotoxicity is needed.

ACKNOWLEDGEMENT

The author would like to thank Drs Anne Schild and O. Zak for their help in performing the experiments shown in Fig. 2.

REFERENCES

1. Davies, G.E. (1982). In "NATO Advanced Study Institute on Immunotoxicology", Nova Scotia, Canada (in press).
2. Wachsmuth, E.D. (1982). In "Advances in Pharmacology and Therapeutics II" (Eds. H. Yoshida, Y. Hagihara, S. Ebashi), Vol.5, pp.7-16. Pergamon Press, Oxford and New York.
3. Vos, J.G. (1977). *Critical Rev. Toxicol.* **5**, 67-101.
4. Dean, J.H., Padarathsingh, M.L. and Jerrels, T.R. (1979). *Drug Chem. Toxicol.* **2**, 5-17.
5. Bradley, S.G. and Morahan, P.S. (1982). *Environmental Health Perspectives* **43**, 61-69.
6. Dean, J.H., Luster, M.I., Boorman, G.A., Leubke, R.W. and Lauer, L.D. (1982). *Environmental Health Perspectives* **43**, 81-88.
7. Dukor, P., Tarcsay, L. and Baschang, G. (1979). *Ann. Reports in Med. Chemistry* **14**, 146-167.
8. Wachsmuth, E.D. and Dukor, P. (1982). In "Immunomodulation by Microbial Products and Related Compounds" (Eds. Y. Yamamura, S. Kotani, I. Azuma, A. Koda and T. Shiba), Int. Congre. Series 563, pp.60-71. Excerpta Medica, Amsterdam, Oxford, Princeton.
9. Davies, G.E. (1982). Uses and limitations of models for predicting hypersensitivity. 1st International Symposium on Immunotoxicology, University of Surrey, Guildford, U.K., this volume p.125.
10. Felix, R.H., Ive, F.A. and Dahl, M.G.C. (1974). *Brit. Med. J.* **4**, 321-324.
11. Dubois, E.L. (1969). *Medicine (Baltimore)* **48**, 217-228.
12. Perry, H.M. (1973). *Am. J. Med.* **54**, 58-72.
13. Balazs, T. and Robinson, C. (1982). *Int. J. Immunopharm.* **4**, 327.

IMMUNOLOGICAL ASPECTS OF GRANULOMA FORMATION

J.L. Turk and D. Parker

*Department of Pathology, Royal College of Surgeons,
Lincoln's Inn Fields, London WC2A 3PN, UK*

When an agent, capable of exciting an inflammatory reaction,
persists at the site, chronic inflammation results. This is
due to the persistence of the agent which causes destruction
and inflammation at the same time as attempting to heal. The
result is a well-circumscribed lesion often referred to as a
"granuloma". The term granuloma or tumour of granulation was
first used by Virchow [1] to cover the lesions that occurred
in a number of chronic infectious diseases. These included
tuberculosis, syphilis and leishmaniasis. At the cellular
level these lesions are characterized by giant cells and epithelioid cells [2], which originate from cells of the mononuclear phagocyte series (MPS) [3]. With the realization
that granuloma formation could occur in lesions of non-
infective origin, it became clear that two types of granuloma
could occur; those that are characterized by epithelioid cells
and those in which the core of the lesion is formed of
actively phagocytosing macrophages. A granuloma may therefore
be redefined in modern terms as a collection of cells of the
mononuclear phagocyte series, with or without the addition of
other inflammatory cell types. The relation of the granuloma
in chronic infections to immunological activity was first
discussed by Dienes and Mallory [4] particularly with respect
to tuberculosis. This was based mainly on the association of
those lesions with a state of delayed hypersensitivity to the
infecting organism. One may therefore divide granulomas into
two main groups; those with an obvious immunological association and those in which there is no clear immunological
relationship.

Immunological granulomas are found in a number of chronic
infectious diseases such as tuberculosis, tuberculoid leprosy,
schistosomiasis and syphilis. They also occur in sarcoidosis
and Crohn's disease and can be induced by the metals zirconium

and beryllium. These granulomas are characterized by an epithelioid cell lesion associated with a lymphocytic infiltration and surrounded by fibroblasts and new collagen formation. Non-immunological granulomas, which contain only phagocytosing macrophages, can be induced by colloidal iron or aluminium and occur in lepromatous leprosy in which there is a specific failure of cell-mediated immunity. The granulomas caused by silica-containing products and muramyl dipeptide [5] are paradoxically highly fibrogenic and may also contain epithelioid cells.

GRANULOMA FORMATION INDUCED BY METALS

Epithelioid cell granulomas which occur in the skin of humans following contact with zirconium salts, have been shown to be a hypersensitivity phenomenon [6,7]. A similar hypersensitivity granuloma can be induced in the skin of guinea pigs immunized and skin tested with sodium zirconium lactate (NaZrL) [8]. These granulomas begin to develop just as the delayed hypersensitivity reactions are dying down, and reach a peak about seven days after skin testing. Histologically, cells of the MPS (mononuclear phagocytic system) with an epithelioid cell appearance are seen, as well as giant cells, fibroblasts and other cell types. Characteristic features of epithelioid cells can best be determined with any certainty by electron microscopy, as these cells have mainly an oval nucleus, a large spherical nucleolus and finely marginated nuclear chromatin. Typical features are the large amount of endoplasmic reticulum, a Golgi apparatus and a fimbriated cell periphery which may show junctional interdigitations with neighbouring cells [9]. Characteristically, epithelioid cells are poorly phagocytic. The early resolution of these lesions is associated with the presence of large numbers of fibroblasts and evidence of considerable fibrosis.

However, not all zirconium-containing compounds induce this type of granuloma, despite the finding that they can induce good delayed hypersensitivity reactions. When guinea pigs are injected with a total of 1 mg of either NaZrL, zirconium aluminium chlorhydrate-glycine complex (ZAG) or aluminium zirconium tetrachlorhydrate (AZT) in Freund's complete adjuvant (containing Mycobacterium butyricum) and skin tested weekly by intradermal injection, good delayed hypersensitivity skin reactions develop. As can be seen from Table 1, AZT would appear to be a better inducer of delayed hypersensitivity than either ZAG or NaZrL. However, it is only in the guinea pigs immunized with NaZrL that allergic type granulomas develop. This occurs, despite the fact that all three compounds contain zirconium. It may be that the aluminium in

Table 1 *Proportion of animals sensitive to sodium zirconium lactate (NaZrL), zirconium aluminium chlorhydrate-glycine complex (ZAG) or aluminium zirconium tetrachlorhydrate (AZT)*

Immunized with	Weeks after immunization			
	6	7	8	9
NaZrL	2/8*	2/8	6/8	7/8
ZAG	1/10	2/10	0/10	4/10
AZT	0/10	2/10	2/9	8/9

* Positive reactions are those with a diameter of erythema > 8 x 8 mm or increase in skin thickness > 6.0×10^{-1} mm 4 hours after skin test.

the other zirconium compounds somehow prevents the development of the allergic granuloma, but cannot alter the ability of the compounds to induce good delayed hypersensitivity reactions.

In marked contrast to the NaZrL granulomas are those produced by the intradermal injection of aluminium hydroxide into normal guinea pigs [10]. These lesions consist of actively phagocytosing macrophages without the addition of other cell types and there is no evidence of any fibroblast activation. Although they persist in the skin for over three months, there is no evidence of the development of a hypersensitivity reaction.

A number of aluminium compounds are extremely damaging to both macrophage and fibroblast cell membranes, causing the release of cytoplasmic enzymes such as lactate dehydrogenase. These compounds have also been shown to cause haemolysis of red cell membranes [11]. A similar mechanism was shown to occur when macrophages were incubated with equivalent amounts of silica [12] and this was also considered to be related to the induction of granuloma formation. However, this is not the only biological action of aluminium compounds that might be related to granuloma formation. A parellelism has been shown between the induction of chronic inflammation by certain compounds, particularly polysaccharides, and their ability to release lysosomal enzymes from macrophages, with their ability to activate the alternative pathway of complement leading to C3 conversion [13] (see page 17). Aluminium compounds were found to activate C3 to the same extent as insulin and zymosan [14]. This was shown by anaphylatoxin production as well as by C3 conversion in two dimensionsal immunoelectrophoresis and CH50 estimations (complement concentration to effect haemolysis of 50% of erythrocytes). C3 conversion did not appear to involve the classical or alternative pathways, and some aluminium compounds were unable to activate C3 in the absence of plasminogen. This indicated that these compounds produced this effect by activating plasminogen through the Hageman factor. Zirconium hydroxide, which did not produce granulomas on direct injection, was neither toxic directly to macrophages or fibroblasts, nor was it able to cause C3 conversion. It is of interest in this connection that *Mycobacterium leprae* which produces a non-immunological granuloma without epithelioid cell formation in lepromatous leprosy patients, who have a specific defect of cell-mediated immunity to the organism, can also activate complement through the alternative pathway [15].

COMPARISON OF IMMUNOLOGICAL AND NON-IMMUNOLOGICAL GRANULOMAS OF MYCOBACTERIAL ORIGIN

The granuloma of tuberculoid leprosy is a typical epithelioid cell granuloma associated with the presence of a strong state of delayed hypersensitivity and the ability to develop epithelioid cell granulomas (Mitsuda reaction) when the individual is injected intradermally with heat killed *M. leprae*. This indicates that the granuloma is produced by a cell-mediated immune response. In contrast, the granuloma of lepromatous leprosy consists solely of macrophages that have ingested "globi" of *M. leprae* and there is an associated specific defect in cell-mediated immunity; patients are unable to develop an epithelioid cell granuloma when injected intradermally with the Mitsuda reagent.

Models of these two types of granuloma have been developed in the auricular lymph node of guinea pigs injected in the dorsum of the ear with Mycobacteria [16]. The intradermal injection of BCG vaccine, live or cobalt-irradiated, produced typical epithelioid cell granulomas in which the epithelioid cells were shown, by electron microscopy, to contain rough endoplasmic reticulum. These cells were similar to those seen in the NaZrL granulomas. There were also considerable numbers of fibroblasts and evidence of new collagen formation. There was little evidence of phagocytosed bacteria in the cells of the mononuclear phagocyte series in the BCG granulomas. In contrast, the granulomas produced by the injection of cobalt-irradiated *M. leprae* consisted mainly of macrophages with ingested organisms. Quantitative evaluation of these granulomas, according to the weight of the lymph nodes and the area of granulomatous infiltration, as measured by planimetry, indicated that the BCG granulomas reached their peak two weeks after induction, whereas the *M. leprae* granulomas peaked at five weeks.

Table 2 *Properties of large cells infiltrating granuloma as compared with peritoneal exudate macrophages*

	Peritoneal exudate macrophages	BCG epithelioid cells (2 week granuloma)	*M.leprae* macrophages (5 weeks granuloma)
Glass or plastic adherence	++ (∿ 60%)	± (∿ 10%)	+++ (∿ 70%)
Fc receptors	+++ (83%)	−	± (∿ 10%)
C3 receptors	+++ (73%)	−	± (∿ 10%)
Peroxidase	+++	−	−
Non-specific esterase	+++	++	++
Fibronectin	++	++	++

The cells of the mononuclear phagocyte series, in these two types of granuloma, were compared with oil induced peritoneal macrophages (Table 2). Both peritoneal and *M. leprae* macrophages were glass adherent, but the epithelioid cells of the BCG granulomas did not adhere to glass. This was consistent with their failure to phagocytose. Erythrocyte-antibody (EA) and erythrocyte-antibody-complement (EAC) rosetting of the peritoneal cells showed that a large proportion of these macrophages carried surface receptors for the Fc component of IgG and C3. A high percentage of these macrophages also exhibited peroxidase and non-specific esterase activity. Immunofluorescence, using fluorescein isothiocyanate (FITC)-conjugated monoclonal antibody against human fibronectin in peritoneal exudate cells, showed the presence of fibronectin in these macrophages. A high percentage of cells of the MPS infiltrating the BCG- and *M. leprae*-induced granulomas were esterase positive and showed the presence of fibronectin. However, these cells did not carry Fc or C3 surface receptors, nor did they exhibit peroxidase activity.

Despite the general acceptance that epithelioid cells are related to mononuclear phagocytes [3] it was important to demonstrate a formal relationship between these two cell types, as the term epithelioid cell has been used to cover all non-lymphoid mononuclear cells in granulomas, whether of an immunological or non-immunological nature. A monoclonal anti-guinea pig macrophage antibody was therefore prepared using guinea pig peritoneal macrophages as antigen. This was found to be specific for macrophages and not just directed

against the Ia antigen or the Fc receptor, as it did not
stain L2C leukaemia cells (a B-cell line with Fc receptors
and Ia antigens). The binding of this monoclonal anti-
macrophage serum to cells of the mononuclear phagocyte series
was compared with that of a guinea pig anti-Ia monoclonal
antibody (kindly given by Dr Ethan Shevac) using immunofluorescence and immunoperoxidase studies [17]. Both BCG
epithelioid cells and *M. leprae* macrophages stained with this
anti-macrophage serum, as did the peritoneal exudate macrophages and the Kupffer cells (Table 3). However, Langerhans

Table 3 *Binding of monoclonal anti-macrophage and anti-Ia to*
cells of the mononuclear phagocyte series in the guinea pig

	Anti- macrophage	Anti-Ia
Peritoneal exudate macrophages	++ (75%)	+ (35%)
Kupffer cells	+++ (∿ 100%)	+++ (∿ 100%)
Skin (Langerhans cells)	- (0%)	+++ (∿ 100%)
BCG granuloma (epithelioid cells)	+++ (100%)	- (0%)
M. leprae granuloma (macrophages)	++ (80%)	++ (80%)

cells in the skin failed to have the specific antigen. Peritoneal macrophages, Kupffer cells, Langerhans cells and the
M. leprae granuloma macrophages were Ia positive, but the epithelioid cells were Ia negative. Thus, it would appear that
epithelioid cells are related antigenically to other cells of
the mononuclear phagocyte series including peritoneal and
other macrophages. However, they differ in that they are
poorly phagocytic, not glass adherent and lack Ia antigen,
indicating that they do not possess an antigen-presenting
function. The presence of rough endoplasmic reticulum would
indicate that these cells have a secretory rather than phagocytic function.
    In order to see whether there was a relationship between
epithelioid cell formation and increased fibroblast activity,
collagen synthesis was examined in explants of auricular
lymph nodes from BCG- and *M. leprae*-injected animals and
compared with that in auricular lymph nodes from animals
painted on the dorsum of the ear with 2,4-dinitrofluorobenzene

(DNFB). Lymph nodes were cut into small pieces and incubated with ^{14}C-proline for 24 hours at 37°C. They were then homogenized in Tris-buffer and divided into two aliquots. One was precipitated directly with cold 10% trichloroacetic acid and the ^{14}C counted to give the total protein, while the other was treated with collagenase at 34°C for 90 minutes and the 10% trichloroacetic acid precipitate (the hydrolysed fraction) which did not contain collagen, was solubilized and counted. The total protein, less the hydrolysed fraction, gave the amount of ^{14}C-proline incorporated into collagen. In these studies it was evident that the nodes from animals injected with BCG synthesize high levels of collagen compared with those from animals sensitized with DNFB or injected with cobalt-irradiated *M. leprae* [18]. There was therefore, a direct association between the presence of secretory epithelioid cells and the subsequent development of fibrosis. One possible explanation for this association between epithelioid cell granulomas and fibrosis is that fibroblast activation results from a release of a specific activating factor from the epithelioid cells with rough endoplasmic reticulum. Further experiments were therefore performed to see whether such a factor was released by granuloma tissues in culture.

Supernatants from both BCG and *M. leprae* granulomas were found to release soluble non-dialysable factors, when incubated in medium alone for 24 hours. These factors stimulated ^{14}C-proline and ^{14}C-leucine incorporation into fibroblasts in culture and depressed their ^{3}H-thymidine uptake. These supernatants did not show any detectable macrophage migration inhibitory activity. On the other hand, supernatants from sensitized lymphocytes incubated with the antigen, and showing positive migratory inhibitory activity, had no effect on fibroblasts. Incubation of DNFB-sensitized lymph nodes in medium also produced supernatants which showed stimulation of ^{14}C-proline incorporation into fibroblasts and depressed ^{3}H-thymidine incorporation. It would appear therefore that fibroblast activation in lymph nodes containing mycobacterial granulomas could result from the release of soluble factors from cells of lymphocyte origin, as well as from those of the mononuclear phagocyte series. These factors appear to be independent of classical lymphokines that act on macrophages *in vitro*. The identification of these factors has, however, not clarified the mechanism of fibroblast activation in BCG granulomas, as compared with *M. leprae* granulomas, nor has it added to our knowledge of the function of the secretory epithelioid cell [19].

Despite this, it is clear that epithelioid cells form a distinct subpopulation of cells of the mononuclear phagocyte

series, that have exchanged their phagocytic role for a
secretory one. They are not glass adherent and lack Ia antigens. As they are recognized in tissues mainly by the typical
appearance under the electron microscope, their presence cannot be determined by light microscopy alone. The role these
cells play in the formation of certain granulomas is intriguing and requires further study.

SUMMARY

Granulomas may be of immunological origin. These granulomas
are usually associated with epithelioid cell formation and
marked fibrosis. Such granulomas are found in a number of
chronic infectious diseases such as tuberculosis, tuberculoid
leprosy, schistosomiasis and syphilis. They also occur in
sarcoidosis and Crohn's disease and can be induced by metals
zirconium and beryllium.

Non-immunological granulomas which contain only phagocytosing macrophages can be induced by aluminium containing compounds, and also occur in lepromatous leprosy. They may be
associated with activation of the third component of complement through the alternative pathway, or through the activation of plasminogen via the Hageman factor. These granulomas
are not associated with epithelioid cell formation or fibroblast activation.

The nature of the epithelioid cell and its relation to
fibroblast activation and increased collagen formation will
be discussed.

REFERENCES

1. Virchow, R. (1865). "Die Krankhaften Geschwulste",
    August Hirschwald, Berlin.
2. Cohnheim, J. (1877). "Vorlesungen über Allgemeinen
    Pathologie", August Hirschwald, Berlin.
3. Metchnikoff, E. (1893). "Lectures on the Comparative
    Pathology of Inflammation", Kegan Paul, Trench, Trübner,
    London.
4. Dienes, L. and Mallory, T.B. (1937). *Am. J. Path.* **13**,
    897-902.
5. Nagao, S., Ota, F., Emori, K., Inoue, K. and Tanaka, A.
    (1981). *Infect. and Immun.* **34**, 993-999.
6. Shelley, W.B. and Hurley, H.J. (1957). *Nature (Lond.)*
    180, 1060-1061.
7. Black, M.M. and Epstein, W.L. (1974). *Am. J. Pathol.* **74**,
    263-274.
8. Turk, J.L. and Parker, D. (1977). *J. Invest. Derm.* **68**,
    336-340.
9. Turk, J.L., Badenoch-Jones, P. and Parker, D. (1978).

J. Path. **124**, 45-49.
10. Turk, J.L. and Parker, D. (1977). *J. Invest. Derm*. **68**, 341-345.
11. Badenoch-Jones, P., Turk, J.L. and Parker, D. (1978). *J. Path*. **124**, 51-62.
12. Allison, A.C., Harington, J.S. and Birbeck, M. (1966). *J. Exp. Med*. **124**, 141-153.
13. Schorlemmer, H.U., Bitter-Suermann, D. and Allison, A.C. (1977). *Immunology* **32**, 929-939.
14. Ramanathan, V.D., Badenoch-Jones, P. and Turk, J.L. (1979). *Immunology* **37**, 881-886.
15. Ramanathan, V.D., Curtis, J. and Turk, J.L. (1980). *Infect. and Immun*. **29**, 30-35.
16. Narayanan, R.B., Badenoch-Jones, P. and Turk, J.L. (1981). *J. Path*. **134**, 253-265.
17. Mathew, R.C., Katayama, I., Gupta, S.K., Curtis, J. and Turk, J.L. (1982). (Submitted for publication).
18. Narayanan, R.B., Badenoch-Jones, P., Curtis, J. and Turk, J.L. (1982). **J. Path**. (in press).
19. Narayanan, R.B., Curtis, J. and Turk, J.L. (1981). *Cell. Immunol*. **65**, 93-102.

THE IMMUNOTOXICITY OF BERYLLIUM

A.L. Reeves

Wayne State University, Detroit, Michigan, USA.

INTRODUCTION

Berylliosis was probably one of the least expected new
diseases to be discovered in this century, and certainly the
least expected new occupational intoxication. The lapse of
time from the first report of its occurrence [1] to its at
least tentative acceptance by industrial physicians [2] took
about 15 years, during which a sceptical medical and chemical
community remained largely unconvinced and expressed its
doubts in sometimes forceful terms [3-5].

The landmark paper which first looked into the epidemiological distribution of berylliosis, and suggested a coherent
theory of pathogenesis, was written by Sterner and Eisenbud
in 1951 [6]. This paper can be credited with making the first
persuasive case for the immunological aetiology of berylliosis,
although the sensitizing property of beryllium salt solutions
had been noted previously [7-10]. Epstein [11] described
berylliosis as a model case of "granulomatous hypersensitivity", a special nosological entity distinct from ordinary
delayed hypersensitivity, or banal chronic inflammation, or
foreign body response to a colloidal substance. Granulomatous
hypersensitivity, according to this classification, is the
specific immune response to tissue contact with a poorly
soluble particle, mediated through the accumulation and proliferation of reticuloendothelial cells. Work accomplished
during the past 30, and particularly the past 15 years to
elucidate the nature and consequences of this response to
beryllium and its compounds is reviewed in this presentation.

THE NATURE OF THE ANTIGEN

Beryllium is an alkaline earth element (Group II A of the
periodic table) but uniquely among the alkaline earths, it is
amphoteric, i.e. readily capable of forming positive or

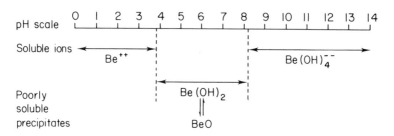

Fig. 1 The ionization of beryllium in aqueous solution.

negative ions in aqueous solutions. The practical consequence
is that common beryllium compounds ionize in both acidic and
basic environments but not at neutrality, where they precipitate to form poorly soluble particles (Fig. 1). This mechanism operates when beryllium salt solutions, in up to moderate
concentration, enter the buffered environment of skin, lung,
or lower gastrointestinal tract.

Several questions emerge at this point. Firstly, is beryllium unique among all metals with this behavior? The answer
is yes and no; amphotericity is certainly the rule in the
periodic table of the elements and is shared by at least one
other light metal (aluminium). Beryllium and aluminium are
in fact frequently regarded as chemical twins and do have a
number of properties in common. However, beryllium is unique
in being by far the lightest of all solid and chemically-
stable substances. The atomic radius of beryllium is 23 times
smaller than that of aluminium and it can fit into positions
on the surface of macromolecules that are far too small for
most other atoms. It is possible that antigenic behavior
depends in part on these fits and/or on complexing capabilities of the substances involved.

Secondly, what is the solid-state chemical form of beryllium
on the surface of the poorly soluble particle? If freshly
precipitated in tissue following entry of beryllium ions, it
is usually the hydroxide. In aged precipitates, as well as
direct inhalants in certain occupational situations, it can be
the oxide. The latter is either intentionally used as
"beryllia" for ceramic formulations, or it can form as a thin
film on the surface of the bare metal upon exposure to air.
Beryllia is manufactured by roasting and sintering beryllium
ores, followed by a number of technological steps, the last
of which is "firing" the mix in kilns to obtain the finished
oxide. Temperature of the firing can be anywhere from 500°
to 1750°C in different manufacturing processes (Fig. 2), and
there is ample evidence that toxicity of beryllium oxides is
inversely related to the temperature of firing [12,13]. Much
of the early disease experience was connected with use of the

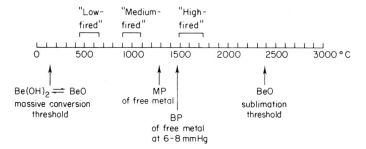

Fig. 2   Temperature scale of beryllia preparation.

"low-fired" compound, which is no longer produced in the
United States. It has been known for some time [14] that
refractive index and birefringence of beryllium oxides were
dependent on firing temperature, even though the crystal form
of the substance was always basically the same — hexagonal,
with a wurtzite-type lattice (Fig. 3). It appeared that the
temperature of firing influenced the frequency of imperfec-
tions in the crystal lattice, known to crystallographers as
the "crystallite size". A "crystallite" is a statistical
concept and describes the average portion of a lattice that
is free from imperfection or irregularity. By X-ray optics,
only the crystallite appears as an isotropic entity and a
macroscopic crystal is a conglomerate of smaller or larger
crystallites. In the case of beryllium oxide, increasing the
firing temperature resulted in larger crystallite size, i.e.
the crystals were the more perfect the higher temperatures
they were fired at. That toxicity should also be governed by
this parameter was certainly a surprise and appears to be
connected with the extent of inner surfaces of a beryllium
oxide particle, reflecting its total adsorptive surface or,
more likely, the density of electrostatic charges on the
outer surface.

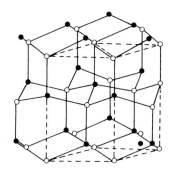

Fig. 3   "Wurtzite-type" crystal lattice.

Thirdly, is beryllium exposure at the tissue level, in view of the amphoteric behavior of the element, always necessarily a solid-state phenomenon? The answer to this question is no — the buffering capacity of tissue fluids can be exhausted by very high concentrations of beryllium, resulting in a shift away from the neutral pH; or precipitation even at neutral pH can be circumvented by complexation. The former mechanism operates in the cases of acute beryllium poisoning formerly encountered in the beryllium extraction industry. The latter situation applies to beryllium citrate or aurintricarboxylate (Fig. 4), both water-soluble but non-ionizable compounds. Aurintricarboxylic acid (ATA) has been successfully used as an antidotal agent against acute beryllium poisoning in experimental animals [15]. ATA proved effective in protecting mice and rats if given parenterally just before or just after an otherwise lethal dose of ionic beryllium. Evidently, ATA tied up beryllium ions, thus preventing the acid burn, result- ing from exhaustion of the buffer system in tissue fluids, which was the direct cause of acute beryllium pneumonitis. It also prevented beryllium hydroxide precipitation, and both beryllium citrate and the beryllium-ATA complex were negative in eliciting any allergic reaction from beryllium sulphate- sensitized guinea pigs [16,17].

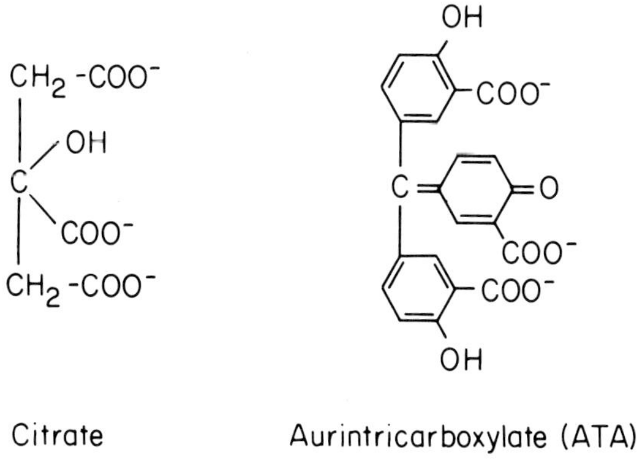

Citrate   Aurintricarboxylate (ATA)

Fig. 4 Beryllium complexing agents.

On the basis of these considerations, an answer of the fundamental question regarding the nature of the antigen in beryllium hypersensitivity can be attempted (Fig. 5). There appears to be no reason to doubt the proposition that the reactive species is always solid-state, and perhaps always the oxide with high density of surface electrostatic charges, determined by inner lattice irregularities. The reactive

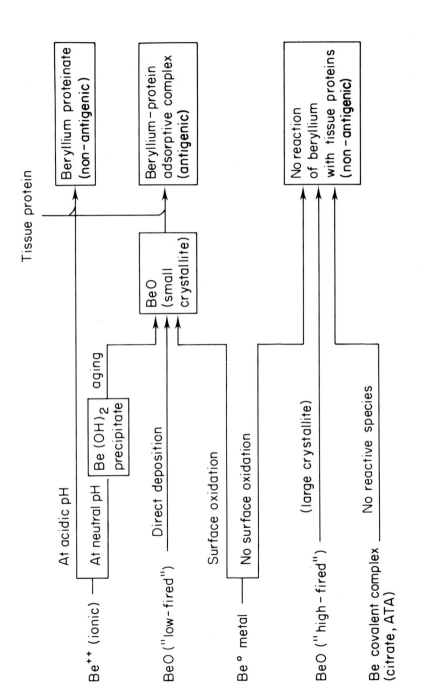

Fig. 5 Antigenicity of chemical forms of beryllium.

particles may enter directly in the course of contact with
beryllium oxide, especially the "low-fired" variety; or with
beryllium metal powder with an oxide film on the surface of
the particles. They may also arise indirectly, through aging
of beryllium hydroxide precipitate formed upon entry of ionic
beryllium into buffered tissue. The reactive species is not
formed when non-ionized soluble beryllium (citrate, aurintricarboxylate) enters the organism; or if timely application
of complexing agents prevented the precipitation or aging of
beryllium hydroxide; or if beryllium concentration at the site
was high enough to upset tissue pH to a point where precipitation of beryllium hydroxide no longer occurred. Beryllium
sulphosalicylate, used in a number of experiments [18,19],
apparently behaves as if it were partially ionized.

Conventional thinking requires that beryllium itself be regarded as a hapten which combines or associates with a tissue
protein to produce the complete antigen. This thinking was
encouraged by our results [16] showing that, in $BeSO_4$-
sensitized guinea pigs, the beryllium complex of guinea pig
serum albumin consistently produced a stronger cutaneous reaction than $BeSO_4$ itself. Binding of beryllium to various
tissue proteins has also been suggested [20-24], but the complexes appeared stable only under non-physiological conditions
of acidic pH. We suggest that an adsorptive association can
exist between proteins and electrostatically charged particles
at physiological pH, and it is these adsorptive complexes
rather than ion-bond proteinates which are identifiable as the
proximate antigen in granulomatous hypersensitivity to beryllium.

TISSUE RESPONSES TO THE ANTIGEN

Humoral Response

After recognition of beryllium as a potential tissue antigen,
efforts were made to interpret ensuing reactions as manifestations of a specific type of hypersensitivity. Increased
concentrations of IgG were found in berylliosis patients as
well as in several healthy beryllium workers, but the specificity of the response remained unproved and no soluble antibody could be isolated [25,26].

Cellular Response

Alekseeva and coworkers produced delay cutaneous hypersensitivity to
beryllium chloride in guinea pigs; showed its passive trans-
ferability with lymphoid cells but not with serum, and established that the hypersensitivity had no immediate component,
did not lead to general anaphylaxis, and did not involve, even

together with homologous protein, humoral antibody formation
[27,28]. Chiappino and coworkers [29,30] found the reaction
in the lungs of guinea pigs intratracheally treated with low-
fired beryllium oxide, morphologically characteristic of
delayed hypersensitivity, and prepared guinea pig-lymphocyte
antiserum from rabbits which could abolish a previously established cutaneous reactivity [31]. These experiments left no
doubt that beryllium hypersensitivity was cell-mediated. The
histopathological reaction in lungs and skin has been described as an accumulation of organized epitheloid cells with
a variable complement of large mononuclear cells and abnormal
giant cells, accompanied by some necrosis and fibrosis [32,11].
The similarity to sarcoidosis was often striking, and there is
at least one other metal, zirconium, which also causes similar
lesions [33].

An interesting question is whether or not there is direct
interaction between the antigen and the cells accumulating in
response to its presence. Phagocytosis of beryllium at least
by alveolar macrophages is well established [13,34] and it was
also shown that phagocytosis was accompanied by lysosomal enzyme release [35]. Beryllium-lysosome interaction in a model
system involving rat livers following intravenous beryllium
phosphate has been studied [36-39]. The particles were taken
up selectively by the Kuppfer cells and caused immediate pronounced swelling with eventual rupture of the lysosomal vesicles. The process was accompanied by distension and vacuolization of the Kuppfer cells, leading to pericanalicular
lobular necrosis. Whether or not this is a pertinent model
system for pulmonary deposits in contact with the granuloma-
forming cells is not certain, although the attribution of the
necrotic component of pulmonary berylliosis tissue to cell
death due to lysosomal disruption is an attractive hypothesis.

Skilleter and Price [40] argue against the nuclear accumulation of beryllium at least in the liver, attributing the
numerous time-honoured results to an artifact. In a variety
of tissues with a variety of techniques, beryllium was
repeatedly found in the nucleus or nucleolus [41-43, 22-24];
and the concept is consistent with the observed effect of
beryllium on DNA transcription [44-47].

Patch Test

The beryllium patch test according to Curtis [9,10] has been
the earliest manifestation of an immunological component in
beryllium disease. It had some early application in human
diagnosis but has been criticized on the grounds that it (a)
gave positive reactions in persons without berylliosis; (b)
caused occasional flare-ups of pulmonary symptoms in persons

with berylliosis; (c) induced contact sensitization in controls [48]. Epstein argued that the beryllium patch test detected conventional delayed contact sensitivity rather than granulomatous hypersensitivity, and was comparable to the tuberculin test which also reflected delayed hypersensitivity to the tubercle bacillus but not tuberculosis [11]. False negatives due to immunosuppression were another obvious possibility. The most troublesome experience with the beryllium patch test was reported by Sneddon [49] in a patient with berylliosis, who developed organized epitheloid cell granuloma at the test site.

Lymphocyte Blast Transformation

Lymphocyte blast transformation can be defined as the morphological enlargement of small lymphocytes into large lymphoblasts *in vitro* [50]. The transformation can be brought about by numerous stimuli including tissue antigens, specific antigens, antisera, and a group of very active stimulants referred to as "non-specific" of which phytohaemagglutinin is the prototype. In 1970, it was shown that among specific antigens, beryllium compounds (including specifically the oxide) caused striking transformation of lymphocytes from beryllium-sensitive subjects only, while the lymphocytes from normal, non-sensitive subjects did not transform [51]. Transformation of beryllium-sensitive and non-sensitive lymphocytes by phytohaemagglutinin was similar. In 1973, Deodhar *et al.*, reported on the exploitation of this discovery for the diagnosis of beryllium disease [52]. Among 35 patients with chronic berylliosis, 25 (71%) showed at least some blast transformation, with 21 patients (60%) showing strong or very strong transformation, even though these patients were treated at the time of the test with prednisone, an inhibitor of immune reactions. There was also a correlation between the severity of the clinical disease and the degree of blast transformation. Incidence of positive results in control groups was low: two out of 28 beryllium workers without the disease; three out of 19 normal healthy subjects; and one out of 11 patients with other lung diseases. These figures show that, practical as the lymphocyte blast transformation may be in the diagnosis of berylliosis, what the positive test shows is not the presence of berylliosis. Rather, it shows the presence of beryllium hypersensitivity which may or may not involve the presence of berylliosis. Nonetheless, in appropriate context, the method has recently become a favourite tool in industrial medicine [53]. An optimized form of the test [54] utilizes purified lymphocytes suspended in 20% serum, with Be^{++} added in the nanomole range. If the beryllium concentration was higher, the transformation became inhibited, apparently due to suppressed DNA bio-synthesis [55-57].

Macrophage Migration Inhibition

Bloom and Bennett [58] demonstrated a soluble factor which could inhibit the free migration of macrophages *in vitro*. The factor was elaborated by sensitized lymphocytes and appeared to be highly antigen-specific but not cell- or species-specific. It appeared possible to culture pure popu-lations of lymphocytes from buffy coat in the presence of an antigen and then test the supernatant of such a culture on guinea pig peritoneal exudate cells. Inhibition of migration of the latter cells was observed if, and only if, the source of the lymphocytes was a sensitized patient. This principle was successfully employed with beryllium as an antigen [59] and it was demonstrated that beryllium oxide-stimulated lymphocytes from patients with berylliosis, but not from normal individuals, produced the inhibitory factor. Marx and Burrell [60] studied seven patients with chronic beryllium disease by means of the macrophage migration inhibition test and found positive results in all, while the results in six normal controls and two non-berylliotic pulmonary patients were negative. On the other hand, Jones Williams *et al.* [61,62] examined seven other chronic berylliosis patients and found positive results only in one, but the other patients were on corticosteroid therapy at the time of testing. In a later paper, Price *et al.* [63] examined 50 healthy beryllium workers, 20 healthy controls, and five chronic berylliosis patients, one of whom was not on steroid treatment. The latter patient had pronounced migration inhibition index which reverted to near-normal when steroid treatment was instituted, while the reverse effect was observed in one patient whose steroid treatment was suspended. It thus seems that macrophage migration inhibition is also a useful indica-tor of beryllium hypersensitivity although it can be abolished by immunosuppressive treatment.

Animal Experiments

Extensive work on experimental animals to reproduce the immunological tissue response to beryllium has been reported [64,65,60,66-68]. The animal of choice in all these studies has been the Hartley guinea pig, which is commercially available as an immunologically "responding" (to poly-L-lysine) substrain. There is one report extending the observations to female rats [69]. The time interval for maximum skin reac-tions following intradermal injection of 0.1 ml aqueous solution of 5 μg Be^{++} (as sulphate) into the shaven abdominal skin of a sensitized guinea pig took 48 to 72 hours, well distinguishable from an irritation reaction which subsided in 24 hours or less. Also, irritation reactions clustered around 2 mm average diameter, whereas hypersensitivity reactions most frequently measured 4 to 5 mm average diameter (Fig. 6).

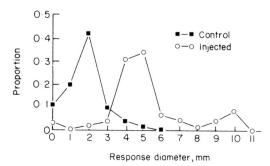

Fig. 6 **Frequency distribution of skin reactions to beryllium sulphate in guinea pigs.** (Reference 67)

After considerable experience it was expedient to establish 3.5 mm diameter as the threshold for a positive skin reaction at 48 hours. It was interesting that a small number of guinea pigs were distinguishable as "heavy responders", with skin reaction diameters of 9 to 10 mm, which appeared to be a specific reaction type rather than the higher end of the size frequency distribution curve peaking at 5 mm [67]. "Heavy responders" were about 10% of all the "responders" and the distinction was not identical to the responsiveness to poly-L-lysine conjugates in the Camm-Hartley strain.

Macrophage migration inhibition proved to be a dependable indicator of beryllium hypersensitivity in experimental animals (Fig. 7). An inhibition of 20% (migration factor of 0.80) was found to be a suitable threshold to define a positive response, and in our experiments it corresponded to a 48-hour skin reaction diameter of 3.5 mm [70]. Marx and Burrell [60] reported positive correlation of the migration inhibitory factor and skin test results in 11 out of 15 cases (73%), and Palazzolo and Reeves [71] calculated a correlation coefficient of -0.45 between skin reaction diameters and per cent macrophage migration (Fig. 8). In the opinion of Salvin *et al.* [72], a correlation between the diameter of induration after skin testing and the degree of migration inhibition of lymphoid cells is non-existent. We suggest that the situation, at least in beryllium hypersensitivity, deserves a second look, especially if optimized conditions for the macrophage migration inhibition test are better defined.

It still remains to be determined whether or not skin

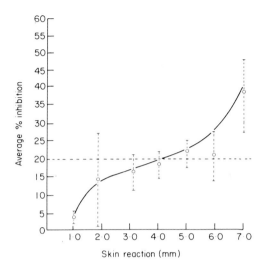

Fig. 7 Correlation of skin reaction diameters to macrophage migration inhibition. (Reference 70)

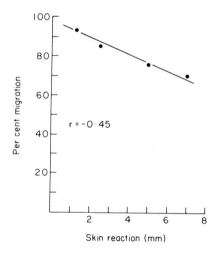

Fig. 8 Regression line of skin reaction diameters and macrophage migration inhibition. (Reference 70)

testing, lymphocyte transformation, and macrophage migration measure basically the same thing. Obviously, all three are assays of delayed hypersensitivity, but each of the tests looks at a different variable and whether or not these are facets of one phenomenon or essentially independent variables, is not known with certainty. The less than perfect

convergence in various animal experiments may have been due
to experimental error.   In human patients, it seemed that
macrophage migration inhibition was more readily reversible
by steroid treatment than lymphocyte blast transformation,
but direct comparisons are yet to be made.

The Genetics of Beryllium Hypersensitivity

One of the interesting side results of experimentation with
animal models in the study of beryllium hypersensitivity was
the finding that ability to respond immunologically to beryllium was genetically controlled (Fig. 9).   Polak *et al.* [73]

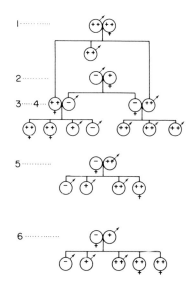

**Fig. 9 Genetic transmission of ability to respond immuno-
logically to beryllium.** (Reference 78)

found that among inbred strains of guinea pigs, only "Strain
II" (responders to 2,4-dinitrophenyl-poly-L-lysine) reacted
to sensitization with beryllium flouride, whereas "Strain
XIII" (non-responders) did not react.   The situation was the
opposite with respect to sensitization to mercuric chloride,
where Strain XIII guinea pigs reacted, whereas Strain II
guinea pigs did not.   The ability to react was transmitted
to progeny as a simple Mendelian dominant, non-sex-linked
characteristic.   In a recent study [68], these observations
were extended, showing that only Strain II animals developed
beryllium granulomas of the lung after intratracheal injections of beryllium oxide, whereas Strain XIII animals did not.
Treated Strain II animals also showed (in comparison to

treated Strain XIII animals or to untreated controls of either
strain) elevated basal chemiluminescence and bacteriocidal
activity of bronchoalveolar lavage cells, and enhanced uptake
of tritiated thymidine in tissue culture by blood, lymph node,
or spleen cells. It is believed that "Strain II" and "Strain
XIII" guinea pigs differ only in the I region of the major
histocompatibility complex, controlled by one allele in a
specific genetic locus.

WAYS TO MODIFY TISSUE RESPONSES TO THE ANTIGEN

Potentiation

Generally, beryllium antigens have been effectively administered without adjuvant, and beryllium itself has been explored
as a possible substitute for mycobacteria in Freund's complete
adjuvant [74]. Beryllium feeding and beryllium inhalation have
been investigated for possible enhancing effects on cutaneous
beryllium hypersensitivity in animal experiments without positive results [64,65], but it was noted that beryllium albumin-
ate of guinea pig serum, prepared according to the method of
Belman [75], consistently gave stronger sensitivity responses
in beryllium sulphate-sensitized guinea pigs than beryllium
sulphate itself [16]. This appears to be the only known
instance of potentiation of beryllium hypersensitivity on
record, although it could be also interpreted as evidence that
the protein complex was immunologically closer to the proximate cutaneous antigen than the beryllium ion. Belman [76]
produced evidence that ionic beryllium applied to the skin
becomes partially bound to epidermal alkaline phosphatase.

Suppression

The general anti-inflammatory effects of corticosteroids have
been successfully exploited in the clinical management of
berylliosis, and it is recognized that those effects included
an immunosuppressant component [62,77]. Experimentally, an
antiserum prepared from rabbits could completely suppress
cutaneous reactivity to beryllium in sensitized guinea pigs
[31], and Turk and Polak [78] could also suppress reactivity
by intravenous injection of high doses of beryllium lactate.
The mechanism of suppression in the latter case appeared to
be related to induced cutaneous anergy (anergy is defined as
the absence of reactions of cell-mediated immunity in a
supposedly primed animal), analogous to what had been observed in a few cases of the Curtis patch test [9,10,79,48].
The state of hypersensitivity in guinea pigs during inhalation exposure to beryllium sulphate was followed in our
laboratory [64,65] and the surprising observation was made

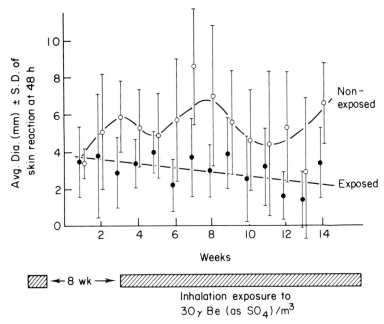

Fig. 10   Skin reaction of guinea pigs during inhalation
exposure to BeSO₄.   (Reference 67)

that inhalation suppressed a previously established cutaneous
reactivity (Fig. 10). The effect could not be attributed to
ingestion of beryllium traces following mucociliary return of
inhaled beryllium into the mouth [80] because, if equivalent
traces of beryllium were directly fed in the drinking water
to sensitized guinea pigs, no immunosuppression could be observed. Suppression of tuberculin reactivity following intradermal injection of beryllium sulphate was observed recently
[17], but this might reflect competition between two antigens
for cutaneous binding sites rather than lack of specificity
of the suppressive effect of beryllium inhalation on beryllium
hypersensitivity. The phenomenon has interesting implications
for the understanding of the epidemiology of distribution of
human berylliosis cases, where it has been frequently the
marginally exposed "neighbourhood case" who suffered gravest
consequences from beryllium, while workers in regular contact
with far greater concentrations sometimes developed apparent
immunity.

THE ROLE OF ALLERGIC TISSUE RESPONSES IN BERYLLIUM DISEASE

Beryllium Dermatitis

Beryllium dermatitis was first described by Van Ordstrand
et al. [81] as edematous papulovesicular lesions, which

appeared particularly on the exposed surfaces of the body of
workers handling soluble beryllium salts.   If insoluble
beryllium compounds became imbedded in the skin, e.g. after
injury with a fluorescent tube containing a beryllium phosphor,
necrotizing ulcerations developed which did not readily heal.
Both conditions have been reproduced in the skin of pigs [82].
In the opinion of Epstein [11], the first reaction is due to
delayed contact hypersensitivity and the second to granulomatous hypersensitivity, two different immunologic entities.

Acute Beryllium Pneumonitis

Acute pulmonary beryllium disease was first encountered in
beryllium extraction plants, with cases resulting from inhalation of aerosols of soluble beryllium compounds (typically
the fluoride) in high concentrations.   All segments of the
respiratory tract were sometimes involved, with rhinitis,
pharyngitis, tracheobronchitis and pneumonitis [83-85].   The
acidity of the beryllium salts was the obvious aetiological
factor and acute disease resulted only if there was exposure
to massive concentrations which would overwhelm the buffer
reserve of body fluids and thus prevent the pulmonary precipitation of beryllium hydroxide.   There is no evidence that
allergic tissue response is involved in acute pulmonary
beryllium disease.

Chronic Pulmonary Granulomatosis (Berylliosis)

A chronic condition among fluorescent lamp workers, different
from acute pulmonary beryllium disease, was first described
by Hardy and Tabershaw [86].   Shortness of breath was the
leading symptom, with pulmonary X-rays showing miliary
mottling.   The onset was frequently insidious, with only
slight cough and fatigue which could occur as early as one
year, or as late as 25 years, after exposure.   Progressive
pulmonary insufficiency with alveolocapillary block, anorexia
with weight loss, and a constant hacking cough with chest pain,
characterized the advanced disease.   Histopathological
examination of lung tissue showed conspicuous interstitial
granulomatosis, similar to that seen in Boeck's sarcoid.
    There can be no doubt today that berylliosis is a manifest-
ation of granulomatous hypersensitivity, but the precise
pathogenesis is very much an open question.   It has been
sometimes described as an "autoimmune" disease on the basis
that the ultimate triggering factor was a body protein, in
combination with, or denatured by, beryllium.   Involvement of
humoral, or of conventional delayed hypersensitivity, factors
was occasionally suggested.   Quite clearly, the lymphocyte
blast transformation, macrophage migration inhibition, or

patch test are diagnostic for the state of beryllium hypersensitivity rather than for the state of berylliosis, and
even though the two are in some kind of causal relationship
to each other they are not the same, and the presence of one
does not require the presence of the other. Beryllium hypersensitivity can and does occur in healthy workers, and
patients with severe berylliosis may not show hypersensitivity
due to topical anergy or immune paralysis. Superimposed on
these uncertainties are the effects of corticosteroid treatment, which explains the false positives and false negatives
to the Curtis test or Jones Williams test. Moreover, it is
important to remember that beryllium inhalation itself suppressed skin reactivity in animal experiments [64]. In a
series of studies on guinea pigs, if cutaneous hypersensitivity
was maintained throughout the course of inhalation exposure by
a program of serial booster shots, the hypersensitive animals
showed an alleviated tissue reaction in the lungs in comparison
to animals whose cutaneous hypersensitivity was not maintained
by booster shots, and whose immune reactivity was allowed to
subside (Fig. 11). On this ground we chose, not without some
debate, the provocative title "Immunity to Pulmonary Berylliosis in Guinea Pigs" for our 1972 paper [65], and we pointed
out that the situation showed some similarity to the relationship of tuberculin sensitivity to tuberculosis where also
controlled induction of sensitivity (e.g., with BCG vaccine)
is thought to confer improved resistance to tuberculosis.

   In an overall correlation of skin reaction diameters to
pulmonary pathologies as quantified by lung weight/body weight

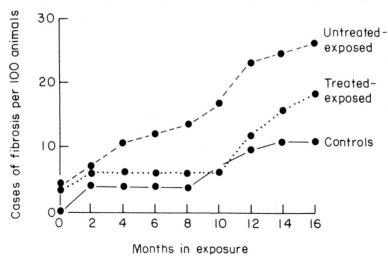

Fig. 11   Pulmonary pathology of guinea pigs during inhalation
exposure to BeSO$_4$.   (Reference 66)

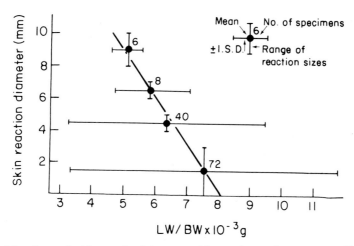

Fig. 12 Correlation of skin reactions to pulmonary pathologies. (Reference 66)

ratios in guinea pigs, we found straight-line reverse relationship clearly showing that skin reactivity and pulmonary vulnerability were mutually inhibitory (Fig. 12) but it was not immediately clear as to which was the cause and which was the effect. Development of the pulmonary lesion might have suppressed skin reactivity; or maintenance of skin reactivity might have modified the development of the pulmonary lesion. These two cause-and-effect sequences are not mutually exclusive but possibly concurrent and inter-dependent. The applicability of these principles to the diagnosis and management of human berylliosis cases has not been sufficiently explored thus far.

Beryllium Neoplasia

Osteosarcoma in the long bones of rabbits after intravenous injection of beryllium oxide was first observed by Gardner and Heslington [87], and adenocarcinoma in the lungs of rats after inhalation of beryllium sulphate was first produced by Vorwald et al. [88]. These basic results have been reproduced, with various modifications, numerous times and it has also been pointed out [89] that guinea pigs did not suffer neoplastic effects from beryllium injection or inhalation. This was ascertained by exposures of the type and duration that were clearly carcinogenic in rats and rabbits, and as guinea pigs, but not rats or rabbits, were also known to develop granulomatous hypersensitivity to beryllium, it has been tempting to speculate on the possible mutual inhibition of the two processes [89]. It was recalled that in the early work on the rabbit bone tumours, prompt concurrent splenic

atrophy was one of the interesting accompanying findings, and
in one study it appeared that splenectomy increased the incidence of bone sarcomas from beryllium in rabbits [90]. These
results were compatible with the hypothesis that some sort of
cellular immunity, with the immunocompetent cells arising from
the spleen, is a possible factor in determining whether the
response to beryllium will be neoplastic or not, and that
various species, or conceivably various individuals of one
species, have resistance to beryllium neoplasia according to
their immunocompetence.

The human cancer experience with beryllium is controversial.
Recent reports claiming a lung cancer prevalence of 1.3 to 1.6
times normal among beryllium workers [91-93] were severely
criticized on numerous grounds, including manipulative use of
input data in order to allow a preordained conclusion [94,95].
Particularly interesting in these studies was the fact that
prevalence of lung cancer among beryllium workers was inversely correlated to the length of occupational exposure; i.e.
workers who were employed in beryllium plants for only a few
weeks or months had a higher lung cancer rate than those
employed for several years. These results, if they allow any
conclusion at all, link beryllium as a presumptive occupational
carcinogen to the hypothesis that continued exposure bolstered
the immunocompetence of the exposed population, resulting in
decreased cancer prevalence.

Clearly, more work is required to clarify this fascinating
possibility. At this time, the assumption that susceptibility
to beryllium cancers also involves an immunotoxicologic factor,
cannot be confirmed or excluded.

SUMMARY

The essential immune reaction to beryllium compounds is
granulomatous hypersensitivity (accumulation and proliferation
of reticuloendothelial cells in response to tissue contact
with a poorly soluble particle). The common denominator in
most or all cases appears to be small-crystallite beryllium
oxide, either in direct exposure to "low-fired" beryllia; or
formed on the surface of the bare metal through atmospheric
oxidation; or formed in situ through aging of beryllium
hydroxide particles precipitated upon entry of ionized beryllium salts into buffered tissues. The proximate antigen is
perhaps an adsorptive protein complex with these particles.
The cellular response includes phagocytosis by macrophages,
leading to swelling and rupture of lysosomes which result in
vacuolization and eventual necrosis of the cells. The process is accompanied by development of delayed cutaneous
hypersensitivity, measurable as patch test, lymphocyte blast

formation, or macrophage migration inhibition. Ability to
respond was genetically controlled in guinea pigs as a dominant non-sex-linked trait, and could be suppressed with lymphocyte antiserum, with large doses of beryllium lactate or,
surprisingly, by inhalation exposure to beryllium sulphate.
  Berylliosis is a manifestation of granulomatous hypersensitivity to beryllium, but the interdependence is complex. The
measurable parameters show the state of beryllium hypersensitivity rather than the state of berylliosis. In guinea pigs,
maintenance of cutaneous hypersensitivity through booster
shots decreased the vulnerability of the lungs from concurrent
beryllium inhalation. Beryllium neoplasia was observed in
those experimental animals not immunologically responding to
beryllium. Cellular immunity may be a factor in determining
whether the response to beryllium will be neoplastic or not,
and various species may have resistance to beryllium tumours
according to their immunocompetence.

REFERENCES

1. Weber, H.H. and Engelhardt, W.E. (1933). *Zentr. Gew.*
    Hyg. **10,** 41-47.
2. Sixth Saranac Symposium (1950). Gardner Memorial Volume,
    (Ed. A.J. Vorwald), pp.3-455. P.B. Hoeber, New York.
3. Hyslop, F., Palmer, E.D., Alford, W.C., Monaco, A.R. and
    Fairhall, L.T. (1943). *U.S.N.I.H. Bulletin* 181.
4. Walworth, H.T. (1949). *Ind. Med. Surg.* **18,** 428-431.
5. Lancet editorial (1951). **i,** 1358.
6. Sterner, J.H. and Eisenbud, M. (1951). *Arch. Ind. Hyg.*
    Occ. Med. **4,** 123-151.
7. DeNardi, J.M., Van Ordstrand, H.S. and Carmody, M.G. (1949).
    Ohio State Med. J. **45,** 567-575.
8. McCord, C.P. (1951). *Ind. Med. Surg.* **20,** 336.
9. Curtis, G.H. (1951). *Arch. Dermat. Syphil.* **64,** 470-482.
10. Curtis, G.H. (1959). *Arch. Ind. Health* **19,** 150-153.
11. Epstein, W.L. (1967). *Progr. Allergy* ii, 36-88.
12. Spencer, H.C., Jones, J.C., Sadek, S.E., Dodson, K.B. and
    Morgan, A.H. (1965). *Toxicol. Appl. Pharmacol.* **7,** 498.
13. Sanders, C.L., Cannon, W.C., Powers, G.J., Adee, R.R. and
    Meier, D.M. (1975). *Arch. Environ. Health* **30,** 546-551.
14. Crossmon, G.C. and Vandemark, W.C. (1954). *Arch. Ind.*
    Hyg. Occ. Med. **9,** 481-487.
15. Schubert, J., White, M.R. and Lindenbaum, A. (1952).
    J. Biol. Chem. **196,** 279-288.
16. Krivanek, N.D. and Reeves, A.L. (1972). *Am. Ind. Hyg.*
    Assoc. J. **33,** 45-52.
17. Kagamimori, S., Williams, W.R. and Jones Williams, W.
    (1981). *Ind. Health* **19,** 139-144.

18. Jones, J.M. and Amos, H.E. (1975b). *Nature* **256**, 499-500.
19. Haard, G.C., Skilleter, D.N. and Reiner, E. (1977). *Exp. Mol. Pathol.* **27**, 197-212.
20. Aldridge, W.N., Barnes, J.M. and Denz, F.A. (1950). *Brit. J. Exp. Path.* **31**, 473-484.
21. Reiner, E. (1971). In "Symposium on Mechanisms of Toxicity" (Ed. W.N. Aldridge), pp.111-125, Macmillan, London.
22. Vasil'eva, E.V. (1969). *Byull. Eksper. Biol. Med.* **iii**, 74-77.
23. Vasil'eva, E.V. (1972). *Byull. Eksper. Biol. Med.* **ii**, 76-80.
24. Parker, V.H. and Stevens, C. (1979). *Chem. Biol. Interact.* **26**, 167-177.
25. Pugliese, P.T., Whitlock, C.M., Ernst, B. and Williams, R.R. (1968). *Arch. Environ. Health* **16**, 374-379.
26. Resnick, H., Roche, M. and Morgan, W.K.C. (1970). *Am. Rev. Resp. Dis.* **101**, 504-510.
27. Alekseeva, O.G. (1965). *Gig. Trud. Prof. Zabol.* **xi**, 20-25.
28. Alekseeva, O.G., Volkova, A.O. and Svinkina, N.V. (1966). *Farmakol. Toksikol.* **iii**, 353-355.
29. Chiappino, G., Barbiano di Belgiojoso, G. and Cirla, A.M. (1968). *Boll. Ist. Sieroter. Milan* **47**, 669-677.
30. Chiappino, G., Cirla, A.M. and Vigliani, E.C. (1969). *Arch. Pathol.* **87**, 131-140.
31. Cirla, A.M., Barbiano di Belgiojoso, G. and Chiappino, G. (1968). *Boll. Ist. Sieroter. Milan* **47**, 663-668.
32. Vorwald, A.J. (1949). *Occup. Med.* **5**, 684-689.
33. Shelley, W.B. and Hurley, H.J. (1958). *Brit. J. Dermatol.* **70**, 75-101.
34. Hart, B.A. and Pittman, D.G. (1980). *J. Reticuloendothel. Soc.* **27**, 49-58.
35. Kang, K.Y. and Salvaggio, J. (1976). *Med. J. Osaka Univ.* **27**, 47-58.
36. Skilleter, D.N. and Price, R.J. (1978). *Chem. Biol. Interact.* **20**, 383-396.
37. Skilleter, D.N. and Price, R.J. (1979). *Biochem. Pharmacol.* **28**, 3595-3599.
38. Skilleter, D.N. and Price, R.J. (1981). *Toxicol. Appl. Pharmacol.* **59**, 279-286.
39. Dinsdale, D. (1982). *Brit. J. Exp. Pathol.* **63**, 103-108.
40. Skilleter, D.N. and Price, R.J. (1980). *Arch. Toxicol.* **45**, 75-80.
41. Firket, H. (1953). *Compt. Rend. Soc. Biol.* **147**, 167.
42. Vorwald, A.J. and Reeves, A.L. (1959). *Arch. Ind. Health* **19**, 190-199.
43. Truhaut, R., Festy, B. and LeTalaer, J.Y. (1968). *Compt. Rend. Acad. Sci. Ser. B.* **266**, 1192-1145.
44. Chèvremont, M. and Firket, H. (1951). *Nature* **167**, 772.

45. Witschi, H.P. (1970). *Biochem. J.* **120**, 623-634.
46. Luke, M.Z., Hamilton, L. and Hollocher, T.C. (1975). *Biochem. Biophys. Res. Comm.* **62**, 497-501.
47. Sirover, M.A. and Loeb, L.A. (1976). *Proc. Nat. Acad. Sci.* **73**, 2331-2335.
48. Hardy, H.L. (1963). *Ann. N.Y. Acad. Sci.* **107**, 525-538.
49. Sneddon, I.B. (1955). *Brit. Med. J.* **1**, 1448-1450.
50. Oppenheim, J.J. (1968). *Fed. Proc.* **27**, 21-28.
51. Hanifin, J.M., Epstein, W.L. and Cline, M.J. (1970). *J. Invest. Dermatol.* **55**, 284-288.
52. Deodhar, S.D., Barna, B. and Van Ordstrand, H.S. (1973). *Chest* **63**, 309-313.
53. Preuss, O.P., Deodhar, S.D. and Van Ordstrand, H.S. (1980). In "Sarcoidosis and other Granulomatous Diseases" (Eds. W. Jones Williams and B.H. Davies), pp.711-714. Alpha Omega, Cardiff.
54. Williams, W.R. and Jones Williams, W. (1982). *Int. Arch. Allergy* **67**, 175-180.
55. Van Ganse, W.F., Oleffe, J., Van Hove, W. and Groetenbriel, C. (1972). *Lancet* **i**, 1023.
56. Jones, J.M. and Amos, H.E. (1974). *Int. Arch. Allergy* **46**, 161-171.
57. Jones, J.M. and Amos, H.E. (1975b). *Nature* **256**, 499-500.
58. Bloom, B.R. and Bennett, B. (1966). *Science* **153**, 80-82.
59. Henderson, W.R., Fukuyama, K., Epstein, W.L. and Spitler, L.E. (1972). *J. Invest. Dermatol.* **58**, 5-8.
60. Marx, J.J. and Burrell, R. (1973). *J. Immunol.* **11**, 590-598.
61. Jones Williams, W., Grey, J. and Pioli, E.M. (1972a). *Brit. Med. J.* **4**, 175.
62. Jones Williams, W., Grey, J. and Pioli, E.M. (1972b). *Lancet* **ii**, 175.
63. Price, C.D., Pugh, A., Pioli, E.M. and Jones Williams, W. (1976). *Ann. N.Y. Acad. Sci.* **278**, 204-211.
64. Reeves, A.L., Swanborg, R.H., Busby, E.K. and Krivanek, N.D. (1970). In "Inhaled Particles III" (Ed. W.H. Walton), pp.599-608. Unwin Bros., Old Woking.
65. Reeves, A.L., Krivanek, N.D., Busby, E.K. and Swanborg, R.H. (1972). *Internat. Arch. Occup. Health* **29**, 209-220.
66. Reeves, A.L. and Krivanek, N.D. (1974). *Trans. N.Y. Acad. Sci.* **36**, 78-93.
67. Reeves, A.L. (1976). *Ann. Clin. Lab. Sci.* **6**, 256-262.
68. Barna, B.P., Edinger, M., Chiang, T., Gautam, S. and Deodhar, S.D. (1982). *Fed. Proc.* (in press: personal communication).
69. Bencko, V., Pekárek, J., Švejcár, J., Beneš, B., Holuša, R., Hurych, J. and Symon, K. (1979). *Česk. Hyg.* **24**, 109-115.

70. Palazzolo, M.J. (1974). Dissertation, Wayne State University, Detroit.
71. Palazzolo, M.J. and Reeves, A.L. (1975). *Soc. Tox. Mtg. Abstr.* **14**, 13.
72. Salvin, S.B., Nishio, J. and Cribik, M. (1970). *Cellular Immunol.* **1**, 62-77.
73. Polak, L., Barnes, J.M. and Turk, J.L. (1968). *Immunology* **14**, 707-711.
74. Salvaggio, J.E., Flax, M.H. and Leskowitz, S. (1965). *J. Immunol.* **95**, 846-854.
75. Belman, S. (1963). *J. Am. Chem. Soc.* **85**, 2154-2159.
76. Belman, S. (1969). *J. Occup. Med.* **11**, 175-183.
77. Preuss, O.P. (1975). In "Occupational Medicine" (Ed. C. Zenz), pp.619-635. Yearbook Med. Pubs., Chicago.
78. Turk, J.L. and Polak, L. (1969). *G. Ital. Dermatol.* **44**, 426-430.
79. Waksman, B.H. (1959). *Arch. Ind. Health* **19**, 154-156.
80. Battisto, J.R. and Chase, M.W. (1955). *Bacteriol. Proc.* **55**, 94-95.
81. Van Ordstrand, H.S., Hughes, R., DeNardi, J.M. and Carmody, M.G. (1945). *J. Am. Med. Assoc.* **129**, 1084-1090.
82. Dutra, F.R. (1951). *Arch. Indust. Hyg. Occup. Med.* **3**, 81-89.
83. Marradi Fabroni, S. (1935). *Med. Lavoro* **26**, 297-303.
84. Gelman, I. (1936). *J. Ind. Hyg.* **18**, 371-379.
85. Van Ordstrand, H.S., Hughes, R. and Carmody, M.G. (1943). *Cleveland Clin. Quart.* **10**, 10-18.
86. Hardy, H.L. and Tabershaw, I.R. (1946). *J. Ind. Hyg.* **28**, 197-211.
87. Gardner, L.U. and Heslington, H.F. (1946). *Fed. Proc.* **5**, 221.
88. Vorwald, A.J., Pratt, P.C. and Urban, E.J. (1955). *Acta Unio Internat. Contra Cancrum* **11**, 735.
89. Reeves, A.L. (1978). In "Inorganic and Nutritional Aspects of Cancer" (Ed. G.N. Schrauzer), pp.13-27. Plenum, New York.
90. Janes, J.M., Higgins, G.M. and Herrick, J.F. (1956). *J. Bone and Joint Surg.* **38A**, 809-816.
91. Infante, P.F., Wagoner, J.K. and Sprince, N.L. (1980). *Environ. Res.*
92. Mancuso, T.F. (1980). *Environ, Res.* **21**, 48-55.
93. Wagoner, J.K., Infante, P.F. and Bayliss, D.L. (1980). *Environ. Res.* **21**, 15-34.
94. Science News Story (1977). **198**, 898-901.
95. Science News Story (1981). **211**, 556-557.

HYPERSENSITIVITY REACTIONS INDUCED BY ANAESTHETIC DRUGS AND PLASMA SUBSTITUTES: INFLUENCE OF PARADIGMS ON INCIDENCE AND MECHANISMS*

W. Lorenz

*Department of Theoretical Surgery,
Centre of Operative Medicine I,
University of Marburg (Lahn), Federal Republic of Germany*

DIFFICULTIES ASSOCIATED WITH THE CLASSIFICATION OF ADVERSE REACTIONS TO ANAESTHETIC DRUGS AND PLASMA SUBSTITUTES AS EITHER HYPERSENSITIVITY REACTIONS OR PSEUDO-ALLERGIC REACTIONS

The involvement of the immune system in adverse reactions to anaesthetic agents and plasma substitutes is not easily demonstrated in clinical conditions. Hypersensitivity reactions [1] and pseudo-allergic reactions [2] can be elicited in different subjects by the same drug (Table 1), although the clinical signs are similar and indistinguishable by a large number of observers [3]. In addition, several exposures to the drug may change the mechanism of the adverse reaction in the same individual. Barbiturates, for instance, can induce a type I pseudo-allergic reaction on first exposure [4], but a type I hypersensitivity reaction after a series of administrations [5]. As, however, pseudo-allergic reactions can be enhanced by high levels of IgE [6], adverse reactions to anaesthetic agents very often cannot be definitely related to the activation of the immune system. The statement of Coombs and Gell 1 should always be considered: "It is an easy error to assume that when one process is demonstrable (e.g. antibody formation against organ antigens), that this and only this is responsible for the whole trouble, or indeed any of it".

However, despite the fact that adverse reactions to

* Supported by grant of Deutsche Forschungsgemeinschaft
(Lo 199/13-6)

IMMUNOTOXICOLOGY
ISBN 0-12-282180-7

Table 1 *Analysis of the mechanisms of adverse reactions to intravenous anaesthetic drugs and plasma substitutes*

A series of tests was performed with plasma of a patient suffering from an adverse reaction to the particular drug. It includes measurement of the consumption and conversion of complement C3 and C4, determination of C3PA and C1 inhibitor level, and estimation of IgE concentration in sequential samples obtained from the subject following the reaction. From Watkins, [5].

		Cases reported	Mechanism analysis possible	Complement involved Classical*	Complement involved Alternative	IgE involved	Probably pharmaco-logical
1974	Althesin	19	5	1	4	2/5	0/5
	Thiopentone	1	0	0	0	0	0
	Methohexitone	1	1	0	1	1/1	0/1
1975	Althesin	16	7	3	4	2/7	0/7
	Propanidid	1	0	0	0	0	0
	Thiopentone	1	1	0	0	0/1	0/1
1976	Althesin	15	12	4	6	1/10	2/12
	Propanidid	2	2	0	2	0/2	0/2
	Thiopentone	2	2	1	1	2/2	0/2
1977	Althesin	12	11	1	5	0/11	5/11
	Thiopentone	6	5	3	1	4/5	0/5
	Dextran	4	2	0	2	0/2	0/2
1978	Althesin	20	18	2	14	1/18	3/18
	Thiopentone	10	9	1	2	2/9	4/9
	Haemaccel	1	1	0	0	0/1	0/1

* Implied immunological memory, often with excessive C3 feedback.

anaesthetic agents and plasma substitutes constitute complex
allergic and pseudo-allergic phenomena, they should be considered in immunotoxicology. These adverse reactions are
clinically relevant [7-11] and in most cases involve stimulation of mast cells which can be regarded as part of the
immune system.

The most common mediator secreted from mast cells is the
biogenic amine histamine. It is released both by allergic
and pseudo-allergic reactions. The measurement of histamine
in patients suffering from adverse reactions to drugs therefore seems to contribute only little to the classification of
these clinical syndromes. However, the development of highly
sensitive and specific plasma histamine assays in man [12-14]
has been rather successful in this particular field provided
quantitative and not qualitative criteria are used for clinical decision making [15]. It is one of the aims of this
presentation to establish mechanisms based on the measurement
of mediators.

PARADIGMS INFLUENCING THE INCIDENCE OF ADVERSE REACTIONS TO ANAESTHETIC DRUGS AND PLASMA SUBSTITUTES

If we are interested in elucidating the mechanisms of adverse
reactions to drugs, we should first know whether we include
all of them or only a relatively small portion. The absolute
number or incidence of clinical observations, however, depends
very strongly on the picture we have of the "disease" [3].
The "syndrome" is not just the simple product of a series of
inductive inferences, but well mixed with hypotheses such as
why should an "anaphylactic reaction" offer a certain cluster
of clinical signs and changes in laboratory parameters?
These hypotheses are derived from work in isolated cells,
animals and human subjects, and the entire scientific picture
is best portrayed as a paradigm according to Kuhn [16].

We were very surprised to see how strongly two different
paradigms influenced the incidence of adverse reactions to
anaesthetics and plasma substitutes (Fig. 1).

The first paradigm which describes the present "standard
opinion" covers the adverse reactions of skin responses,
hypotension and bronchospasms. Of these adverse reactions,
skin responses must be considered the most important, as
cardiovascular and respiratory symptoms are so common in
anaesthesia and surgery and therefore judged as rather un-
specific.

In the second paradigm as a transformation [16] of the first
one (Fig. 1), any clinical sign occurring early after drug
administration is accepted as an indication for a pseudo-
allergic (anaphylactoid) or hypersensitivity reaction. A

Paradigm 1

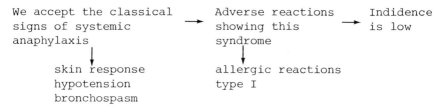

Paradigm 2

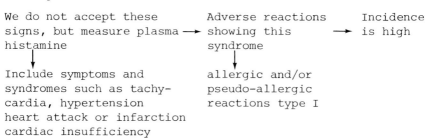

Fig. 1 Influence of paradigms on the incidence of adverse reactions to anaesthetic drugs and plasma substitutes. For illustrations of this problem see the text dealing with polygeline and the review of Lorenz et al. [20].

series of such symptoms has been described by Ring [17] in Fig. 29 of his monograph of adverse reactions to plasma proteins and dextran and by Lorenz et al. [3] for histamine-release responses to polygeline (Haemaccel(R)). If each of these symptoms is used as a single indication of "disease" (independently from the others), then far too many "reactions" are diagnosed. The sensitivity of such a procedure is high, but the specificity low. However, the latter can be improved by the measurement of mediators (especially histamine). This biogenic amine can now be determined with convenience [18] and high reliability [15] in human plasma.

Clinicians who accept the first paradigm will find only a low incidence of adverse reactions, mainly type I hypersensitivity reactions (Fig. 1). Those, however who accept the second paradigm will detect a high incidence of both type I hypersensitivity reactions and type I pseudo-allergic reactions. To illustrate these rather theoretical reflections, the results of several clinical trials on polygeline have been compiled (Table 2).

The study of Ring and Messmer [21] was a multicentre trial

Table 2 *Incidence of adverse reactions to polygeline: comparison of five clinical trials.*

The studies of Schöning and Koch [9] and Lorenz et al. [23] were carried out in patients, those of Lorenz and Doenicke [15] and Lorenz et al. [24] in human volunteers. The trial of Ring and Messmer [21] was a multicentre study, some details of which are described in the text. From Lorenz et al. [20].

Number of infusions (n_1)	Number of infusions complicated by reactions (n_2)	Incidence (n_1/n_2) (%)	Trial
6151	9	0.15	Ring and Messmer [21]
150	45	30	Schöning and Koch [9]
25	9	36	Lorenz et al. [24]
40	21	53	Lorenz and Doenicke [15]
600	187	31	Lorenz et al. [23]

in 31 Southern German hospitals. All anaphylactoid reactions which the clinicians observed in 1975 and reported spontaneously to the coordinators were registered and analyzed. In the year of the study, the vast majority of doctors accepted paradigm 1 which they had acquired during graduation and clinical training. Very probably they reported only those reactions occurring during their routine work which resembled the classical syndrome of systemic or local anaphylaxis. The incidence of anaphylactoid reactions to polygeline (Haemaccel) was only 0.15%.

Paradigm 2 was created in several controlled clinical trials [3]. Exogenous histamine was injected into human volunteers in a dose (600 ng/kg) which elevated plasma histamine levels to the same extent as an average histamine-release response to the plasma substitute polygeline or to several anaesthetic drugs [22]. Polygeline was infused into volunteers and patients and the set of clinical indications with the highest incidence ratio were used to define the adverse reaction elicited in conscious human subjects (Table 3). Applying paradign 2 (Fig. 1), the incidence of hypersensitivity

Table 3 *Clinical signs and plasma histamine level in a systemic type I allergic or pseudo-allergic reaction (SAR) in conscious human subjects.*

Values obtained from three controlled clinical trials in volunteers and patients receiving exogenous histamine and polygeline (Haemaccel) in its now outdated formulation. From Lorenz et al. [3].

Group of subjects	Indicants for SAR	Incidence ratio (%)
Volunteers after i.v. histamine injection	Tachycardia	97
	Plasma histamine > 1 ng/ml	78
	"Metallic" taste	75
	Flush	69
	Congestion of head	67
	"Wet eyes", tears	64
	Hypertension	58
	Headache	58
Volunteers with SAR following Haemaccel (R)	Plasma histamine > 1 ng/ml	93
	Tachycardia	83
	Wheals	58
	Sensation of heat	50
	Narrowness of throat	50
	Hypertension	50
	Headache	42
	"Wet eyes", tears	42
Patients with SAR following Haemaccel (R)	Tachycardia	93
	Plasma histamine >1 ng/ml	87
	Erythema	70
	Wheals	60
	Cough	50
	Flush	43
	Stuffy nose	30
	Facial oedema	30

reactions and/or pseudo-allergic reactions to polygeline was about 200 to 300 times higher than in the multicentre trial (Table 2). Similar findings were obtained with several anaesthetic drugs such as propanidid, althesin and thiopentone [5]. The incidence of adverse reactions which demand treatment are now in the order of magnitude of 0.5 to 1%. As several million administrations are recorded every year, the clinical relevance of the problem is obvious.

INVOLVEMENT OF MAST CELLS IN VARIOUS TISSUES IN ADVERSE REACTIONS TO ANAESTHETIC DRUGS AND PLASMA SUBSTITUTES

Adverse reactions to several anaesthetic drugs and plasma substitutes involves the stimulation of mast cells which play an important role in type I hypersensitivity reactions by binding IgE at the Fc-receptors of their plasma membrane. Histamine secretion and mast cell degranulation by these drugs can best be demonstrated in dogs since many tissues and blood from several circulatory regions can easily be obtained during the reactions or immediately after the death of the animals [20].

Dogs develop pseudo-allergic reactions to cremophor EL, the solvent of many anaesthetic and hypnotic drugs, on first exposure [25,26], whereas pigs show these reactions on a second exposure about seven days after the first exposure [27]. These reactions correspond very closely to those of many drug combinations in man in which cremophor EL is used as a solubilizer [20,25,26]. The question which cannot be answered yet is whether these adverse reactions are pseudo-allergic reactions, hypersensitivity reactions including antibodies and complement, or a mixture of both.

The tissues from which histamine is released by cremophor EL correspond only partly to those which are also affected in type I hypersensitivity reactions [30] or in pseudo-allergic reactions elicited by the classical histamine liberators such as compound 48/80 [31] (Table 4). The strong histamine release within the skin which is associated with generalized urticaria is observed not only in adverse reactions to cremophor EL, but also in IgE-mediated and 48/80-induced reactions. Mast cells in the liver, however, seem to be only marginally involved, in contrast to anaphylactic reactions and 48/80 intoxication reactions.

The most surprising effect of cremophor EL, however, is exerted on mast cells in the gastrointestinal tract. Histamine is released in gastric and intestinal mucosa and especially in the pancreas and the mast cells disappear as the consequence of degranulation. There is no other known agent that exhibits such a specific and dramatic effect on the mast cell stores of histamine in the gastrointestinal tract [32, 33]. This is reflected in the clinical picture, too, as the animals regularly suffer from immediate diarrhoea.

The cremophor EL-induced adverse reaction in dogs cannot be explained as a type I hypersensitivity reaction on the basis of these findings. Adverse reactions to the anaesthetic agents propanidid, althesin, flunitrazepam and diazepam [20] are either produced by a mechanism in man which is different from that in dogs [5,26] or the adverse reactions in dogs,

Table 4 *Histamine content and mast cell density in several tissues of dogs following treatment with cremophor EL.*

Tissue	Histamine content (µg/g)			Mast cell density (cells/mm^2)		
	NaCl	Cremophor EL	Decrease (%)	NaCl	Cremophor EL	Decrease (%)
Abdominal skin	18.5 ± 7.0	3.2 ± 0.3	83**	86 ± 39	11 ± 3	87**
Liver, parenchyma	41.0 ± 15.3	45.4 ± 16.7	0	85 ± 21	54 ± 14	37*
Diaphragm	12.1 ± 4.7	11.3 ± 4.3	7	–	–	–
M. quadriceps	5.4 ± 2.2	3.7 ± 0.9	32	–	–	–
Gastric mucosa						
– fundus	101 ± 15	81 ± 22	20	156 ± 6	79 ± 36	51**
– corpus	117 ± 37	102 ± 24	13	111 ± 38	68 ± 27	39*
– antrum	69 ± 25	44 ± 18	36*	125 ± 17	45 ± 15	64**
Jejunum	145 ± 26	88 ± 21	39**	123 ± 10	66 ± 33	46**
Ileum	84 ± 17	57 ± 19	32*	–	–	–
Colon	77 ± 19	49 ± 18	37*	–	–	–
Pancreas	11.4 ± 3.6	2.8 ± 2.1	75**	–	–	–

– = not determined. $\bar{x}$ + S.D. (n = 6).   Student t-test: * p < 0.05, ** p < 0.005

pigs and human subjects are caused by the same mechanism in
many of the cases. The definition of these reactions as type I
pseudo-allergic reactions would then be most appropriate, in
the present state of our knowledge. To investigate this concept we have studied a number of the components of cremophor
EL (Fig. 2). The original data can be studied in our previous
communications [25,26], but a qualitative analysis of the
effects on blood pressure and histamine release are compiled
in Table 5. From these data is has to be concluded that the
effect of cremophor EL and its components to induce type I
pseudo-allergic reactions is connected with distinct chemical
features: the most potent compounds are oxethylated and
additionally esterified, unsaturated or hydroxylated fatty
acids [26]. 12-Hydroxystearinic acid was a less toxic compound than cremophor EL in our studies in dogs, and this has
been confirmed in large trials in cattle, which showed considerably less reactions to vitamins dissolved in oxethylated
12-hydroxystearinic acid than to vitamins dissolved in
cremophor EL [34].

Legend to Table 4 (opposite)

Histamine values (mean ± S.D.) as histamine dihydrochloride.
For the experiments in conscious dogs, 6 pairs of animals
(14-22 kg, both sexes) were chosen as pairs of the same litter
to reduce biological variation. One animal of the pair was
treated by 0.1 ml/kg cremophor EL administered i.v. into a
fore-paw vein once a day for three days (B), the other dog
received saline in the same volume as cremophor EL and under
the same circumstances (A). The dogs received ear clips and
were allocated to the two treatment groups by simple random-
ization with random digits. Only two dogs (treatments AA,
AB, or BB) were used for one experiment. One hour after the
last injection, and following pentobaritone anaesthesia, the
animals were killed by arterial bleeding and aliquots of
tissue removed quickly for histamine assay and estimation of
mast cell density according to Lorenz et al. [28]. For count-
ing the cells, three different methods of fixation (lead acetate, Susa and Carnoy solution) were applied, but staining
with toluidine blue was always accomplished at pH 4.0. There
was no significant difference between the number of cells
counted after the three fixation procedures. Data collected
from Lorenz et al. [29].
- = not determined. Student's t-test for means of two independent samples: * < 0.05, ** < 0.005.

Table 5 *Qualitative analysis of hypotensive and histamine-releasing actions of solubilizing agents and fatty acids*

Group of solubilizing agents and fatty acids	Data arranged in classes[a]	
	Hypotension (0 - +++)	Histamine release (incidence $\geq$ 10 ng/ml)
Preparations of cremophor EL		
Cremophor EL (several batches[b])	+++	8/8
Mulgophen EL (technical quality[c])	+++	8/8
Cremophor EL (purified[d])	+++	8/8
Components of cremophor EL and Tween 80		
Hydrophilic components	0	0/8
Glycerol, polyglycol ethers[e]	0	0/8
Hydrophobic components[f]	+++	8/8
Unreacted castor oil	0	0/8
Unreacted ricinoleic acid	++	1/8
Unreacted oleic acid	++	0/8
Unreacted esters of ricinoleic acid and oleic acid	?	?
All oxethylated products of the hydrophobic part	?	?
Oxethylated ricinoleic acid	+++	0/8
Oxethylated glycerol esters of ricinoleic acid	?	?
Oxethylated oleic acid	+++	3/8
Oxethylated glycerol, monooleate ester	+++	8/8
Tween 80 (oxethylated sorbitol oleate esters)[g]	+++	8/8
Chemically modified components of cremophor EL		
Hydrogenated, oxethylated castor oil (Arlatone G)	+++	8/8
Hydrogenated, oxethylated castor oil (RH 40)[h]	+++	8/8
Hydrophilic components of RH 40	0	0/8
Hydrophobic components of RH 40	+++	8/8
12-Hydroxysteric acid (HSA)[i]	+++	0/8
Oxethylated 12-HSA (several batches)	++	1/8
Oxethylated 12-HSA (bleached)	+++	7/8
Oxethylated glycerol esters of 12-HSA	?	?
9(10)-HSA[j]	?	?
Oxethylated 9(10)-HSA	+++	2/8
Oxethylated glycerol esters of 9(10)-HSA	+++	8/8
Detergents on a non-fatty acid base		
Lensodel NP 40	+++	0/8
Lutensol AP 10	+++	0/8
1-*n*-propoxy-2-hydroxypropane	++	0/8
1-methoxy-2-hydroxybutane	+	0/8
Pluronic F 68	0	0/8

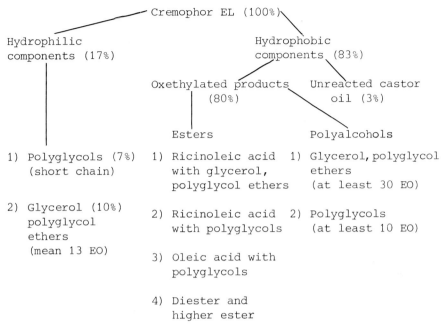

Fig. 2 Composition of the solubilizer cremophor EL.
EO = ethylene oxide (from Lorenz *et al.* [25])

Legend to Table 5 (opposite)

^a Arrangement in classes. Hypotension 0 = no hypotension,
+ = 1-30, ++ = 31-60, +++ $\geq$ 61 mmHg. This classification
was chosen as blood pressure responses were observed quite
regularly. Histamine release was quantitated by its incidence of clinically relevant responses ($\geq$ 10 ng/ml increase
in whole blood histamine levels); this criterion appeared
best for discrimination.

^b Several batches of cremophor EL produced since 1970 were
shown to be rather similar in their toxicity [26].

^c Technical quality means very crude quality.

^d Purification by extraction procedures.

^e Oxethylated glycerol.

^f Micellophor^(R) = ORPE [22].

^g Tween 80 is also a mixture of various compounds. The en-
hancement of histamine release by sorbitol as ligand instead
of glycerol was remarkable [25].

^h Cremophor RH 40 consists mainly of esters of 12-hydroxy-
stearic acid. Arlatone G contains 25 EO, RH 40 contains
45 EO.

ⁱ Derived from ricinoleic acid.

^j Derived from oleic acid.

[?] Not investigated.

Dogs also develop type I pseudo-allergic reactions to the plasma substitute polygeline (Haemaccel) [35]. The tissues from which histamine is released in these reactions are very similar to those which are affected in type I hypersensitivity reactions or during intoxication with compound 48/80 (Table 6). No distinction can be made between allergic and pseudo-allergic reactions to Haemaccel by studying the involvement of mast cells in various tissues in adverse reactions to this drug.

Table 6 *Histamine content in canine tissues following treatment with polygeline (Haemaccel).*

Histamine values (mean ± S.D.) as histamine dihydrochloride. Statistical evaluation of the t-test for paired data.
* $p < 0.05$. The increase of the histamine content in the ileum is explained by histamine up-take under the circumstances of the experiment. (From Lorenz et al. [36]).

Tissue	Histamine content ($\mu g/g$)		Changes
	before infusion	after infusion	(±%)
Skin, neck	36.2 ± 18.0	27.6 ± 14.5	−24*
abdomen	30.5 ± 15.2	15.6 ± 12.4	−49*
Muscle, diaphragm	18.1 ± 13.8	12.2 ± 10.6	−33*
Stomach, fundus	90.5 ± 38.2	91.2 ± 40.7	0
corpus	66.0 ± 27.1	62.9 ± 21.8	−5
antrum	45.7 ± 15.9	41.3 ± 11.7	−10
Ileum	45.8 ± 8.5	65.7 ± 18.0	+43*
Liver	66.6 ± 24.7	36.2 ± 17.0	−46*
Lung	45.6 ± 21.4	47.8 ± 25.1	+5

THE ATOPIC STATUS — AN EPIPHENOMENON IN ADVERSE REACTIONS TO ANAESTHETIC AGENTS?

In about 50% of incidents (Table 7), the adverse reactions to barbiturates, especially thiopentone, are likely to be caused by type I hypersensitivity reactions [5,10,37]. This very plausible hypothesis is well founded by several findings. Reactions to thiopentone were observed very often in patients who received the drug several times for induction of anaesthesia [5,37,38]. The patients showed a history of atopy [38] which was supported in about half of them by elevated serum IgE levels exceeding the upper limit of the normal

Table 7 *Reaction mechanisms in "immediate" adverse reactions involving two commonly used anaesthetic drugs (Sheffield study for 1974-1980). From Watkins* [37]

Drug	No. of cases	Idiosyncratic reactions involving:			
		Antibody	Complement (all pathways)	Complement (C3) alone	Pharmacological reasons
Althesin	75	25(33%)	61(81%)	35(47%)	15(20%)
Thiopentone	40	20(50%)	12(30%)	3(7%)	17(43%)

range (200 i.u./ml) [5]. Intradermal testing was conducted in many of these patients [39,40]. Positive results were obtained in a variety of them using both the Prausnitz-Küstner test in human subjects and the PCA test in monkeys [40].

However, about 40% of the reactions to thiopentone seemed to be elicited by pharmacological actions of the drug involving neither antibodies nor complement consumption and conversion (Table 7). This finding is supported by results obtained in human volunteers in whom plasma histamine levels [41], or stimulation of gastric acid secretion as an *in vivo* test for histamine release, were measured. The incidence of histamine-release responses to thiopentone and methohexitone was 90 and 75%, respectively (Fig. 3).

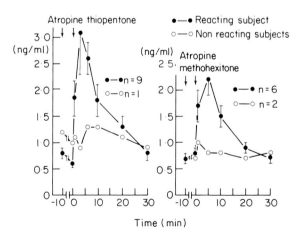

Fig. 3 Histamine release in human volunteers following i.v. administration of thiopentone and methohexitone. x̄ ± S.E.M., O = time of injection. Histamine values as histamine base/ml plasma. From Lorenz and Doenicke [41].

Paradigm 1:

A subject with atopic
status (case history,   Plasma histamine
total IgE in serum   > 1 ng/ml,   Type I hypersensi-
> 200 i.u./ml) has an → several exposures → tivity reaction to
anaphylactoid reaction   to the drug   thiopentone
to thiopentone

Paradigm 2:

The same findings as   Type I pseudo-
in (1), but thio-   The same findings _ allergic reaction
pentone releases   → as in (1)   ‾ to thiopentone,
histamine in "normal"   enhanced by an
subjects directly   atopic status

**Fig. 4 Influence of paradigms on the mechanism of adverse
reactions to barbiturates.** For illustration of this problem
see text in section on The Atopic Status — an Epiphenomenon
in Adverse Reactions to Anaesthetic Agents?

If we apply the Coombs-Gell statement in the first para-
graph of this article to the observations collected here it
seems reasonable to ask whether the atopic status may just
be an epiphenomenon in adverse reactions to anaesthetic
agents. Two paradigms form the background for the arguments
(Fig. 4) which are complementary to each other and may nevertheless both be true. Support for the second paradigm comes
from animal experiments which are compiled in an excellent
review of Stanworth [42] and the Ph.D. thesis of Sydbom [6]:
"Immunization increased the spontaneous histamine release
and the sensitivity to other non-immunological stimuli, such
as phosphatidylserine and changed the cyclic nucleotide
status". It is supported by experiments with human lung *in
vitro* [43]. According to the second paradigm (Fig. 4) the
adverse reactions to barbiturates are considered as type I
pseudo-allergic reactions enhanced by an atopic status. Is
amplification an epiphenomenon? Very probably not. But
this discussion demonstrates how complex the situation is.

ELUCIDATION OF MECHANISMS VIA MEASUREMENT OF MEDIATORS

Since the discoveries of Lewis [44] and Dale [45] it was a
paradigm to associate histamine with allergic reactions.
However, when serotonin, slow-reacting substance of anaphylaxis (SRS-A), kallidin and bradykinin, prostaglandins and
leukotrienes were found to mimic inflammatory and hypersensitivity responses in various pharmacological systems, it

Table 8 *Biologically active substances (AS) which may be in-*
volved as mediators in allergic and pseudo-allergic reactions.
5-HT serotonin, ECF-A eosinophil chemotactic factor of anaphylaxis, NCF-A neutrophil chemotactic factor of anaphylaxis, PAF
platelet-activating factor.

AS acting at receptors	Histamine, catecholamines, 5-HT, kinins, anaphylatoxins, leuko-trienes, ECF-A, NCF-A, PAF, prosta-glandins, thromboxanes, tachykinins (e.g. substance P)
Releaser or former of AS	Anaphylatoxins (C3a, C4a, C5a), arginine esterase, Cl-esterase, kallikreins
Stimulator or modulator of second-messenger systems	Acetylcholine, ATP, cyclic nucleo-tides, Ca^{2+}

became a paradigm *not* to assign any distinct pathological
function to histamine or any of the other mediators in question (Table 8) [46].

The development of highly sensitive and specific histamine
assays in tissue and body fluids (for a review see [47] and
the discovery of histamine H_2-receptor antagonists by Black
et al. [48] created a new paradigm [49]:

Plasma histamine determination led to a much better
understanding of histamine-induced reactions in human
subjects than other techniques and — which is a most
important advantage — increase the possibility to
differentiate between histamine-induced reactions and
anaphylactoid reactions caused by other mediators.

The earlier suggestion that histamine might be involved in
all types of "allergic" reactions induced a histamine philos-
ophy. Differentiation, however, gives histamine its place at
least in human pathophysiology.

Applying the new paradigm to studies on the mechanisms of
allergic and pseudo-allergic drug reactions we were surprised
to recognize how much it influenced their interpretation
(Fig. 5). There are plenty of data which demonstrate histamine release by antigen-antibody reaction involving IgE at the
mast cell surface, but these data do not unequivocally include
measurements in man *in vivo*. From studies in whole animals
[30,50,51], it is evident that type I hypersensitivity reactions involving reaginic antibodies release large amounts of

Paradigm 1:

	Plasma histamine	Allergic reactions
IgE, C3a and C5a	highly elevated	type I-III to poly-
release histamine →	following poly- →	geline, pseudo-
	geline, but not	allergic reaction
	after dextran	to dextran

Paradigm 2:

IgE releases con-		Type I allergic
siderable amounts		reaction or pseudo-
of histamine,	Findings as in (1)	allergic reaction
C3a and C5a only →	→	to polygeline
small amounts		type III allergic
in vivo		reaction to dextran

**Fig. 5 Influence of paradigms on identifying mechanisms of
adverse drug reaction via measurement of histamine.** For
illustration of this figure see text in section on elucidation
of mechanisms via measurement of mediator.

histamine *in vivo* and it is reasonable to suggest that this
also happens in man.

However, such evidence cannot be provided for histamine
release by complement. Anaphylatoxins are potent histamine
liberators from human basophils *in vitro* and from human skin
when injected locally (for review see Stanworth [42], but it
remains uncertain whether they do so' *in vivo*, i.e. when they
are generated in the systemic circulation. Studies in whole
animals suggests that complement activation and formation of
anaphylatoxins release smaller amounts of histamine in guinea-
pigs than antigen-antibody reactions involving reaginic antibodies [50,51]. Actually, no histamine release at all was
measurable in aggregate anaphylaxis in the monkey (type III
allergic reaction) when two of the new specific assays for
plasma histamine are used [52]. It is conceivable that
anaphylatoxins are rapidly inactivated by enzymes in plasma
(carboxypeptidase B-like enzymes or amino peptidase activities
[42] which lower their efficiency *in vivo*. Very similar findings were obtained with kinins which are potent histamine
releasers *in vitro* [53], but were rather ineffective in the
whole dog [54]. Kallikrein which decreased the blood pressure
for a long time did not show any significant histamine
release.

The consequences of paradigms 1 and 2 with regard to histamine release by complement *in vivo* (Fig. 5) are very remarkable. For polygeline (Haemaccel) which released considerable
amounts of histamine in patients *in vivo* [3], allergic

reactions type I-III could not be excluded by paradigm 1. In addition, a type III allergic reaction to dextran could not be suggested as this reaction would include complement activation and, as a consequence of this, a measurable histamine release. This, however, could not be shown in volunteers and patients with clinical reactions — even in a lethal case [20, 55]. Paradigm 2 alters the possibilities to interpret the mechanisms of adverse reactions to the two plasma substitutes. Only two likely pathways remain for polygeline, and for dextran the type III allergic reaction cannot be excluded, and this is the most likely explanation for a number of other reasons (see next section).

ELUCIDATION OF MECHANISMS VIA ANIMAL MODELS — FALSE-POSITIVE AND FALSE-NEGATIVE ASSOCIATIONS

As systemic type I hypersensitivity reactions and pseudoallergic reactions always carry the risk of a life-threatening clinical situation, animal models were desired in which the mechanisms of adverse drug reactions could be studied with more reliability than in man.

For anaesthetic drugs dissolved in cremophor EL or the Tweens, the dog model [26] and pig model [26] have already been mentioned. Both models differ from the clinical situation since cremophor EL did not release histamine in man except in combination with some other drugs [8,20,26]. However, there are also striking similarities, including the fact that cremophor EL is necessary both in animals and in man to elicit a substantial histamine release, and that some reactions in patients occur on first exposure as in the dog model and on second exposure as in the pig model.

With respect to plasma substitutes, models in several species have also been developed. Polygeline (Haemaccel) was successfully studied in dogs [35,56] and monkeys [56]. The similarity of the adverse reactions of polygeline in patients and dogs was so great that the animal model could be used to improve the drug. "Purified" polygeline (Haemaccel-35) contains only a slight excess of the cross-linking material hexamethylene diisocyanate over the stoichiometrically necessary amount. It no longer produces immediate systemic adverse reactions in dogs and in patients [56]. The excess of crosslinking material is chemically transformed in blood to hexamethylene diamine which has been shown to be a histamine liberator in dogs (unpublished data). Both in human subjects and in dogs the adverse reaction to polygeline was blocked by premedication with H_1- and H_2-receptor antagonists [15,23,24, 57]. For this reason the dog model proved excellent for the elucidation of the mechanism of Haemaccel-induced adverse

Table 9 *The most likely mechanism of polygeline (Haemaccel)*
induced immediate adverse reactions in man

Polygeline (Haemaccel[R])
Type I pseudo-allergic reaction by direct release of histamine

- about 30% of individuals show reactions, severity dose-
  dependent, frequency distribution of histamine values
  corresponding to one population

- depending on the amount of cross-linking material.
  Haemaccel-35 free of systemic responses

- reactions completely prevented by H_1- + H_2-receptor
  antagonists (even urticaria)

- no correlation between reactions and antigelatin titres

- findings in man in agreement with those in dogs

reactions. All arguments compiled in Table 9 support the
hypothesis that polygeline (Haemaccel) elicits adverse reactions by a type I pseudo-allergic reaction by direct (chemical,
pharmacological) histamine release [56].

Dextran was also successfully studied in dogs [58]. An
"aggregate anaphylaxis" (type III allergic reaction) could be
elicited in this species by a dextran-protein conjugate and
could be prevented by monovalent hapten. In contrast to this
reaction in dogs, dextran unequivocally produces a type I
pseudo-allergic reaction in rats, including a massive histamine
release. This reaction, however, has never been demonstrated
in any adverse reaction to dextran, neither in human volunteers nor in patients. All arguments compiled in Table 10
support the hypothesis that dextran (Macrodex) elicits adverse
reactions by a type III allergic reaction including complexes
between dextran and IgG antibodies [58].

SUMMARY

The involvement of the immune system in adverse reactions to
anaesthetic agents and plasma substitutes in man is not easily
demonstrated. Hypersensitivity reactions and pseudo-allergic
reactions can be elicited by the same drug in different individuals, such as by propanidid, althesin, thiopentone and
other barbiturates. In addition, several exposures to the
drug may change the mechanism of drug reaction in the same
individual, although the clinical picture cannot be distinguished. In adverse reactions to dextran and gelatin, the

Table 10 *The most likely mechanism of dextran (Macrodex)-
induced immediate adverse reactions in man*

Dextran (Macrodex[R])
Type III allergic reaction including complexes between dextran and IgG antibodies

- no significant histamine release, consistent with findings in monkey "aggregate anaphylaxis"

- intensity of reactions largely proportional to the level of circulating precipitating antibody

- findings in man in agreement with those in dogs, but not in rats (pseudo-allergic reaction including massive histamine release)

mechanisms of drug response are the subject of considerable controversy. As polygeline is a chemically modified poly-peptide, hypersensitivity reactions are expected to occur but evidence in animals and man strongly confirms a pseudo-allergic mechanism (pharmacologically-induced histamine re-lease). Dextran is assumed to cause anaphylactoid reactions by releasing histamine as shown in rats, but in man, monkey and dog, circulating immunocomplexes seem to cause hyper-sensitivity reactions (type III) without histamine release. Cremophor EL as the solvent for anaesthetic agents seems to elicit pseudo-allergic reactions as shown in dogs and hyper-sensitivity reactions including a short-term memory of only one to two weeks as shown in pigs. In man, both types of reactions can be observed. In the development of new anaes-thetic agents it is mandatory to avoid as far as possible cremophor EL as a solubilizer. New detergents have to be developed which show a markedly reduced toxicity.

REFERENCES

1. Coombs, R.R.A. and Gell, P.G.H. (1975). In "Clinical Aspects of Immunology" (Eds. P.G.H. Gell, R.R.A. Coombs and P.J. Lachmann). 3rd edn, pp.761-781. Blackwell Scientific Publications, Oxford.
2. Dukor, P., Kallós, P., Schlumberger, H.D. and West, G.B. (1980). In "PAR, Pseudo-Allergic Reactions. Involvement of Drugs and Chemicals" Vol.1, pp.1-307. S. Karger, Basel.
3. Lorenz, W., Doenicke, A., Schöning, B., Ohmann, Ch., Grote, B. and Neugenauer, E. (1982). *Klin. Wochenschrift* **60**, 896-913.

4. Lorenz, W., Doenicke, A., Leier, R., Reimann, H.-J.,
    Kusche, J., Barth, H., Geesing, H., Hutzel, M. and
    Weissenbacher, B. (1972). *Eur. J. Pharmacol*. **19**, 180-190.
5. Watkins, J. (1981). In "Adverse Reactions to Anaesthetic
    Drugs" (Ed. J.A. Thornton). Vol.8, pp.137-167. Excerpta
    Medica — Elsevier North Holland Biomedical Press,
    Amsterdam.
6. Sydbom, A. (1982). Anaphylactic histamine release from
    isolated rat mast cells. Methodological and pharmacolog-
    ical studies. Ph.D. thesis, Karolinska Institutet, pp.1-53.
7. Doenicke, A. and Lorenz, W. (1970). *Anaesthetist* **19**,
    413-417.
8. Lorenz, W., Doenicke, A., Meier, R., Reimann, H.-J.,
    Kusche, J., Barth, H., Hutzel, M. and Weissenbacher, B.
    (1972). *Bri. J. Anaesth*. **44**, 355-369.
9. Schöning, B. and Koch, H. (1975). *Anaesthetist* **24**, 507-
    516.
10. Watkins, J., Udnoon, S., Appleyard, T.N. and Thornton, J.A.
    (1976). *Br. J. Anaesth*. **48**, 457-461.
11. Ring, J. and Messmer, K. (1977). *Lancet* **i**, 466-469.
12. Lorenz, W., Benesch, L., Barth, H., Matejka, E., Meier, R.,
    Kusche, J., Hutzel, M. and Werle, E. (1970). *Z. Analyt.
    Chem*. **252**, 94-98.
13. Lorenz, W., Reimann, H.-J., Barth, H., Kusche, J., Meier,
    R., Doenicke, A. and Hutzel, M. (1972). *Hoppe-Seyler's
    Z. Physiol. Chem*. **353**, 911-920.
14. Beaven, M.A., Jacobsen, S. and Horáková, Z. (1972). *Clin.
    Chim. Acta* **37**, 91-103.
15. Lorenz, W. and Doenicke, A. (1978). *Mount Sinai J. Med.*
    45, 357-386.
16. Kuhn, T.H.S. (1970). The structure of scientific revolu-
    tions, 2nd edn, Vol.2, No.2 (Eds. O. Neurath, R. Carnap
    and Ch. Morris). Internat. Enzyklopedia of Unified
    Science, The University of Chicago Press, Chicago.
17. Ring, J. (1978). Anaphylaktoide Reacktionen nach Infusion
    natürlicher und künstlicher Kolloide. In "Anaesthesiology
    and Intensive Care Medicine" Vol.111 (Eds. R. Frey, F. Kern
    and O. Mayrhofer), pp.1-202. Springer Verlag, Berlin.
18. Lorenz, W., Neugebauer, E. and Schmal, A. (1982). *Ann.
    Anesth. Franc*. (in press).
19. Kazimierczak, W. and Diamant, B. (1978). *Progr. Allergy*
    24, 295-365.
20. Lorenz, W., Doenicke, A., Schoning, B. and Neugenauer, E.
    (1981). In "Adverse Reactions of Anaesthetic Drugs"
    Vol.8 (Ed. J.A. Thornton). pp.169-238. Excerpta Medica —
    Elsevier North Holland Biomedical Press, Amsterdam.
21. Ring, J. and Messmer, K. (1977). *Anaesthetist* **26**, 279-287.
22. Doenicke, A., Lorenz, W., Beigl, R., Bezecny, H., Uhlig, G.,

Kalmar, L., Praetorius, B. and Mann, G. (1973). *Br. J. Anaesth.* **45**, 1097-1104.

23. Lorenz, W., Doenicke, A., Schöning, B., Mamorski, J., Weber, D., Hinterlang, E., Schwarz, B. and Neugenauer, E. (1980). *Agents Actions* **10**, 114-124.

24. Lorenz, W., Doenicke, A., Dittmann, I., Hug, P. and Schwartz, B. (1977). *Anaesthetist* **26**, 644-648.

25. Lorenz, W., Reimann, H.-J., Schmal, A., Dormann, P., Schwarz, B. and Neugebauer, E. (1977). *Agents Actions* **7**, 63-67.

26. Lorenz, W., Schmal, A., Schult, H., Lang, S., Ohmann, Ch., Weber, D., Kapp, B., Lüben, L. and Doenicke, A. (1982). *Agents Actions* **12**, 64-80.

27. Glen, J.B., Davies, G.E., Thomson, D.S., Scarth, S.C. and Thomson, A.V. (1979). *Br. J. Anaesth.* **51**, 819-827.

28. Lorenz, W., Schauer, A., Halbach, St., Calvoer, R. and Werle, E. (1969). *Naunyn Schmiedeberg's Arch. Pharm.* **265**, 81-100.

29. Lorenz, W., Thermann, M., Hamelmann, H., Schmal, A., Maroske, D., Reimann, H.-J., Kusche, J., Schingale, F., Dormann, P. and Keck, P. (1973). In "International Symposium on Histamine H -Receptor Antagonists" (Eds. C.J. Wood and M.A. Simkins). pp.151-168. Deltakos (UK Ltd.) London.

30. Rocha e Silva, M. (1966). In "Histamine and Antihistaminics", Part 1 (Eds. M. Rocha e Silva and H.A. Rothschild). Vol.18/1, pp.431-480. Springer Verlag, Berlin.

31. Rothschild, A.M. (1966). In "Histamine and Antihistaminics", Part 1 (Eds. M. Rocha e Silva and H.A. Rothschild). Vol. 18/1, pp.386-430. Springer Verlag, Berlin.

32. Ennis, M. and Pearce, F.L. (1980). *Eur. J. Pharmacol.* **66**, 339-344.

33. Lorenz, W., Parkin, J.V., Rohde, H., Barth, H. Troidl, H., Thon, K., Hinterlang, E., Weber, D., Albrecht, R. and Röher, H. (1981). In "Gastric Secretion — Basic and Clinical Aspects" (Eds. St.J. Konturek and W. Domschke), pp.29-51. Georg Thieme Verlag, Stuttgart.

34. BASF (Personal communication).

35. Messmer, K., Lorenz, W., Sunder-Plassman, L., Klövekorn, W. and Hutzel, M. (1970). *Naunyn Schmiedeberg's Arch. Pharmacol.* **267**, 433-445.

36. Lorenz, W., Thermann, M., Messmer, K., Schmal, A., Dormann, P., Kusche, J., Barth, H., Tauber, R., Hutzel, M., Mann, G. and Uhlig, R. (1974). *Agents Actions* **4**, 336-356.

37. Watkins, J. (1982). In "Trauma, Stress and Immunity" (Eds. J. Watkins and M. Salo). pp.254-291. Butterworth Scientific, London.

38. Clarke, R.S.J. and Dundee, J.W. (1981). In "Adverse

Reactions of Anaesthetic Drugs" (Ed. I.A. Thornton).
Vol.8, pp.30-46. Elsevier-North Holland Biomedical Press,
Amsterdam.

39. Fisher, M. McD. (1978). In "Adverse Response to Intravenous Drugs" (Eds. J. Watkins and A.M. Ward). pp.137-
144. Academic Press, Grune & Stratton, London.

40. Fisher, M. McD. (1980). *Anaesthesiology* **52**, 318-324.

41. Lorenz, W. and Doenicke, A. (1978). In "Adverse Response
to Intravenous Drugs" (Eds. J. Watkins and A.M. Ward).
pp.83-112. Academic Press, Grune & Stratton, London.

42. Stanworth, D.R. (1980). In "Genetic Aspects and Anaphylactoid Reactions, PAR Pseudo-Allergic Reactions. Involvement of Drugs and Chemicals" Vol.1 (Eds. P. Dukor,
P. Kallos, H.D. Schlumberger and G.B. West). pp.56-107.
S. Karger, Basel.

43. Kaliner, M. (1977). *J. Clin. Invest.* **60**, 951-959.

44. Lewis, T. (1926). *Heart* **13**, 153-191.

45. Dale, H.H. (1929). *Lancet* **216**, 1232-1285.

46. Anonymous (1981). Histamine and Antihistamines in
Anaesthesia and Surgery *Lancet* 74-75.

47. Neugebauer, E. and Lorenz, W. (1981). *Behring Inst. Mitt.*
68, 102-133.

48. Black, J.W., Duncan, W.A.M., Durant, C.J., Ganellin, C.R.
and Parsons, E.M. (1972). *Nature* **236**, 385-390.

49. Lorenz, W. (1975). *Agents Actions* **5**, 402-416.

50. Giertz, H., Hahn, F., Schmutzler, W. and Kollmeier, J.
(1964). *Inter. Arch. Allergy Appl. Immunol.* **25**, 26-45.

51. Giertz, H., Hahn, F., Seseke, G. and Schmutzler, W. (1967).
Naunyn Schmiedeberg's Arch. Pharmacol. Exp. Pathol. **256**,
26-39.

52. Smedegard, G. (1980). Anaphylactic shock. Pathophysiology
of aggregate and cytotropic anaphylaxis in the monkey.
Thesis, Acta Universitatis Upsaliensis.

53. Johnson, A.R. and Erdös, E.D. (1973). *Proc. Soc. Exp.
Biol. Med.* **142**, 1252-1256.

54. Tauber, R., Lorenz, W., Schmal, A., Dormann, P., Mann, G.,
Uhlig, R. and Maroske, D. (1974). *Langenbecks Arch. Chir.
Suppl. Chir. Forum* pp.135-137.

55. Lorenz, W., Doenicke, A., Messmer, K., Reimann, H.-J.,
Thermann, M., Lahn, W., Berr, J., Schmal, A., Dormann, P.,
Regenfuss, P. and Hamelmann, H. (1976). *Br. J. Anaesth.*
48, 151-161.

56. Lorenz, W., Doenicke, A. Schoning, B., Karges, H. and
Schmal, A. (1981). In "Joint WHO/IABS Symposium on the
standardization of albumin, plasma substitutes and plasma
pheresis" Genf 1980. Development Biol. Standardization
48, pp.207-234. S. Karger, Basel.

57. Schöning, B., Lorenz, W. and Doenicke, A. (1982). *Klin. Wochenschrift* **60**, 1048-1055.
58. Hedin, H., Richter, W., Messmer, K., Renck, H., Ljungström, K.-G. and Laubenthal, H. (1981). In "Joint WHO/IABS Symposium on the Standardization of Albumin, Plasma Substitutes and Plasma Pheresis" Genf 1980. Develop. Biol. Standardization **48**, pp.179-189. S. Karger, Basel.

THE PATHOLOGY OF IMMUNE-MEDIATED DISEASES
OF THE PERIPHERAL AND CENTRAL NERVOUS SYSTEMS

M.L. Cuzner

The Multiple Sclerosis Society Laboratory,
Department of Neurochemistry,
Institute of Neurology, London WC1N 2NS

The central nervous system (CNS) differs from other organs in
that it has no lymphatics and access of soluble or cellular
agents of the systemic immune response to the brain is
greatly restricted by virtue of the blood-brain barrier.
Morphologically this barrier consists of tight junctions
between the endothelial and epithelial cells of the capillaries which prevent intercellular diffusion. Such junctions
are missing in certain parts of the brain and this physiological gap allows for a limited exchange of proteins and
lymphoid cells between the blood circulation and the CNS.
For example, in normal cerebrospinal fluid (CSF) the cell
count which is largely mononuclear is about $2-3/mm^3$, thus
there are somewhere between 10^5 and 10^6 lymphocytes in the
total CSF volume of approximately 150 ml. Although under
normal conditions it is largely separated from the effects
of systemic immune reactions, the CNS is able to mount a
local immune response when it is damaged by infections or
autoimmune disease. The same does not apply to the peripheral nervous system (PNS) which is not separated from normal
immune surveillance.

There are three central questions to be answered about
immune disorders of the nervous system, namely (a) against
what antigens of the CNS is the immune response directed,
(b) what is the mechanism of immune damage and (c) what is
initiating or triggering the immune response?

One of the most common immune-mediated diseases of the
peripheral nervous system, is myasthenia gravis. The responsible antigen in myasthenia gravis is the acetylcholine
receptor (AChR) [1]. In most patients with this disease
there is an antibody in the serum against the AChR, and using

monoclonal antibodies it has been demonstrated that there are
multiple determinants [2]. The antibody levels do not
directly correlate with disease, but it has been shown that
the mechanism of damage at the motor end-plate of the neuro-
muscular junction is an antibody-mediated dysfunction of the
receptor. Direct experimental evidence comes from transfer
of the disease to animals using the IgG fraction of serum
from patients with myasthenia [3]. The triggering of disease
in myasthenia is considered to be associated with abnormalities of the thymus gland. There is a surface antigen on
thymocytes which cross-reacts with the AChR [4]. It is also
associated with HLA-B8. There is no evidence of a virus in
myasthenia and furthermore there are no abnormalities in
immunoregulatory cells.

A second immune-mediated condition of the PNS, which is
representative of the acute inflammatory demyelinating polyneuropathies, is the Guillain-Barré syndrome. In contrast to
most membrane systems there are only three or four major
proteins in both PNS and CNS myelin. Ultrastructurally, PNS
and CNS myelin are very similar, but they have only one protein in common. In the PNS the most antigenic protein is a
basic protein, P2, which is the responsible antigen in the
experimental model of the acute polyneuropathies. The antigen in Guillain-Barré syndrome is considered to be the P2
protein, but cell-mediated immunity has only been demonstrated
against crude peripheral nerve extracts [5]. If the P2 protein is purified from PNS myelin, the antigenic properties
are lost. The mechanisms of demyelination in the more common
neuropathies is a macrophage-mediated demyelination [6].
Macrophages penetrate the basement membrane of the peripheral
nerve and strip off the myelin, by insinuating between the
lamellar structure of the myelin sheath. There is little
known about humoral factors in the peripheral neuropathies,
but some recent experiments show that serum from patients
with Guillain-Barré syndrome can induce demyelination in
experimental conditions [4]. In this condition the trigger
of the disease appears to be a viral infection which precedes
the onset of the disease. In at least 70% of people with
Guillain-Barré syndrome, a prior non-specific viral infection
takes place. Experimentally a wide variety of viruses can
provoke an identical specific autoimmune reaction against the
PNS myelin. They must act via a final common pathway, by
either triggering some underlying mechanism, or having a
shared antigen with PNS myelin.

One end result of most viral infections and autoimmune
diseases of the CNS is demyelination [7]. White matter
appears to be the target, secondary if not primary, of an
immune attack on the CNS. In virus infections of the CNS,

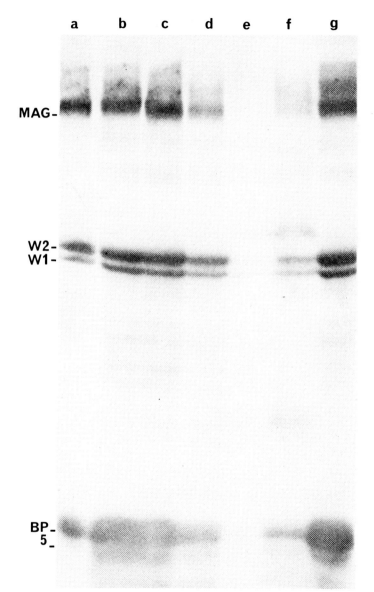

Fig. 1 Immunoblot of SDS-treated membrane proteins separated
on a polyacrylamide slab gel, incubated with antiserum to
basic protein (BP), Wolfgram protein doublet of molecular
weight 43-46K (W1, W2) and myelin-associated glycoprotein
(MAG). (a) standards, (b) and (g) control white matter,
(c) MS white matter, (d) plaque rim, (e) plaque, (f) SSPE
white matter.

the ensuing demyelination may be caused through direct damage
of the host tissue by the virus, or by incorporation of virus
genome material into brain cells. A third possibility may be
a shared common antigen, and fourthly the demyelination may
be the result of "bystander" demyelination. The structure of
the myelin sheath may give some clue as to why it appears to
be a primary target for immunocompetent cells. Figure 1
shows a polyacrylamide gel electrophoresis (PAGE) pattern of
CNS myelin, stained by immunoperoxidase, following incubation
with antibodies against the specific myelin proteins, which
are degraded during demyelination [8]. They are a high
molecular weight myelin-associated glycoprotein, which is one
of the first proteins to disappear in a demyelinating lesion,
a protein-doublet of the first proteins to disappear in a
demyelinating lesion, a protein-doublet of M.W. 43-46K, and
the myelin basic protein which is very susceptible to proteo-
lytic digestion by cells of the phagocytic series, and is
almost completely lost from demyelinated lesions [9].

The basic protein is the immunogen which is responsible for
the induction of experimental autoimmune encephalomyelitis
(EAE) which has been put forward as a model for the human
demyelinating disease, multiple sclerosis (MS). EAE is the
prototype autoimmune demyelinating disease of the CNS. It
results in an inflammatory demyelination and has a human
counterpart in such conditions as post-measles or post-rabies
vaccinal encephalomyelitis. It is not the virus that causes
the demyelination, but an immune response mounted against
myelin basic protein. EAE is characterized pathologically
by inflammatory cell infiltrates, particularly in the spinal
cord, which precipitate hind-limb paralysis in the animals in
the acute form of the disease, which occurs ten days after an
intradermal inoculation of homologous or heterologous spinal
cord or purified basic protein, incorporated into Freund's
adjuvant [10]. It is an acute monophasic disease and very
few animals survive. In the acute form of the disease the
myelin destruction is mediated by macrophages, which can be
seen in EM studies to separate the lamellae of the myelin
sheath and engulf the myelin debris. The trigger in this
disease is a delayed-type hypersensitivity reaction to basic
protein and this can be demonstrated in the circulating
lymphocytes of animals as early as seven days after inoculation, before clinical symptoms appear. In the acute disease
there is minimal involvement of the humoral immune system.

In recent years a chronic form of EAE has been induced by
manipulating the proportions of immunogen and adjuvant. If
young animals are inoculated, a chronic relapsing form of EAE
is induced (CREAE), which resembles more closely multiple
sclerosis [11]. The clinicopathological features of CREAE

Table 1 *Chronic relapsing experimental autoimmune encephalo-myelitis (CREAE)*.

(CREAE):   A model for Multiple Sclerosis?

  Induction:

  Inoculation of young (3 week) strain 13 guinea pigs with
    homogenate of spinal cord in Freund's adjuvant contain-
    ing mycobacterium tuberculosis.

  Symptoms:

  Attributable to CNS conduction block, paralysis,
    incontinence, etc.

  Clinical course:

Phase	Days post-inoculation
Acute	(17-29)
1st remission	(30-50)
1st relapse	(60-90)
2nd relapse	(120-130)
* Chronic remission	(170-310)
** Chronic relapse	(170-310)

  Post-mortem histology (especially spinal cord)

  Acute phase: inflammation with mononuclear cell
    infiltrates

  Chronic relapse: inflammation with mononuclear cell
    infiltrates

              + macroscopic plaques.

---

*   in remission   2 months
** in relapse   2 months

are illustrated in Table 1. In CREAE there is an increased
IgG/albumin ratio in the CSF, and antibody against basic
protein can be demonstrated. The same oligoclonal IgG band
spectrum is present in both the serum and CSF of animals with
CREAE, indicating that there is an identical humoral response
both inside and outside the CNS compartment. However if the
humoral immune response in CREAE is quantified, only 1% of
the total IgG is directed against the basic protein. The
majority of the antibody is directed against the major component of the adjuvant, *mycobacterium tuberculosis*, which is
essential for disease induction [12]. The humoral immune
events in CREAE are summarized in Table 2. The direction of

Table 2 *Humoral events in CREAE induced by inoculation with spinal cord homogenate in adjuvant-containing mycobacterium tuberculosis.*

1. Polyclonal B cell activation by M. tuberculosis, raised serum IgG, persists at 6 months p.i.

2. Raised IgG/albumin ratio in CSF - especially in relapse phases, therefore secretion of IgG by plasma cells within CNS.

    Identical oligoclonal IEF spectra of IgG in CSF and serum. Therefore (grossly) identical humoral response by plasma cells inside and outside CNS.

3. Antigenic specificity of oligoclonal IgG in CREAE sera.

Antigenic specificity	% Total (approx.)
Anti-M. tuberculosis	10%
Anti-basic protein	1%
Anti-whole spinal cord homogenate	1%

    i.e. majority of oligoclonal IgG does not react with components of the (native) sensitizing inoculum.

the disease to the CNS in EAE is via the delayed hypersensitivity reaction to the basic protein, and in the acute form this is reflected in inflammation with little demyelination. As the disease progresses and the humoral component emerges, plasma cells may be drawn into the CNS accompanying the T cells. Once in the CNS the plasma cells may be released from immunoregulatory control and synthesize antibody which, regardless of the specificity, results in antibody-dependent cell-mediated demyelination.

The only consistent laboratory finding in multiple sclerosis (MS) is oligoclonal banding of IgG in the CSF of more than 90% of patients accompanied by a raised CSF IgG/albumin ratio in 75% of the cases. The humoral immune reaction appears to be restricted to the CNS and the oligoclonal band pattern remains constant throughout the course of the disease. Thus IgG of restricted heterogeneity is synthesized within the CNS of most MS patients but the responsible antigen has not been identified. The pathology of MS is represented by discrete areas of demyelination, surrounded by perivascular cuffs of inflammatory cells. Macrophages containing myelin are present in actively demyelinating plaques but they do not penetrate the sheath or split the lamellae as in EAE [13]. IgG is present in macrophages and also appears to be taken

Table 3 *Yields of immunoglobulin G in supernatants and acid extracts of particulate fractions from control, MS and SSPE brains.*

Tissue sample	Supernatant IgG (µg/g tissue)	Particulate IgG (µg/g tissue)
Control; white/grey matter	18.5	0.72
MS; macroscopically-normal white matter	51.3	1.55
MS; white matter near ventricular plaque	196.3	7.05
MS; ventricular plaque	71.5	5.13
MS; fibrous plaque	170.0	15.6
SSPE brain; white/grey matter	167.4	26.0
SSPE brain; white/grey matter	147.9	128.1

up by reactive astrocytes in the vicinity of the plaque.

The mechanism of demyelination in MS is unclear and progress in this line is hindered by the lack of a specific antigen. One possibility is that immune complexes are formed in the plaque, but if the IgG is extracted from a plaque the large majority of it is not particulate-bound, but is in the supernatant fraction [14]. On the other hand, in subacute sclerosing panencephalitis (SSPE), which results from persistent measles infection of the CNS with widespread demyelination, the proportion of bound IgG in the CNS is an order of magnitude greater than in extracts of MS brain (Table 3). The IgG extracted from all MS plaques displayed an oligoclonal pattern in IEF and corresponding supernatant and particulate extracts showed a large number of common IgG bands. A different oligoclonal pattern was observed for each MS brain but within any single MS brain, plaques from different areas displayed an underlying common band pattern, with quantitative differences in IgG spectra (Fig. 2). In the case of SSPE, where measles antigen-antibody complexes have been identified, the oligoclonal band pattern is considerably clearer and probably represents the product of a smaller number of lymphocyte clones. No brain-specific antibodies can be identified in CSF or brain extracts from cases of MS or SSPE using immunoblotting techniques, although in the SSPE extracts there is strong staining against measles antigen (Fig. 3) [15]. There is no clear-cut evidence of

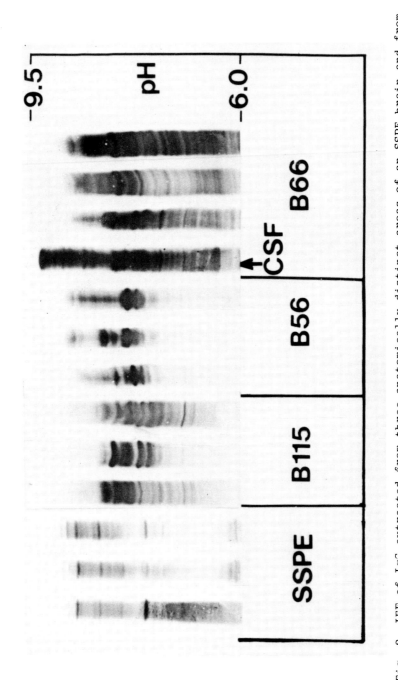

Fig. 2 IEF of IgG extracted from three anatomically distinct areas of an SSPE brain and from three individual plaques from each of three MS brains.

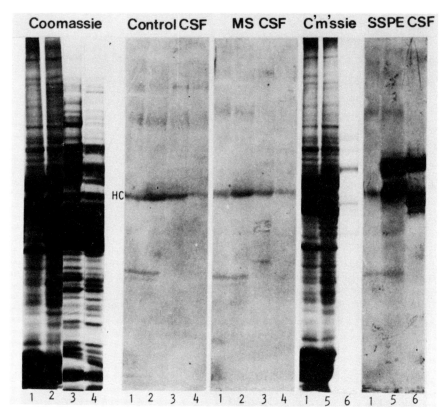

Fig. 3 Analyses by immunoblotting of reactivity of IgG with human brain proteins in MS and SSPE.   Representative human SDS-treated proteins in Coomassie blue-stained polyacrylamide slab gels and corresponding immunoblots incubated in control, MS or SSPE CSF, followed by immunoperoxidase staining are shown.   Lanes (1) and (3) control white matter, particulate and soluble proteins respectively.   Lanes (2) and (4) MS white matter, particulate and soluble proteins respectively. Lane (5) SSPE white matter, particulate proteins.   Lane (6) SDS-solubilized measles virus.

cell-mediated immunity in MS, but recently a number of investigators have shown independently that there are marked changes in immunoregulatory cells in the peripheral blood of MS patients, during active disease [16]. The predominant immune reaction within the CNS appears to be humoral, but the overproduction of antibody may be the result of abnormal immunoregulation of plasma cells which persist in the CNS for long periods of time.

REFERENCES

1. Drachman, D.B. (1978). *N. Engl. J. Med*. **298**, 136-142 and 186-193.
2. Mittag, T., Kornfeld, P., Tormay, A. and Woo, C. (1976). *N. Engl. J. Med*. **294**, 691-694.
3. Toyka, K.V., Drachman, D.B., Griffin, D.E. and Pastronk, A. (1977). *N. Engl. J. Med*. **296**, 125-131.
4. Feasby, T.E., Hahn, A.F. and Gilbert, J.J. (1980). *Neurology* (NY) **30**, 363.
5. Rocklin, R.E., Sheremata, W.A., Feldman, R.G., Kies, M.W. and David, J.R. (1971). *N. Engl. J. Med*. **284**, 803-808.
6. Prineas, J.W. (1981). *Ann. Ncurol*. **9** (Suppl.) 6-19.
7. DalCanto, M.C. and Rabinowitz, S.G. (1982). *Ann. Neurol*. **11**, 109-127.
8. Newcombe, J., Glynn, P. and Cuzner, M.L. (1982). *J. Neurochem*. **38**, 267-274.
9. Cuzner, M.L. and Davison, A.N. (1979). *Mol. Aspects Med*. **2**, 147-248.
10. Paterson, P.Y. (1980). In "The Suppression of Experimental Allergic Encephalomyelitis and Multiple Sclerosis" (Eds. A.N. Davison and M.L. Cuzner), pp.11-30. Academic Press.
11. Wisniewski, H.M. and Keith, A.B. (1977). *Ann. Neurol*. **1**, 144-148.
12. Mittag, T., Kornfeld, P., Tormay, A. and Woo, C. (1976). *N. Engl. J. Med*. **294**, 691-694.
13. Prineas, J.W. and Graham, J.S. (1981). *Ann. Neurol*. **10**, 149-158.
14. Glynn, P., Gilbert, H.M., Newcombe, J. and Cuzner, M.L. (1982). *Clin. Exp. Immunol*. **48**, 102-110.
15. Newcombe, J., Glynn, P. and Cuzner, M.L. (1982). *J. Neurochem*. **38**, in press.
16. Weiner, H.L. and Hauser, S.L. (1982). *Ann. Neurol*. **11**, 437-449.

THE IMMUNOLOGICAL PROTECTION OF THE GUT: STUDIES ON THE PHYSIOLOGY OF IgA TRANSPORT

J.G. Hall

*Institute of Cancer Research,
Clifton Avenue, Sutton, Surrey, UK*

INTRODUCTION

The pathogenic bacteria and viruses that afflict the gut, or
cause systemic disease by entering through its wall, must
first gain a foothold by attaching themselves to the enterocytes that constitute the epithelium. This attachment depends often upon the precise steric relationships between the
surfaces of the micro-organisms and complementary receptors
on the enterocytes. It is apparent that a molecule as large
as an immunoglobulin, possessing an affinity for the critical
region of the micro-organism's surface would be able to inter-
vene and prevent the initial attachment and the undesirable
consequences that would otherwise follow. Thus the first line
of immunological defence of the gut, and other vulnerable
epithelia in the respiratory and genito-urinary tracts, is
represented by immunoglobulin antibodies present in the
boundary layer of mucus that covers them. In strict anatomical terms this is an "external" situation, where the physical
and chemical conditions are quite different from the standard
milieu intérieur and which are inimical to the function, or
indeed the survival, of cellular defences such as macrophages
and granulocytes. This anatomical distinction leads to a
physiological conundrum. How does a serum protein molecule
as large as an immunoglobulin manage to escape from the
circulating protein pool and get onto the external surface of
the gut? The answer is that a very specialized trans-cellular
transport system has been evolved. The general features of
this transport system are common to many species but, even
among mammals, each species seems to have its own peculiar-
ities and only a few species have been the subject of detailed
investigation. What is written below summarizes what we
know now, but it describes only the tip of the iceberg. The

facts that are presently submerged may, when they surface,
differ from our expectations.

THE BASIC SYSTEM

In many animals, including man, rats, mice and rabbits the
principal immunoglobulin found in the external secretions
and on mucous membranes is IgA. This immunoglobulin has the
general structure of all immunoglobulins, the two heavy (α)
chains being antigenically distinct from those of the other
classes. A distinguishing feature of IgA is that it is
usually secreted from the plasma cells which produce it in a
dimeric form; two entire immunoglobulin molecules are joined
together by a joining or "J" chain (Fig. 1). In addition to
the IgA dimers small amounts of both monomers and higher
polymers are produced. Man is unusual in producing significant amounts of monomeric IgA and this, as we shall see
later can complicate the picture.

The dimeric IgA that is secreted by the submucosal plasma
cells diffuses through the interstitial fluid of the gut and
through the basement membrane of the epithelium until it
reaches the enterocytes. These display on their surfaces a
receptor known as secretory component (SC) which unites
avidly with dimeric or polymeric IgA. It does not unite with
IgG or monomeric IgA but may unite, rather less avidly, with
IgM if IgA is absent. It is important to stress that SC is
a part of the epithelial cell and its evolution is quite distinct from that of the immunoglobulins, it is present in
foetal epithelia long before the lymphoid system has developed.

Once the dimeric IgA has united with the SC on the baso-
lateral aspects of the enterocyte, an endocytic vesicle is
formed and the whole SC-IgA complex is engulfed and transported across the cytoplasm and discharged onto the external
surface of the cell. The IgA so secreted is still firmly
bound to SC and is referred to as "secretory IgA" (S-IgA).
By collecting and purifying S-IgA it has been established
that SC is a glycoprotein of about 70,000 daltons, though
when the SC is in the intact enterocyte membrane it may be
somewhat larger. The exact nature of the bond between dimeric
IgA and SC is unclear and may differ between species and between subclasses of IgA. Although the J chain is essential to
make the crucial dimeric structure there is no evidence that
J chain, as such, actually unites with the SC. At low temperatures the bond between SC and IgA dimer is reversible but
under physiological conditions it is not, and once IgA has
united with SC the union, for practical purposes, is permanent.

The outline shown diagrammatically in Fig. 1 is well documented and generally accepted [1-3] but it leaves two

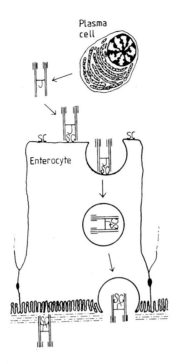

Fig. 1 Diagram to show how IgA is transported across entero-cytes. The submucosal plasma cell secretes IgA, dimerized by J chain, into the interstitial fluid. This dimeric IgA unites with the secretory component (SC) which is displayed on the baso-lateral aspects of the enterocytes, which internalize the IgA-SC complexes in endocytic vesicles. Each vesicle is trans-ported across the cytoplasm and discharges its contents across the luminal aspect of the enterocyte. Once in the lumen of the gut the SC helps to anchor the IgA molecule with which it is combined in the boundary layer of mucus which overlies the epithelium.

important questions unanswered. First, where do the sub-mucosal plasma cells which produce the IgA come from? Second, what happens to the IgA that does not succeed in uniting with SC before it is absorbed into the intestinal lymphatics?

LOCAL AND SYSTEMIC PRODUCTION OF IgA

The immunoglobulin-producing plasma cells that are so abun-dant in the *lamina propria* beneath the intestinal epithelium are "end-cells" with a half life of three to six days [4]. Accordingly, they must be replaced continually. The details of this process are complicated and have been reviewed [5-8].

Briefly, antigens which penetrate the gut wall react with
macrophages and lymphocytes of the gut-associated lymphoid
tissue (G.A.L.T.) either in the wall of the gut or in the
mesenteric lymph nodes. The result of this interaction is
the generation of large numbers of lymphoid blast cells
(immunoblasts) which are discharged into the intestinal lymph
and carried to the blood. These immunoblasts do not remain
long in the blood for they have the intriguing property of
extravasating selectively in the *lamina propria* of the small
gut, where they differentiate into plasma cells [9]. This
process ensures that a localized antigenic stimulus in the
gut produces the cellular wherewithal for specific IgA antibody formation to become distributed over the entire length
of the gut (and also to the mammary gland in lactating
animals). It follows that apparently local IgA responses
always have a systemic component and some conventional IgG
and IgM antibodies are nearly always formed as well [10].
The IgA responses also exhibit immunological memory [11] and
the same range of thymus dependency [10] as do conventional
immune responses. The systemic nature of IgA responses is
not always appreciated and is sometimes denied. This is
probably because while it has been possible to identify IgA
antibodies in secretions it has often not been possible to
find them in the blood. The false conclusion drawn from this
was that IgA production was a totally local event. In fact,
very large amounts of IgA antibody do pass through the blood
but because they are so rapidly and efficiently extracted
from the blood by the liver they have often escaped detection.

THE HEPATO-BILIARY ROUTE OF IgA SECRETION

Not all the IgA produced by the submucosal plasma cells of
the gut is able to reach the enterocytes. After all, the net
fluid flow in the interstitium of the gut is, in health, in-
wards rather than outwards and it is inevitable that much of
the IgA is swept up into the intestinal lymphatics. Indeed,
it is easy to demonstrate relatively large amounts of IgA in
intestinal lymph [5,12]. However, although large volumes of
intestinal lymph are continually entering the blood the
levels of IgA in the blood serum of most species is very low.
This apparent paradox could only be reconciled by postulating
that some organ was extracting the IgA from the blood.
Quantitative considerations dictated that such an organ must
have both a large blood supply and a discontinuous vascular
endothelium that would not impede the egress of macromolecules
of the size of dimer IgA. Clearly, the only organ that meets
this specification is the liver and its function in clearing
IgA from the blood has been amply proved in experiments on

rats. First, it was found that IgA is virtually the only
intact immunoglobulin in rat bile where it accounted for at
least 25% of the total protein. Also, ligation of the common
bile duct caused the concentration of IgA in the blood, to
increase nearly tenfold in three to four days. These observations set in train studies of the dynamics of the transport
process. By injecting dimeric IgA labelled with ^{125}I intravenously into rats which had a cannula in the common bile
duct, it was shown that 25 to 50% of the injected dose
appeared in the bile in an intact form within 5 h [12,13].
Electron microscope studies showed that the IgA united with
the sinusoidal facet of the hepatocyte and was transported
across the cytoplasm and discharged into the biliary cana-
liculi [14]. Immunochemical and biophysical experiments
showed that rat hepatocytes have SC on their surfaces [15]
and that the IgA was transported in endocytic vesicles [16].
In other words, the transport of IgA by the hepatocytes was
in the rat entirely analogous to that which occurs in enterocytes. Although these experiments all involved the use of
myeloma IgA, normal polyclonal IgA antibodies were found to
behave in the same way [17]. Again, only dimeric or polymeric
IgA can be transported into the bile; monomeric IgA, S-IgA and
the IgGs have not the ability to unite with SC and so cannot
be transported.

    After deliberate antigenic stimulation of the G.A.L.T. of
rats, large numbers of IgA-producing cells are generated and
impressive titres of antibodies appear in the bile. These
are almost exclusively of the IgA class, whereas those in the
blood are IgG and IgM, never IgA [10,11,17,18].

    In considering the titres of antibodies in bile, or indeed
in any secretion, it must be remembered that the system is
"open-ended". The antibodies cannot progressively accumulate,
as they do in the blood, to give the very high titres that
are encountered often in traditional serology. However, in
spite of this the titres of antibody in secretions sometimes
approximate to those in blood, and this must surely mean that
IgA is being produced at a much greater rate than IgG or IgM.
Probably, in many animals, much more IgA is produced than any
other class of immunoglobulin but exact quantification is
difficult. It is not easy to assess how much IgA gets into
the gut via the enterocytes on the one hand or via the bile
on the other.

    The provision of douches of biliary IgA antibody to coin-
cide with the entry into the duodenum of freshly ingested
food and bacteria seems a priori a good way of neutralizing
pathogens in the ingesta and protecting the biliary apparatus
from ascending infections. There may be other functions too.
Inevitably, small amounts of dietary macromolecules are

liable to be absorbed intact and there is always the potential
risk of allergic reactions to dietary constituents. Luckily,
polymeric or dimeric IgA that has united with its specific
antigen is also cleared rapidly from the blood [19,20]. In
this way immune complexes involving dietary antigens that
become systematized can be excreted into the bile with none
of the damaging allergic reactions that can be caused by antibodies of the IgG, IgM and IgE classes. Those other antibodies do not usually enter the lumen of the gut in any quantity and they are in any case more susceptible to proteolysis
than IgA. They do however represent a second line of defence
in situations where the mucosa has been penetrated or damaged.
Figure 2 shows a scheme of how these antibodies may be called
into play if the lumenal IgA fails to prevent the ingress of
antigen. In the example shown antibodies of the IgE class
have sensitized the local mast cells which degranulate when
the antigen impinges on them. The resulting vasoactive amines
cause increased blood flow and hyperpermeability of the

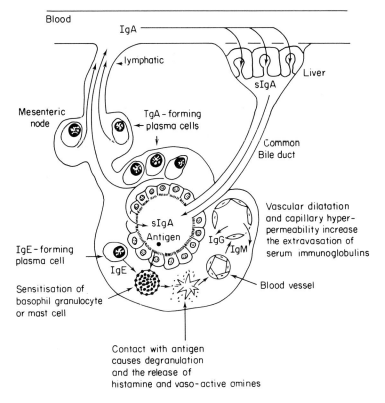

Fig. 2 Diagram to show how immunoglobulins of various
classes may cooperate in protecting the gut.

vascular system so that increased amounts of IgG and IgM antibodies accumulate in the local tissue fluid. Such antibodies
could, after uniting with antigen, activate complement (which
IgA cannot do) and so further increase the local inflammatory
response. Under these conditions it seems that the gut epithelium itself may become more permeable, perhaps by the de-
stabilization of inter-cellular junctions, and some humoral
serum factors enter the gut lumen. It seems that the triggering of this immunological "cascade" may be the mechanism of
the "self-cure" episodes during which animals are able to rid
themselves suddenly of the burden of intestinal helminthic
parasites.

COMPARATIVE ASPECTS OF THE HEPATO-BILIARY TRANSPORT OF IgA

When the experiments of the transport of ^{125}I-dimeric rat
myeloma IgA from blood to bile in rats had been completed they
were repeated using ^{125}I-dimeric human myeloma IgA. It was
found that rats transported human IgA just as well as they did
their own, and rabbits transported both human and rat material
with equal facility [21]. These studies have been extended
[22,23] and it seems that the hepatocytes of animals like
rats, mice and rabbits can transport a wide range of heterologous IgAs, whereas in guinea pigs, sheep, pigs, cattle and
dogs only homologous IgA is transported from blood to bile.
Ruminants like sheep present a special problem because,
although they possess IgA it occurs in relatively small
amounts and IgG_1 is the principal immunoglobulin in the external secretions.

These experiments indicate that IgA is capable of reacting
with the SC from widely differing species and suggests that
these molecules must be highly conserved in evolutionary
terms. The phenomenon is not restricted to mammals; the
domestic fowl transports human dimeric IgA from blood to bile
just as efficiently as does the rat [4] but chicken SC has
yet to be identified as a biochemical entity.

THE SITUATION IN MAN

Although human IgA dimers are rapidly and actively transported from blood to bile by several mammals it is not known
for certain how much IgA is transported by the human hepatobiliary system, or which cells carry out the transport process.
It is very difficult to obtain normal human bile, and bile
obtained from inflamed tissues by, e.g., "T" tube drainage
has a grossly abnormal composition and may give misleading
values. Such evidence as we have on normal human bile shows
that it contains much more IgA, per unit of protein, than
does blood [23]. It has been known for years that obstructive

jaundice is accompanied by elevated levels of serum IgA [25], and the blood biochemistry of patients with liver disease is consistent with a substantial role for hepatobiliary IgA transport in normal people [26]. Although a claim has been made for the presence of SC on human hepatocytes [27] this has not been confirmed in studies which indicated that a specialized hepatobiliary epithelial cell is responsible for the transport of IgA into the bile of man [28]. Thus, although there is a substantial amount of circumstantial evidence for IgA transport from blood to bile in man, we can say little about it in quantitative or kinetic terms.

The problem is complicated further by the fact that man differs from all the common laboratory animals in that 75 to 80% of the IgA in human serum is monomeric. This fact itself suggests that the dimeric or polymeric forms are being preferentially excreted, because there is evidence that most of the IgA produced is, in fact, dimeric or polymeric. For example, when lymphocytes from normal human peripheral blood were stimulated *in vitro* with a polyclonal B-cell activator like pokeweed mitogen, the analysis of the IgA produced showed that much more of it was in the form of polymers and dimers than would have been predicted from the polymer/monomer ratio in the blood serum [29]. Similarly, the IgA in the sera of most patients with IgA myeloma is predominantly dimeric or polymeric [23]. The balance of evidence, then indicates that most of the IgA produced in man is dimeric or polymeric but because this is cleared so rapidly by the liver, most of the IgA that remains circulating in the blood is of the monomeric form. Clearly, though, much more evidence is required before any conclusive assessment can be made.

PATHOLOGY OF THE IgA SYSTEM

Perhaps the most common defect is IgA deficiency. However, one must be suspicious of diagnoses of IgA deficiency which rest purely on analyses of blood serum. For example, an individual who produced little IgA monomer would have a very low concentration of IgA in the blood even though his epithelia might be adequately protected by normal amounts of polymeric IgA. Undoubtedly, though, cases of genuine IgA deficiency do exist. Some of the patients do have an increased incidence of infections of the upper respiratory tract and other epithelia but others remain apparently healthy, at any rate in temperate, developed countries. This is probably because IgM can substitute for IgA. IgM is a pentamer and, in the absence of IgA, can apparently unite with SC and undergo trans-epithelial transport. There are anecdotal reports of such patients showing a relative increase in blood

levels of monomeric IgM, presumably because their normal penta-
meric forms were being secreted.

The basic cause of congenital or acquired IgA deficiency is
unknown and few drugs or toxins seem to act selectively on the
IgA system. The lymphoid tissues of the G.A.L.T., which produce the IgA, are, of course, susceptible to irradiation,
cytotoxic drugs and steroids, as are all lymphoid tissues, but
none of these agents show any selectivity for the G.A.L.T.

Obviously, hepatotoxic agents or drugs which cause choles-
tasis may impair the liver's ability to transport IgA into
the bile. Under these circumstances, although IgA levels in
the blood would build up and could, conceivably, exert feedback inhibition on IgA plasma cells, the epithelia would still
be able to protect themselves by transporting IgA to their
external surfaces.

Certain drugs like phenytoin [30] and penicillamine [31] do
seem to induce a selective IgA deficiency but they take a long
time to produce an effect which is very far from complete.

It is possible to imagine that drugs which affect vesicle
formation and the movement of intracellular organelles would
also have an affect on IgA transport but their acute toxic
effects *in vivo* would probably be manifested in other much
more disastrous ways.

Some quasi-malignant diseases do seem to preferentially
involve the G.A.L.T. Alpha-chain disease is a paraprotein-
aemia caused by proliferation of abnormal lymphoid cells in
the G.A.L.T. [32]. The disease occurs commonly in under-
developed Mediterranean countries and is thought to be due to
a combination of poor diet and continual gastrointestinal infections and infestations. In its early stages it is apparently reversible by antibiotics but if untreated it may
become frankly malignant. Even then the disease usually
remains confined to the G.A.L.T. Similarly, it is intriguing
that lymphoproliferative diseases involving superficial nodes
may metastasize to other nodes but not to the G.A.L.T. In
other words the malignant lymphoid cells retain the migratory
characteristics of their normal counterparts [33].

ACKNOWLEDGEMENT

The Institute of Cancer Research is supported by grants from
the Medical Research Council and Cancer Research Campaign.
Figure 1 is produced by courtesy of the African Journal of
Clinical and Experimental Immunology.

REFERENCES

1. Brandtzaeg, P. and Savilahti, E. (1978). *Adv, Exp. Med.
    Biol.* **107**, 219-226.

2. Brown, W.R. (1978). *Gasteroenterol.* **75**, 129–138.
3. Nagura, H., Nakane, P.K. and Brown, W.R. (1979). *J. Immunol.* **123**, 2359,2368.
4. Mattioli, C.A. and Tomasi, T.B. (1973). *J. Exp. Med.* **138**, 452–460.
5. Hall, J.G. (1979). *Blood Cells* 5, 479–492.
6. Hall, J.G. (1980). *Monographs in Allergy* **16**, 100–111.
7. Lamm, M.E. (1976). *Adv. Immunol.* **22**, 223–290.
8. Bienenstock, J. and Befus, A.D. (1980). *Immunology*, **41**, 249–270.
9. Hall, J.G., Parry, D. and Smith, M.E. (1972). *Cell. Tissue Kinet.* 5, 269–281.
10. Andrew, E. and Hall, J.G. (1982). *Immunology* 45, 169–176.
11. Andrew, E. and Hall, J.G. (1982). *Immunology* 45, 177–182.
12. Orlans, E., Peppard, J., Reynolds, J. and Hall, J.G. (1978). *J. Exp. Med.* **147**, 588–592.
13. Jackson, G.D.F., Lemaitre-Coelho, I., Vaerman, J-P., Bazin, H. and Beckers, A. (1978). *Eur. J. Immunol.* **8**, 123–126.
14. Birbeck, M.S.C., Cartwright, P., Hall, J.G., Orlans, E. and Peppard, J. (1979). *Immunology* **37**, 477–484.
15. Orlans, E., Peppard, J., Frey, J.F., Hinton, R.H. and Mullock, B.M. (1979). *J. Exp. Med.* **150**, 1577–1581.
16. Mullock, B.M., Hinton, R.H., Dobrota, M., Peppard, J. and Orlans, E. (1979). *Biochim. Biophys. Acta.* **587**, 381–391.
17. Reynolds, J., Gyure, L., Andrew, E. and Hall, J.G. (1980). *Immunology* **39**, 463–468.
18. Hall, J.G., Orlans, E., Reynolds, J., Dean, C., Peppard, J, Gyure, L. and Hobbs, S. (1979). *Int. Arch. Allergy Appl. Immun.* **59**, 75–84.
19. Peppard, J., Orlans, E., Payne, A.W.R. and Andrew, E. (1981). *Immunology* **42**, 83–89.
20. Peppard, J., Orlans, E., Andrew, E. and Payne, A.W.R. (1982). *Immunology* **45**, 467–472.
21. Hall, J.G., Gyure, L.A. and Payne, A.W.R. (1980). *Immunology* **41**, 899–902.
22. Hall, J.G., Gyure, L.A., Payne, A.W.R. and Andrew, E. (1981). In "The Mucosal Immune System" (Ed. F.J. Bourne), pp.31–44. Martinus Nijhoff, The Hague.
23. Orlans, E., Peppard, J., Payne, A.W.R., Fitzharris, B.M., Mullock, B.M., Hinton, R.H. and Hall, J.G. (1982). *Annals N.Y. Acad. Sci.* **409**, 411–427.
24. Rose, M.E., Orlans, E., Payne, A.W.R. and Hesketh, P. (1981). *Eur. J. Immunol.* **11**, 561–564.
25. Thompson, R.A., Carter, R., Stokes, R.P., Geddes, A.M. and Goodall, J.A.D. (1973). *Clin. Exp. Immunol.* **14**, 335–344,
26. Kutteh, W.H., Prince, S.J., Phillips, J.O., Spenney, J.G.

and J. Mestecky (1982). *Gasteroenterology* **85**, 184–193.

27. Hsu, S.M. and Hsu, R.L. (1980). *Gut* **21**, 985–989.
28. Nagura, H., Smith, P.D., Nakane, P.K. and Brown, W.R. (1981). *J. Immunol.* **126**, 587–595.
29. Kutteh, W.H., Koopman, W.J., Conley, M.E., Egan, M.L. and Mestecky, J. (1980). *J. Exp. Med.* **152**, 1424–1429.
30. Seager, J., Wilson, J., Hamison, D.L., Hayward, A.R. and Soothill, J.F. (1975). *Lancet* **ii**, 632–635.
31. Hjalmarson, O., Hanson, L.A. and Nilsson, L-A. (1977). *Br. Med. J.* **26 Feb**, 549.
32. Seligmann, M. (1975). *Br. J. Cancer* **Suppl.II**, 356–361.
33. Hall, J.G., Hopkins, J. and Orlans, E. (1977). *Biochem. Soc. Trans.* **5**, 1581–1583.

IMMUNOTOXICOLOGY:
THE PROSPECTS FOR IMMUNORESTORATION

J.W. Hadden

Immunopharmacology Program,
University of South Florida, Medical College,
12901 North 30th Street, Tampa, Florida 33612, U.S.A.

INTRODUCTION

Immunotoxicity is a well known phenomenon in iatrogenic immunosuppression for organ transplantation. In this circumstance, the immunosuppression is intentional and carefully designed to inhibit cellular immune response involved in graft rejection. Generally, the acceptance of the organ can be gained with minimal risk for the patient; however, significant sequelae do exist in the form of increased incidence of cancer, particularly of skin, gut and lymphoid tissues, and an increase in the number of infections, particularly with facultative intracellular pathogens, fungi and herpes-related viruses. In dire circumstances of infection, the immunosuppression can be reversed by discontinuation of therapy, however, at the risk of graft rejection. All in all, the risks of this form of calculated immunotoxicity are considered tolerable.

In cancer, immunotoxicity is evident even in the absence of therapy. In addition to nutritionally defined immune deficiences, the tumour itself may elaborate toxic components which impair the function of cellular immune responses, in particular. The introduction of multi-drug chemotherapy or wide field irradiation imposes immunotoxicity which frequently can be life threatening. Most chemotherapy regimens involve suppression of the granulocyte-macrophage lineages to the limits of tolerance. The impairment of these primary bulwarks of defence against pathogens opens the door for a variety of infections. Additional impairment of cellular immune responses contributes to the significant incidence of virus infections most commonly with the herpes-cytomegalo viruses

IMMUNOTOXICOLOGY
ISBN 0-12-282180-7

(CMV). In cancer, the long lasting effects of the intense immunotoxicity is of secondary concern to survival from the cancer itself; however, increasingly evident are higher incidences of infection and secondary cancers in long-term survivors of such therapy. The current effort at immunotherapy of cancer has as its aim the eradication of residual tumour, however, as a second benefit, reduced incidence of infection is a calculated but less well documented goal.

In both of these clinical circumstances the immunotoxicity resulting from therapy is intentional and its study has contributed much concerning the role that various types of immunosuppression have in inducing particular defects in resistance and giving rise to particular types of infection. For example, depressions of granulocyte function give rise to infections with pyrogenic pathogens gaining access particularly by the oral/respiratory route, e.g. streptococci, staphylococci and pneumococci. Monocyte/macrophage defects contribute to susceptibility to fungi and intracellular pathogens, like the mycobacteria. T-lymphocyte defects give rise to reduced resistance to a wide variety of viruses, bacteria and parasites. B-lymphocyte defects are mostly manifested in pyrogenic infections of the respiratory and gastrointestinal tracts. The elucidation of these defects has significantly improved the management of such patients; however, immunorestoration therapies have a long way to go before they are effective, safe and generally employed.

Increasingly, immunodeficiency resulting from immunotoxicity is being recognized as a circumstance of life. Transient cellular immunodeficiency is common with acute viral infections and probably is the major cause of the frequent secondary bacterial infection commanding such extensive antibiotic use. Perhaps the most insidious and pervasive of immunodeficiences occurs with ageing. In this circumstance it is not clear whether immunotoxicity is part of the picture. One of the most profound and perplexing immunotoxicity syndromes appears to be the recently described gay-related immunodeficiency (GRID or AID). In this syndrome, progressive depletion of both T- and B-cells occurs and 60% of the patients die of infections with such pathogens as *pneumocystis carinii* or with a strange, aggressive form of Koposi's sarcoma. The cause of the destruction of the immune system is not known; however, drug (amyl nitrite)-virus (CMV) interactions have been suggested as one possibility.

A number of toxic environmental exposures have been implicated in immunotoxicity. Notable examples include polychlorinated biphenyls, polybrominated biphenyls, dioxane, and asbestos, all of which have been discussed at this conference (see Bekesi and Dean in this text). With these

exposures the fundamental question arises. If we can identify
a population exposed to a particular immunotoxicant, immunosuppressed, and vulnerable to infection and cancer, are there
rational approaches to treating these patients to prevent the
predicted sequelae?

The idea of treating a dysfunctional or failing immune system, while relatively new, has direct parallel to each of the
other organ systems for which we have a therapy for dysfunction
(e.g. the heart, pulmonary, renal, gastrointestinal and CNS,
etc.). While not generally ready for widespread clinical use,
such therapies do exist in experimental forms and their development so far warrants their consideration for ultimate clinical use. Such therapy is termed immunoprophylaxis as it
involves pretreating an immunosuppressed host and demonstrating
that resistance is restored. Examples of such therapy include: thymic hormone therapy which has been employed in a
variety of immunodeficiencies and there is a strong clinical
impression that reduced infection results [1]. Thymosin α_1
has been given to mice immunosuppressed with 5-fluorouracil
pretreatment and shown to prevent the high mortality which
normally results from parenteral exposure to pathogens like
herpes virus, *candida, Listeria* and *pseudomonas* [2]. Muramyl
dipeptide, a macrophage activator, has been introduced in a
similar setting and has been shown to increase resistance to
a variety of pathogens [3]. Isoprinosine has been shown to
restore immune responsiveness in cancer patients, to ameliorate infections, and reduce tumour incidence [4]. Bestatin,
levamisole and tuftsin have been employed to treat ageing
mice prone by way of progressive immune deficiency to develop
a high incidence of tumours [5,7]. Such treated mice lived
longer and failed to develop the expected tumours. Reticulo-
endothelial system expanders in the form of polyglycans (e.g.
krestin, lentinan, levan, schyzophyllan, glucans) have been
generally effective in reducing the mortality and morbidity
of infectious challenge [8]. Interferon and various interferon inducers have been useful in preventing virus infection
[9]. These present only a few examples of possible therapeutic agents employed in an immunoprophylactic mode.

In this review I would like to enumerate some of the agents
available and to develop the possible target cells of various
immunotherapy agents so that in circumstances of immunotoxicity where the immunologic defect is defined, a therapeutic strategy could be envisaged for the treatment of the
immunosuppression. It should be emphasized that these are
experimental therapies developed principally for immunorestoration in cancer patients and they have yet to be applied
experimentally in a meaningful way in this context. For this
reason standard therapy involving vaccination, gamma globulin

administration, and avoidance of epidemic infections remains
the only currently available approach to manage such patients.

Immunotherapy Agents

Thymic hormones. A number of hormones have been isolated
from the thymus and have been demonstrated to induce the
maturation of T-cell precursors and to promote the differentiated and proliferative functions of mature T-cells [1,8,10].
These hormone preparations include thymosin fraction V,
thymosin α_1, thymopoietin, thymulin (previously facteur thy-
mique serique), and thymic humoral factor, to name a few. Of
these, thymosin α_1, thymopoietin and thymulin have been purified, sequenced, and synthesized chemically or by genetic
engineering techniques. With the exception of thymic humoral
factor each of these factors has been shown to derive from
thymic epithelial cells based on immunofluorescence studies.
The biological role of these secretory factors has not been
fully established; however, they are thought to regulate the
progressive maturation of T-cells and to contribute through
their heterogeneity to differential regulation of various
T-cell functions. While their intrathymic role remains unclear, their presence in the circulation and the correlation
of their declining levels with ageing and with the development of various immune-based diseases lends strong support to
their role as hormonal regulators. In a variety of circumstances in which animals have been made thymus-deficient, by
thymectomy or other means, these hormone preparations have
been shown to restore, at least partially, deficient T-cell
function. Based upon this experimental rationale these substances, particularly thymosin fraction V or equivalent extracts, have been employed clinically to treat both primary
and secondary immunodeficiency. The results to date have
been encouraging and while they are not specifically indicated
or licensed to treat any particular disease, their consideration for use in treating the deficits arising from thymus
atrophy, as occurs in PBB and asbestos exposure, seems
reasonable.

Lymphokines. While a large variety of T-cell produced soluble
mediators termed lymphokines have been described, space
limitations do not allow an elaboration here. Perhaps the
three lymphokines most relevant to consider in immunologic
reconstitution of immunosuppressed patients are T-cell growth
factor (TCGF), macrophage growth factor/colony stimulating
factor (MGF/CSF), and interferon (IFN).
 a) TCGF T-cell growth factor has an action to participate
in clonal expansion of T lymphocytes by acting as a second

signal in the initiation of proliferation and by perpetuating
repeated subsequent cell divisions [11]. It also has been
implicated as an inducer of natural killer (NK) cell activity.
Very recently, we [12] have found it to be a promoter of
differentiation of immature intrathymic lymphocytes and have
suggested that in concert with thymic hormones it is an essential factor in T-lymphocyte maturation and exit from the
thymus to replenish the peripheral T-cell pool. Defects in
TCGF production and action have been described in ageing and
autoimmune disorders in mice. While therapy with TCGF *per se*
has not been attempted, it seems logical to predict that as
chemically pure, genetically engineered TCGF becomes available its therapeutic use in T-cell lymphopenic disorders with
deficient delayed hypersensitivity will be attempted. Its
use in conjunction with thymic hormones will be rational and
may yield synergistic reconstitution.

   b) MGF/CSF. this factor acts to promote monocyte/macro-
phage proliferation both at the levels of the bone marrow and
in the periphery [13,14]. It is complemented in its action
by CSFs which act on both granulocyte and macrophage precursors. Collectively and individually, CSF will promote the
reconstitution of these two phagocytic populations. In addition, MGF/CSF has been described to activate macrophage bactericidal capacity [14]. Again, therapeutic application has
not been attempted in man; however, as purified, inexpensive
molecular preparations become available their use to re-
constitute the number and function of these cell populations
will be warranted. The MGF/CSF will be particularly relevant
in application to macrophage-mediated resistance to facultative intracellular pathogens including tubercle bacilli,
leprosy bacilli, salmonella and brucella and various viruses,
fungi and parasites.

   c) IFN. the interferons represent a group of antiviral
proteins which inhibit the intracellular replication of many
but not all viruses, inhibit both normal and malignant cell
proliferation, and promote killer cell functions of T-cells,
macrophages and NK cells [9]. With quantities of partially
purified IFN available, therapy of infections and tumours in
both animals and humans has been attempted. It is apparent
from these studies that pretreatment with interferon may
prevent certain viral infections, and to a lesser extent,
treatment after the onset of infection may ameliorate the
course of infection. γ or immune interferon is a lymphokine
selectively produced by T-cells and although the most extensive clinical experience with interferons has involved α or
leukocyte interferon, the therapeutic application of immune
interferon would be calculated, based on animal experiments
to be, at least, as effective and perhaps less toxic than

α interferon. Within the context of treatment of patients
suffering immunotoxicity, general application of IFN would
not be recommended since its antiproliferative effects may
inhibit immune reconstitution. The most appropriate applications would be in the context of specific infections, viral
and otherwise, to which macrophage and NK cells are critical
in resistance.

Levamisole. Levamisole (2,3,4,6-tetrahydro-6-phenylimidazo
(2,1-b) thiazole) was one of the first chemically-derived
immunostimulants [15-17]. Its immunopharmacology includes
actions directly on lymphocytes, macrophages and granulocytes
to modify their mobility, secretion and proliferation. It
can be augmenting or depressing in its effect depending on
the dose and timing of administration. *In vivo* levamisole
augments the expression of cellular more than humoral immunity,
and the latter effect is probably dependent on its action on
T-cells and macrophages. Its action is generally that of an
immunopotentiator in that demonstrable positive effects
usually require the concomitant administration of a primary
stimulus such as antigen. The magnitude of effects appears
to depend on the degree to which the stimulus is optimal and
the normality of the responding immune system. For this
latter characteristic, levamisole has been termed an "immuno-
normalizing" agent. In general, its action is weak and non-
responder strains of mice and individual humans exist for
reasons which are not yet clear. Its use has been relatively
safe with mild side effects of metallic taste, nervousness,
nausea and vomiting; however, occasional more severe side
effects are dermatitis and agranulocytosis (particularly in
individuals with HLA B 27 and rheumatoid arthritis).

In murine and human tumours when used in adjunctive protocols in which the primary tumour was decreased by chemotherapy,
radiation or surgery, levamisole showed some increase in mean
survival time or the number of individuals surviving. The
effect in humans with cancer, when observed, has been a small
increase (15%) in the number of patients remaining in remission following primary tumour reduction by other therapies.
Clinical efficacy in rheumatoid arthritis comparable to
penicillamine has been reported by a number of investigators.
Numerous reports have appeared of efficacy in such diverse
disorders as chronic and recurrent viral infections, *herpes*,
chronic and recurrent bacterial infections including leprosy,
aphthous stomatitis, erythema multiforme and lupus erythematosus. Each of these disorders is immune based and, almost
without exception in each, immunological disturbance has
been demonstrated which can be interpreted as contributing
to its pathogenesis. While the clinical applications can be

justified and supported, the issues of less than moderate
efficacy, prolonged periods to achieve a response, and certain
non-responder frequency in any particular disease category,
and our inability to monitor effects of drugs on the immune
system simply and consistently, has accounted for its slow
acceptance. Within the context of immunorestoration, a number of reports support the ability of levamisole to increase
defective delayed hypersensitivity and, in an animal study
[6], to reverse the effect of ageing on the immune response
and to prevent the otherwise high incidence of spontaneous
tumour development. Thus while active in the context of
immunorestoration, toxicity and inconsistent efficacy make
it not the first agent to consider.

Sulphur-containing agents. a) NPT 16416:   (7,8-dihydro-
thiazole-3,2,4-hypoxanthine) was first synthesized by us to
produce a nontoxic drug similar in structure and action to
levamisole [18]. NPT 16416 is considerably less toxic than
levamisole. Its immunopharmacologic effects to increase
active rosetting of T lymphocytes and to induce T-cell
differentiation in the Komuro and Boyse assay are evident *in
vitro* at 0.01 µg/mℓ. Like levamisole, only small effects are
observable on T-cell lymphoproliferative responses; however,
at 5-200 µg/mℓ, B-cell responses to endotoxin and pokeweed
are augmented. In mice, antibody responses to sheep erythrocytes are augmented by low doses of NPT 16416. The immunotherapeutic effects of this compound remain to be determined.
   b) DTC (sodium diethyldithiocarbamate) has been developed
by Renoux as a less toxic sulphur-containing compound based
on the premise that part of levamisole's *in vivo* activity
results from its sulphur moiety [19]. Like levamisole, DTC
induces *in vivo* a thymic hormone-like factor (hepatosin)
which is thought to derive from the liver rather than the
thymus. The cellular targets of action are presumed to be
T-cells based upon effects of DTC to induce hepatosin and,
in turn, of this substance to induce T-cell differentiation
in vitro. Other actions remain to be investigated. DTC has
been used safely as a treatment of human patients with metal
poisoning. In addition to pharmacologic effects to protect
animals against certain carcinogens and ionizing radiation,
DTC augments both humoral and cellular immune responses. *In
vivo* administration to humans has been demonstrated to modify
T-cell proliferative responses to mitogens and to restore
depressed T-cell rosetting to sheep erythrocytes, actions
shared by the thymic hormones. The therapeutic effects of
this compound remain to be determined.
   c) Other sulphur-containing compounds of interest include
thiabendazole, thiazolobenzimidazole (WY 18251-(3-(p-chloro-

phenyl(thiazole(3,2-a)benzimidazole-2-acetic acid), and
Cimetidine (N"-cyano-N-methyl-N'-2 (-methylimidazole-4yl)
methylthio ethyl guanidine).

Isoprinosine. Isoprinosine (a complex of p-acetoamidobenzoic
acid, N,N-dimethylamino-2-propanol and inosine (3:1 molar
ratio) is under development as an antiviral agent [4,21,22].
The components of isoprinosine form a complex by a variety of
physico-chemical criteria and as a complex, display biological
activities either not apparent or weakly so when the components are employed alone. Isoprinosine is virtually non-toxic
with only hyperuricaemia reported consistently as a side
effect. It has been applied in 57 countries to several
thousand humans for the treatment of viral or virus-related
disorders. In carefully controlled or double blind studies,
significant, mild to moderate efficacy to reduce symptoms
and/or shorten disease period or recurrences have been reported in subacute sclerosing panencephalitis (SSPE), and in
herpes simplex type II, influenza and rhinovirus infections.

While antiviral activity might be involved to explain these
clinical results, it seems much more likely that known effects
of this compound on the immune system make a more plausible
explanation. The immunopharmacology of isoprinosine includes
actions to induce lymphocyte differentiation in a way comparable to thymic hormones and actions to augment lymphocyte,
macrophage, and NK cell functions in a potentiator mode of
action. In general, the activity, both *in vitro* and *in vivo*,
of isoprinosine has been more consistently reproducible and
of greater magnitude than that of levamisole. While most of
the clinical studies have been for viral infections, a substantial amount of data supports effects of isoprinosine to
augment, in patients, virus-specific immune parameters,
mitogen and lymphokine responses, active rosettes and skin
test responses.

Isoprinosine has been shown to be active in murine tumour
systems to potentiate vaccine protection in L1210 leukaemia,
to potentiate interferon therapy in sarcoma 180, and to
reduce tumour development in NZB mice with autoimmune disease.
Isoprinosine therapy has promoted restoration of depressed
immunologic responses in humans with cancer treatment with
radiation and decreased infections in chemotherapy-treated
leukaemia patients. Within the context of immunoprophylaxis
two features of isoprinosine are particularly notable; the
first is that it has been taken continuously for up to 13
years without significant side effects, and the second is
that unlike other agents, it has not shown immunosuppression
based either on dose or frequency of administration. These
data, in addition to the animal studies, should justify the

immunoprophylactic application of isoprinosine in immunosuppressed patients. Such trials are being planned for patients with the recently described gay-related immunodeficiency
(GRID) also called acquired immunoregulatory disease (AID).

NPT 15392. A structurally similar (non-complex) compound,
NPT 15392, (9-erythro-2-hydroxy-3-nonylhypoxanthine) has been
developed by us [20,21]. This compound shares each of the
immunopharmacological activities of isoprinosine. A number
of differences in the degree of activities suggests that NPT
15392 may have clinical activities which will be complementary
to those of isoprinosine. Specifically, NPT 15392 at 0.01-1
µg/mℓ induces T-cell differentiation and augments active
rosettes of T-cells and modulates their proliferative, helper
and suppressor functions. It also potentiates lymphokine
effects on macrophages. At therapeutic doses of 0.1-1 mg/kg,
side effects in animals and humans have been negligible and
animal toxicity studies indicate an oral LD50 of more than
500 mg/kg. *In vivo* immunopharmacologic effects have included
significant augmentation of antibody and cellular immune responses in mice. NPT 15392 augments NK cell activity in mice
in vivo but not *in vitro*. This effect is apparently not
mediated by interferon and the effect of the combination of
interferon and NPT 15392 on NK cell activity is additive.

In murine models NPT 15392 has shown effects to partially
reverse tumour, virus and chemotherapy-induced immunosuppression in a number of studies. Correlation of immunorestoration with increased survival or decreased metastasis
formation has been observed in these studies. In immunopharmacologic trials in humans with cancer, under the aegis
of the EORTC, NPT 15392 showed effects to augment lymphocyte
counts, active rosettes, and NK cells in most, but not all,
patients. It also reduced elevated IgG levels. In the
immunotherapeutic perspective, it would appear necessary to
administer NPT 15392 intermittently rather than continuously.

Muramyl Dipeptide. Muramyl dipeptide (N-acetylmuramyl-L-
alanyl-D-isoglutamine, MDP) is a water-soluble substance
representing the smallest active component of the mycobacterial cell wall having adjuvant activity characteristic
of complete Freunds Adjuvant (CFA) [3]. A large series of
analogues have been prepared, particularly by French and
Japanese investigators, and it appears that the immunopharmacology of the MDP analogues depends on their particular
structure. MDP itself has both adjuvant potential when
administered with antigen and protective potential in bacterial challenge when given before and, to an extent, after
antigen. Based upon structure-function studies with the

analogues, these two activities appear to be dissociable.
The side effects of MDP, fever and prostaglandin production,
have been obviated by analogue formation. The n-butyl ester
derivative under development by Chedid and co-workers does
not induce fever and shows both adjuvant and protective
activity. Many of the published immunopharmacological studies
have been performed with MDP itself and the critical features
of action include promotion of macrophage activation for
tumouricidal and bactericidal activity and for secretion of
enzymes and monokines. The effect of MDP is a direct one not
requiring lymphokine or other influence. With oil and antigen,
MDP can augment both humoral and cellular immunity. *In vitro*
studies indicate action of MDP on T helper and suppressor
function and on B cell proliferation as well. The particip-
ation of monokines and other macrophage-derived mediators in
these functions has not been completely ruled out.

As a 3-substituted sugar, MDP is interesting in offering
insight into the immunostimulating mechanisms of polyglucoses
and glycans [8]. The various immunologically active glycans
(lentinan, krestin, levan, schizophyllan, etc) require a
1,3-β link to be active, suggesting that the chemical modification at the 3 position is critical. The various glycans
also appear to act via effects on the macrophage. The MDPs
may, therefore, offer a more specific approach to macrophage-
oriented immunotherapy without the problems of persistent
retention of high molecular weight antigens and without prolonged reticuloendothelial system expansion. While the major
focus on the MDPs has been on uses related to adjuvancy with
vaccines, their immunopharmacology strongly suggests useful
applications in infections in which the macrophage plays a
role in the resistance. A complementary therapeutic action
might well be observed with levamisole or isoprinosine.

Azimexon. Azimexon (BM12,531),2-(2-cyanaziridinyl)-(1)-(2-
carbamolyaziridinyl)-(1)-propane, is an orally active
immunostimulating compound [22]. Its immunopharmacology,
from *in vitro* studies, shows direct action on both lymphocytes and macrophages. *In vivo* studies show augmented cell-
mediated immunity, T-cell dependent humoral immunity and NK
cell activity. It also induces an expansion of the reticulo-
endothelial system with splenomegaly. It induces leukocytosis
and hastens recovery from leukopaenia. In animal studies with
cancer, the drug is more active in increasing survival and
longevity in adjuvant protocols with irradiation and chemotherapy than is levamisole. In human patients, a variety of
depressed immune parameters were improved following clinical
administration of azimexon. Its only significant side effect
known to date is a dose-related toxic haemolytic anaemia

which may limit clinical indications.

Bestatin. Bestatin ((2S, 3R)-3-amino-2-hydroxy-4-phenyl-butyryl-1-leucine) is a non-toxic, orally active immuno-stimulating compound extracted from *Streptomyces olivo-reticuli* [23]. Cellular targets of its action appear to be the macrophage, the bone marrow precursors for granulocytes, NK cells, and possibly T lymphocytes. *In vivo* injection in mice of 5-50 mg/kg increases DNA synthesis in the spleen, thymus, and bone marrow but not in other organs tested. *In vivo* treatment of mice is associated with up to 3-fold in-creases in antibody production to sheep erythrocytes (SRBC) and delayed hypersensitivity to SRBC or oxazolone. Immuno-restoration in tumour-bearing or chemotherapy-treated mice was also observed. Some tumour growth inhibition was observed by bestatin treatment in animals bearing slow growing tumours IMC and Gardner's lymphosarcoma and increased survival was observed in L1210 leukaemia or Erhlich's ascites tumour following chemotherapy. Prophylactic therapy inhibited spontaneous tumour development in aged mice in association with immunorestoration [5]. Human toxicity has been neglig-ible and efforts to increase NK cell activity and E rosette forming T-cells have been observed in some patients. Clari-fication of immunopharmacologic mechanisms is needed but additional clinical studies appear warranted.

Tuftsin. Tuftsin (Thr-Lys-Pro-Arg) represents residues 289-292 of the heavy chain of γ-globulin and is thought to be liberated by selective cleavage with tuftsin-endocarboxy-peptidase [24,25]. Tuftsin acts to stimulate motility, phagocytosis, processing of antigen, and tumouricidal activity in macrophages. Tuftsin increases neutrophil chemotaxis, phagocytosis, and killing. Reportedly, NK cell activity is increased. As a biological peptide, it is non-toxic and without significant side effects. *In vivo* administration of tuftsin in mice produces macrophages activated for tumour-icidal activity and increases T-cell dependent or independent antibody production and antibody-dependent cytotoxicity. In murine tumour models, tuftsin prolonged survival in L1210 leukaemia and in the Cloudman S-91 melanoma. In addition, immunoprophylactic therapy in aged mice reduced the incidence of spontaneous neoplasms, presumably a result of immuno-restoration [7].

Pyrimidinoles. In general, interferon inducers have been limited in their development by their toxicity and the refractory state to interferon induction which develops following their administration [26]. The 6-phenyl-

pyrimidinoles represent an interesting group of compounds in
this regard. Two compounds of this group 2-amino-5-bromo-
6-phenyl-4-pyrimidinol (ABPP) and 2-amino-5-iodo-6-phenyl-
4-pyrimidinol (AIPP) both show antiviral and antitumour
activity. While both agents activate macrophages and NK cells,
only ABPP is an inducer of interferon; the mechanisms of
their protective effects remains, therefore, to be fully
clarified. On the basis of its ability to induce interferon
ABPP has been emphasized and Stringfellow [26] has recently
reported that weekly administration can be used without losing
protection. The comparative effects of AIPP remain of great
interest since it apparently has potent immunomodulating
effects without interferon induction as a side effect.

CONCLUSION

The foregoing represents only a partial list of biologically-
and chemically-defined agents potentially useful in the
immunotherapy of patients who are immunosuppressed as a result of toxicological exposures. These agents can presently
be envisaged to be employed to reduce the frequency of infection resulting from immunosuppression, and hopefully to prevent the expected increase in cancer. In the development of
new strategies, already it is apparent that combinations of
immunotherapeutic agents offer potentiative interactions
(e.g. isoprinosine and interferon, MDP or endotoxin and
lymphokines, endotoxin and cell wall skeleton, etc) these
potentiative interactions need to be more fully explored.
With more potent immunorestoration, new, safe strategies to
overcome immunosuppression will be forthcoming.

REFERENCES

1. Goldstein, A.L., Lowe, T.L.K., Thurman, G., Zata, M.,
    Hall, N.R., McClure, J.E., Hu, S-K. and Shuloff, R.S.
    (1982). In "Immunological Approaches to Cancer Thera-
    peutics" (ed. E. Mihich), pp.137-190. John Wiley and
    Sons, New York.
2. Ishitsuka, R. Presented in symposium "Biological Res-
    ponse Modifiers in Human Oncology and Immunology"
    Tampa, July 1982. In press, Plenum Press, New York.
3. Lederer, E. and Chedid, L. (1982). In "Immunological
    Approaches to Cancer Therapeutics" (ed. E. Mihich),
    pp.107-136. John Wiley and Sons, New York.
4. Ginsberg, T. and Hadden, J.W. (1982). In "Frontiers in
    Immunomodulation" (eds. H. Fudenberg and F. Ambrogi).
    In press, Plenum Press, New York.
5. Bruley-Rosset, M., Hercend, T., Martinez, J., Rappaport,
    H. and Mathé, G. (1981). J. Natl. Cancer Inst. 166,
    1113-1119.

6. Bruley-Rosset, M., Florentin, I., Kiger, N., Schulz, J.
    and Mathé, G. (1979). *Immunol.* **38**, 75-83.
7. Bruley-Rosset, M., Florentin, I., Kiger, N., Schulz, J.
    and Mathé, G. (1982). *Cancer Treat. Rep.* in press.
8. DiLuzio, N. and Chihara, G. (1981). In "Advances in
    Immunopharmacology" (eds. J. Hadden *et al.*), pp.477-490.
    Pergamon Press, Oxford.
9. Johnson, H.M. (1982). In "Immunological Approaches to
    Cancer Therapeutics" (ed. E. Mihich), pp.241-256. John
    Wiley and Sons, New York.
10. Schuloff, R.S. and Goldstein, A.L. (1981). In "The
    Lymphokines" (eds. J.W. Hadden and W.E. Stewart II), pp.
    397-422. Humana Press, Clifotn, N.J.
11. Watson, J., Mochizuki, D. and Gillis, S. (1980). *Immunol.*
    Today **1**, 113-117.
12. Chen, S.S., Tung, J.S., Gillis, S., Good, R.A. and
    Hadden, J.W. (1982). *Int. J. Immunopharmac.* **4**, 381.
    (In press, *Proc. Natl. Acad. Sci.*).
13. Sadlik, J. and Hadden, J.W. (1983). In "Advances in
    Immunopharmacology II" (eds. L. Chedid, J. Hadden *et al.*).
    In press, Pergamon Press, Oxford.
14. Hadden, J., Englard, A., Sadlik, J.R. and Hadden, E.M.
    (1981). In "Lymphokines and Thymic Hormones" (eds. A.
    Goldstein and M. Chirigos), pp.159-172. Raven Press,
    New York.
15. Renoux, G. (1978). *Pharmac. Ther.* **2**, 397-421.
16. Symoens, J. and Rosenthal, M. (1977). *J. Retic. Endothel.*
    Soc. **21**, 175-194.
17. Amery, W. (1979). *Int. J. Immunopharmacol.* **1**, 65-70.
18. Hadden, J., Giner-Sorolla, A., Hadden, E., Ikehara, S.,
    Pahwa, R., Coffey, R., Castellazzi, A., Jones, C.,
    Maxwell, K. and Simon, L. (1982). *Int. J. Immunopharmacol.*
    4, 287.
19. Renoux, G. and Renoux, M. (1981). In "Augmenting Agents
    in Cancer Therapy" (eds. E. Hersh, M. Chirigos and M.
    Mastrangelo), pp.427-440. Raven Press, New York.
20. Hadden, J. and Giner-Sorolla, A. (1981). In "Augmenting
    Agents in Cancer Therapy" (eds. E. Hersh, M. Chirigos and
    M. Mastrangelo), pp.497-522.
21. Simon, L., McKensie, D. and Hadden, J. (1983). In
    "Biological Response Modifiers in Human Oncology and
    Immunology" (ed. H. Friedman). In press. Plenum Press,
    New York.
22. Chirigos, M. and Mastrangelo, M. (1982). In "Immuno-
    logical Approaches to Cancer Therapeutics" (ed. E. Milich),
    pp.191-240. John Wiley and Sons, New York.
23. Umezawa, H. (1981). "Small Molecular Immunomodifiers of
    Microbial Origin", Pergamon Press, New York

24. Najjar, V. and Schmidt, J. (1980). *Lymphokine Reports* **1**, 157-167.
25. Nishioka, K., Amoscoto, A., Babcock, G. (1981). *Life Sci*. **28**, 1081-1090.
26. Stringfellow, D. (1983). In "Advances in Immunopharmacology II" (eds. L. Chedid, J. Hadden *et al*.). In press, Pergamon Press, Oxford.

PROBLEMS IN IMMUNOTOXICOLOGICAL ASSESSMENT: EXAMPLES WITH DIFFERENT CLASSES OF XENOBIOTICS

F. Spreafico, A. Vecchi, M. Sironi and S. Filippeschi

INTRODUCTION

As repeatedly emphasized in this volume, immunotoxicology has to be considered as still a very young sub-speciality. This youth is reflected by a number of still unresolved problems of both practical and conceptual relevance, ranging from the definition of an immunotoxic substance to the best choice of experimental systems for both the initial recognition of immunoactivity of xenobiotics and for permitting a sound extrapolation of animal results to man. A number of these problems have recently been discussed elsewhere [1]. Accordingly, the objective of this chapter is to review a series of results obtained by this group, investigating the immunological activity of various representative xenobiotics and focusing on those aspects which can be regarded as being of more general significance.

Steroid Contraceptives

Our interest in investigating the possible immunological activity of steroid contraceptive drugs was stimulated essentially by the lack of direct information on this point, despite the large human use of such compounds and the fact that both estrogenic and progestagenic hormones have been reported to influence immune reactivity. For these studies three estrogen-progestin combinations were chosen which, at the time the study was initiated, were representative of those most used clinically. In order to simulate realistic clinical conditions, these contraceptive combinations were used at the minimal dose giving 100% antifertility effect in rodents. Conversely, it should be noted that most previous studies of immune effects of natural or synthetic hormones have been

IMMUNOTOXICOLOGY
ISBN 0-12-282180-7

Table 1 *Immunological effects of estrogen-progestin contraceptive combinations in rodents*

Drug	Dose (mg/kg /day)	anti-SRBC PFC mouse	anti-SRBC PFC rat	EAE rat	Auto-abs. mouse	Con A mouse	LPS mouse	anti-SIII PFC % mouse	Thy 1+ cells mouse
norethindrone + mestranol	4 0.2	↓↓	–	↓↓	↓↓	↓↓	–	–	↓
norethynodrel + mestranol	4 0.06	↓	–	↓↓	↓	–	–	–	↓
lynestrenol + mestranol	5 0.3	–	–	↓↓	–	–	–	–	–

SRBC, decreased mouse antibody formation to T-dependent antigen sheep erythrocyte; PFC, plaque-forming cells; EAE, experimental allergenic encephalomyelitis; auto-abs., anti mouse-erythrocyte autoantibodies; Con A, concanavalin A mitogenesis; LPS, lipopolysaccharide mitogenesis; Thy 1+ marker thymus cells; ↓, decreased response or number; –, no effect.

performed with non-physiological, indeed frequently supra-
pharmacological doses. These results have been detailed elsewhere [1,2] and are summarized in Table 1. In the conditions
employed, contraceptive treatment was associated with significant depression of both humoral and cell-mediated reactivities
as for instance revealed by decreased antibody formation in
mice to the T-dependent antigen sheep erythrocytes (SRBC),
decreased titre and proportion of animals forming anti-mouse
erythrocyte autoantibodies, and reduced duration, severity and
proportion of affected animals in another autoimmunity model,
i.e. experimental allergic encephalomyelitis (EAE) in rats.
As analysed in depth in the mouse primary anti-SRBC response,
immunodepression was relatively moderate, entailing only 50-
70% reduction in antibody-forming splenocyte numbers, seen
only after repeated contraceptive treatments (at least 8-day
treatment with the most active norethindrone-mestranol combination and 30 days with lynestrenol - mestranol) and was
readily reversible upon treatment discontinuation.

In addition, no significant effects were observed by reducing the contraceptive dose by 50% or when the progestin
or the estrogen components were given alone at the same dose
present in the active combination. In an attempt to define
the possible cellular target of oral contraceptive immune
activity, it was observed that at doses capable of inhibiting
the anti-SRBC response, the mouse humoral response to a T-
independent antigen (type III pneumococcal polysaccharide)
was unaffected. Splenocytes of mice given immunodepressive
contraceptive treatment showed a reduced responsiveness to
the T stimulant Con A, whereas their reactivity to the B mitogen LPS was unimpaired. Although any contraceptive effects
on other immunocytes (e.g. macrophages, suppressor cells) were
not investigated, these data together with the effects on EAE
and anti-erythrocyte autoantibodies (both T-dependent reactivities), support the hypothesis that T-lymphocytes are, if
not the exclusive, at least a primary target of oral contraceptive immunodepression. This contention is also supported
by the finding that in mice given immunodepressive contraceptive regimens, and in which total spleen cellularity is unchanged, lowered proportions of T but not B cells could be seen.

Table 1 also shows two findings of possibly more general
significance in relation to immunotoxicological testing and
evaluation. Firstly, significant differences in the potency
of the immunological effects were present among the three oral
contraceptive combinations tested, the norethindrone-mestranol
combination proving in our conditions, to be the most active
one, whereas lynestrenol-mestranol was effective only in one
of the model conditions investigated. Although our experiments
provide no direct clues as to the basis for this inter-drug

difference, this observation draws attention to the possibility
that xenobiotics of similar classes may significantly vary in
their immunotoxicological potential. Secondly, the differential susceptibility to a given oral contraceptive of the same
immune reactivity (i.e. the primary anti-SRBC response) in
mice and rats, underlines the possibility that even closely
related animal species may differ in their sensitivity to
exogenously-induced immuno-modulation. This point has obvious
relevance to the choice of animal species for immunotoxicological screening and to the extrapolation of animal results
to man. In connection with the latter point, it is worth
noting that reports describing an SCD-dependent immunodepressive activity in humans have been published [3]. These
effects include lowered mitogen reactivity, changes in immunoglobulin and autoantibody levels, altered humoral responses to
standard vaccines and improvements in patients with autoimmune
pathologies, i.e. all immunological effects paralleling those
observed in animals. The finding that T-cell function is
reduced in animals given pharmacological doses of oral contra-
ceptives, and the relatively moderate immunodepression found
in our study, may also have a bearing on the higher incidence
of viral infections observed in chronic oral contraceptive
users of the Third World countries, but apparently not seen
in the Western World [3]. Cells of the T-lineage are tradi-
tionally believed to be more important in the defence against
viral infections. Relatively minor immune derangements may
combine with other immunodepression-causing factors, such as
a low nutritional status, to produce overt pathological consequences, especially in areas where certain infectious agents
are endemic.

Saccharin

The main reasons for investigating the possible immunological
activity of saccharin were the following. Firstly, this
artificial sweetener (1,2-benzisothiazol-3(2H)-one-1,1-dioxide)
is widely employed in the Western World, as reflected by the
fact that at least one fourth of the U.S.A. population uses
products containing this chemical for a total consumption
estimated in 1976 in the range of 3 million kilograms. In
addition, saccharin has been reported to be a carcinogen or
cocarcinogen in rodents, primarily inducing bladder tumours
[4-8], although the existence of an oncogenic risk for man
with this chemical is still a matter of debate [9-12]. Considering that the mechanism(s) of animal oncogenicity of
saccharin are still obscure and that immune disturbances may,
in principle, play a role in carcinogenesis, it was therefore
of interest to examine whether the chemical possessed

immunological reactivity in experimental conditions. In view
of the fact that saccharin is apparently not biotransformed
in vivo [13], the first studies were conducted *in vitro*,
focusing on cells currently credited with a major role in the
control of neoplastic cell emergence, i.e. macrophages and NK
cells. As detailed elsewhere [14-16], *in vitro* exposure of
rat and mouse cells to at least 99.5% pure saccharin in the
0.1 - 2 mg/ml concentration range did not significantly modify
(in either direction) macrophage or NK-cell dependent cytotoxicity capacity. However, a significant and marked (up to
90%) inhibition in responsiveness to PHA and LPS was observed
when rodent lymph node cells were exposed throughout the test
to saccharin concentrations at and above 0.5 mg/ml, whereas
lower concentrations (0.05 - 0.2 mg/ml) were essentially ineffective (Table 2). It should be noted in this connection
that the inhibitory concentrations found in these conditions
are realistic in the rat (i.e., the species in which bladder
tumours after saccharin feeding were first described), since
a 5% saccharin diet in this species results in circulating
levels of this chemical of the order of 0.06 mg/ml, whereas
in the urine they can be as high as 30 mg/ml.

In agreement with the *in vitro* results, no changes in macrophage and NK-cell cytotoxicity were found in rats and mice
tested after 30 days feeding with 1-5% saccharin-containing
diets. On the other hand, this same treatment produced in
both rats and mice a clear decrease in the number of splenocytes producing antibody after primary immunization with sheep
erythrocytes, a reduction already evident with a 1% diet and
which was progressively stronger with higher doses of the
chemical (Table 2). At variance with this finding, a 30 days
feeding period with 5% saccharin did not significantly affect
delayed-type hypersensitivity to the same antigen, and was
not associated with detectable changes in lymphoid cellularity,
nor indeed with any obvious untoward health effect. It may
also be mentioned that in our hands no differences in the
sensitivity to *in vitro* or *in vivo* saccharin were seen between
male and female rodents, whereas in some studies [4,8], males
have been reported as having a greater susceptibility to
saccharin-associated carcinogenicity. Results described above
could in principle support the possibility that repeated exposure to high doses of saccharin may be associated in experimental animals with an immunotoxicological risk. Although
macrophage and NK-cell dependent activities appeared resistant to this chemical, saccharin reduced the responsiveness
to both T and B mitogens *in vitro*. Saccharin given *in vivo*
decreased primary antibody production while leaving unchanged
the cell-dependent reactivities. The possible biochemical
basis for such apparently selective immunological effects are

Table 2 *Immunological effects of saccharin in rats*

IN VITRO				IN VIVO		
Saccharin mg/ml	Mitogenesis PHA %			Saccharin in diet %	Anti-SRBC.PFC per spleen[a]	Splenocyte number (x 10^6) (mean ± S.E.)
	0	3	cpm			
–	2531 ± 366	32053 ± 2480		–	19925 (18535-21430)	497 ± 94
0.1	4067 ± 881	58064 ± 7425		1.0	3255 (2740-3865)**	426 ± 96
0.2	2439 ± 395	56319 ± 508		2.5	1400 (1325-1480)**	366 ± 103
0.5	3604 ± 409	26903 ± 2789*		5.0	865 (635-1185)**	494 ± 107
2.0	3309 ± 873	22680 ± 2227*				

[a] anti-SRBC haemolytic plaque-forming cells (PFC) were evaluated at peak primary response, immunization being performed after a 30 days saccharin diet at the indicated concentrations.

* p < 0.05

** p < 0.01

PHA, phytohaemagglutinin

unresolved, and also undetermined is whether this activity is of relevance in the animal oncogenicity of saccharin. As the concentrations of this chemical that are to be inhibitory for lymphocyte mitogen reactivity *in vitro* are well within those found in the urine of animals fed a carcinogenic diet, and *in vivo* antibody depression was seen at doses below (i.e. 1%) the minimal ones reported [4] to be carcinogenic in rodents (i.e. 5%), one may speculate that a local impairment of at least some lymphocyte-mediated defences might occur.

As with many animal toxicology studies the question can be raised as to the relevance of the preclinical results to man, a question reinforced by the finding that the immune changes seen in our studies were selective and observed only at high but not at lower saccharin doses or concentrations. A 5% saccharin diet (i.e., the allegedly minimally effective one as carcinogenic in rats) corresponds to a daily intake of 5 g/kg for a 300 g rat, whereas it has been estimated that the average daily intake of this sweetener for the U.S.A. population is between 0.4 and 3 mg/kg, depending on age and diet [11]. However, simple comparisons of exposure, although informative, are not necessarily the correct approach in such animal-man extrapolation problems, since differences in pharmacokinetics or metabolism among species may markedly influence bioavailability and thus the biological effects of xenobiotics.

Table 3 gives the main kinetic parameters obtained in a recent study from this Institute in rats given a 5% saccharin diet and in adult volunteers receiving "normal" daily intakes (130 mg/60 kg) of this chemical [17]. It was observed that rats given a carcinogenic 5% saccharin diet have in their body fluids, concentrations of saccharin several orders of magnitude higher than seen in humans "normally" exposed to this sweetener. As in rats fed this compound, tumours arise preferentially if not exclusively in the bladder, urinary saccharin levels may be of greater interest and Table 3 shows that the mean saccharin urinary levels in rats were 200 times higher than in man, this rat/man differential reaching a value of over 700 if the 24 h excretion/kg parameter is considered. Rats given a 1% saccharin diet (which decreased humoral but not cellular reactivities in our tests) excreted approximately 70 and 200 times greater quantities of this compound in the urine than "normally" exposed humans, considering the above-mentioned parameters.

On the basis of these bioavailability data, it would appear likely that a standard human dietary exposure to this sweetener should be associated with a relatively wide margin of safety in terms of immunotoxicological risk, if it is assumed that rodent and human lymphoid cells are equally sensitive to

Table 3 *Saccharin pharmacokinetic parameters in rats fed a carcinogenic 5% saccharin diet, and in human volunteers given a "standard" dietary intake of this sweetener.*

Parameter	Rat (5 g/kg)	Man (2.2 mg/kg) [a]	Rat/Man ratio
Peak urinary concentration (μg/ml)	34,670	175	198
Mean urinary concentration (μg/ml)	24,600	120	205
24 h urine excretion (μg/kg)	$1,380 \times 10^3$	1,880	735
Peak plasma concentration (μg/ml)	54	0.35	155
AUC[b] of plasma (mg/ml/h)	836	2.24	385

[a] Daily for 5 days

[b] Area under the curve

saccharin. In connection with the latter point, it should however be added that in a series of tests, human lymphocytes were not affected in their responsiveness to mitogens even when exposed *in vitro* to saccharin concentrations which were markedly and consistently inhibitory for rodent cells in the same conditions, thus suggesting the existence of a further safety factor for man. Whether this susceptibility difference between rodent and human lymphocytes also applies to other cells, and other biological effects of saccharin, is still unknown. In a more general immunotoxicological perspective, our findings described herein not only illustrate again the possibility that xenobiotics may be quite selective in their immunological effects, but may be viewed as re-emphasizing the importance of considering basic pharmacological tenets (such as the use of bioavailability data) and of conducting multi-species analysis in the performance of immuno-toxicological investigations with the objective of obtaining information more relevant to the assessment of human risk potential of xenobiotics.

TCDD and TCDF

Polychlorinated dibenzodioxins and dibenzofurans are persistent environmental pollutants and their 2,3,7,8-tetrachloro
isomers (TCDD and TCDF, respectively) are known to possess
very high toxicity in all animal species investigated. TCDD
can be formed in the industrial synthesis of 2,4,5-trichloro-
phenol and thus occur as a contaminant of widely-used chemicals such as herbicides, and accidental poisoning of animals
and humans has occurred in a number of instances as a consequence of the production and/or use of chlorophenol and chloro-
benzene compounds [18,19]. TCDF is present in polychlorinated
dibenzofuran mixtures detectable in polychlorinated biphenyls
(PCBs) which have also been responsible for a series of large-
scale animal and human poisoning [20,21]. In addition, the
potential for wide human exposure to these chemicals is increased by the presence of TCDD and TCDF in the exhaust
products of municipal and industrial heating facilities and
incinerators [22].

Although various aspects of the toxicology of these compounds are still unclear, an immunological activity has been
well documented in animals in the case of TCDD [23,24], but
to a much lower extent for TCDF which is considered to be
generally 15-30 times less toxic than TCDD [25]. In our hands
[15,26-29], TCDD induced in mice a profound and long-lasting
depression of humoral responses to T-dependent and independent
antigens; repeated exposures by either oral or parenteral
routes requiring lower quantities for effective suppression
than single administrations. For instance, a single 6 µg/kg
TCDD dose inhibited, by over 80%, the number of primary anti-
SRBC antibody-producing splenocytes in C57Bl/6 mice for a
period exceeding 40 days (Table 4). Secondary responses,
which are generally more resistant to modulation by drugs or
chemicals, were also markedly suppressed, a point of possible
concern for humans, for instance in relation to defence
against infections. A depression in humoral immunity was
also seen in mice born and fostered by mothers given TCDD
during pregnancy and lactation; indeed, evidence has been obtained that TCDD is markedly more damaging to a developing
immune system, as *in utero* or during the first days after
birth. As similar higher sensitivity has also been documented
for other xenobiotics, the point appears of general importance
for immunotoxicological evaluation.

Also of relevance to the problem of the choice of experimental conditions in immunotoxicity testing is the finding
that antibody depression by TCDD in the mouse is markedly
strain-dependent, the susceptibility directly paralleling the
TCDD capacity to bind to specific cytosol receptors and to

Table 4 *Immunodepressive effects of TCDD and TCDF in C57B1/6 mice*

DOSE RESPONSE*			TIME-COURSE**		
Substance	Dose (µg/kg)	PFC/spleen (% of control)	Substance	Day of treatment	PFC/spleen (% of control)
–	–	100	–	–	100
TCDD	0.5	42	TCDD	-7	14
	1.2	38		-21	16
	6.0	14		-42	20
	30.0	3			
TCDF	11	67	TCDF	-7	17
	45	49		-21	45
	180	17		-42	73
	900	9			

*TCDD or TCDF were given i.p. 7 days before antigen (SRBC).

**6 µg/kg TCDD or 180 µg/kg TCDF were given i.p. at days reported.

SRBC (4 x 10^8) were given i.p. on day 0 and test was performed 5 days later.

induce arylhydrocarbon hydroxylase (AHH), an enzymic complex known to be involved in the biotransformation of a variety of aromatic xenobiotics including carcinogens. Since the locus controlling AHH expression is involved in the function of other genes, it has been hypothesized that the nuclear trans-location of the receptor-ligand complex may result in changes in gene expression or repression [30]. In line with the finding that in all species investigated the thymus is the organ most affected by TCDD, this chemical also affects cell-mediated immunity. Although in our experiments the capacity of lymphocytes to respond to mitogens and to recognize allo-antigens in a graft-versus-host assay was not affected, an evident and persistent cell depletion in central and periph-eral lymphoid organs occurred after TCDD administration to adult mice of a sensitive strain. In other words, under these conditions there was no functional inhibition on a unit cell number basis, although a reduction in the total organ

capacity to mount cellular reactivities was present. Similarly, young adult rodents given otherwise immunodepressive TCDD
doses had no impairment in NK and macrophage-mediated cytotoxicity, although cellular depletion which also included
cells of the monocyte-macrophage lineage resulted in a reduction in total capacity to express both activities. It should
be mentioned however that TCDD administration to mice in the
pre- and post-natal period was found to be associated not only
with lowered numbers of cells involved in natural resistance,
but also with their functional impairment. These effects contribute to the decreased resistance to infection and tumour
challenges seen after TCDD treatment [24] and, possibly, also
play a role in its animal carcinogenicity [31,32].

   The effects of TCDD on humoral reactivity are qualitatively
paralleled by TCDF [33], single injections of doses above
20 μg/kg being significantly depressive of the primary anti-
SRBC response (Table 4). The duration of humoral depression
was also significantly shorter with TCDF, possibly in relation
to its shorter half-life in the body (2 days versus 17 for
TCDD), whereas the strain-dependency of this effect was comparable to that of TCDD. The decrease in thymus cellularity
was also markedly strain-dependent, which suggests that
T-dependent reactivities may also be impaired with TCDF,
although detailed results on cell-mediated responses are not
yet available. The strain-dependency of the effects observed,
and the finding that TCDF is *in vitro* the most potent inhibitor of TCDD binding to specific receptors [34], support the
possibility that these receptors also play a role in the *in
vivo* biological activity of TCDF, although the binding may be
weaker and/or of shorter duration as suggested by the shorter
$T_{\frac{1}{2}}$ of this chemical in the body and its shorter immune effects.

Plant Toxins

Not only man-made chemicals but also natural substances may
have an immunotoxicological potential. Although little attention has so far been paid to such xenobiotics, one may find
potent immunomodulators in plant toxins as, for instance,
shown by the immunological activity of plant lectins such as
PHA [35] or of aflatoxins [36], as well as that of fungal
products such as Lentinan [37]. With this background it was
of interest to investigate [38] the possible immune effects
of two protein synthesis inhibitors of vegetable origin, the
so-called *Momordica charantia* inhibitor (MCI) and *Phytolacca
americana* antiviral protein (PAP-S); both are approximately
30,000 daltons proteins representative of toxic proteins
widely distributed in the vegetable kingdom, including plants
of major interest such as oat, barley, etc. Interest in

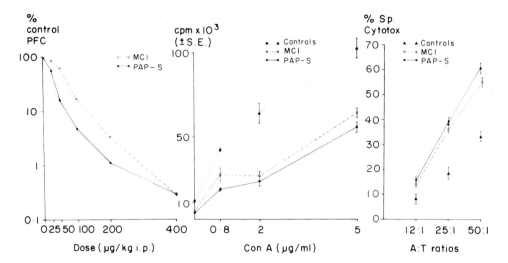

Fig. 1 **Effect of the *in vivo* administration of MCI and PAP-S
on murine immune reactivities.** Left panel: primary immune
response to SRBC evaluated in the spleen 4 days after immunization. Centre panel: splenocyte response to Con A, results
expressed as ^{3}H-TdR uptake after 72 h culture. Right panel:
spleen macrophage-mediated cytotoxicity against tumour target
cells evaluated after 72 h culture at different Attacker:
Target (A:T) cell ratios. Substances were injected 2 days
before antigenic stimulation or *in vitro* testing.

these products derives from their close structural and biochemical similarity to ricin chain A, i.e. that part of the
ricin molecule (a substance known for its extreme toxicity)
which blocks protein synthesis by irreversibly binding to the
60S ribosomal subunit.

In mice, single injections of MCI and PAP-S in perfectly
tolerated doses can markedly suppress antibody formation to
T-dependent antigens, while totally sparing that to T-
independent stimuli. In addition (Figure 1), these substances reduced *in vitro* and *in vivo* lymphocyte responsiveness to T-cell polyclonal activators while affecting that to
B cell mitogens only at concentrations resulting in a decrease
in cell viability, thus suggesting that B cells are not a
primary target for MCI and PAP-S. The involvement of T cells
is further supported by the capacity of these substances to
reduce delayed-type hypersensitivity, to prolong skin allograft survival and to inhibit NK-cell mediated cytotoxicity.
On the other hand, the injection of clearly immunodepressive
doses was associated with very evident increases in macrophage

functional capacity (Fig. 1), an enhancement also seen *in vitro* employing pure macrophage preparations. The precise relationship between the latter effect and the apparent T cell inhibition induced by these substances, and thus the recognition of the primary cell target(s) for MCI and PAP-S, is still in need of clarification.

On a more general level, the findings described reiterate the possibility that the immunological activity of xenobiotics can be quite complex with the possible coexistence of effects of opposite sign. In addition to emphasizing that substances active on the immune system, even in minute doses, are widely distributed in our environment, these results draw attention to the possibility that damage to immunity can be a very sensitive indicator of toxicity. Immune effects induced by the above toxins were in fact seen at doses not associated with other organ-specific or general toxicity.

ACKNOWLEDGEMENTS

This work was supported by CNR Progetto Finalizzato "Chimica Fine e Secondaria" Contract No. 81.01747.95, Euratom Contract No. B10-C-355-81-I, and a grant of the Gustavus and Louise Pfeiffer Foundation.

REFERENCES

1. Vecchi, A., Tagliabue, A., Mantovani, A., Anaclerio, A., Barale, C. and Spreafico, F. (1976). *Biomedicine* **24**, 231-237.
2. Spreafico, F., Vecchi, A., Anaclerio, A., Moras, M.L., Tagliabue, A., Barale, C., Mantovani, A., Sironi, M. and Polentarutti, N. (1977). In "Pharmacology of Steroid Contraceptive Drugs" (eds. S. Garattini and H.W. Berendes), pp.267-276. Raven Press, New York.
3. Royal College of Practitioners (1974). A Report from the Oral Contraception Study, pp.176-179. Pitman Medical Publications, London.
4. Arnold, D.L., Charbonneau, S.M., Moddie, C.A. and Munro, I.C. (1977). *Toxicol. Appl. Pharmacol.* **41**, 164.
5. Mondal, S., Brankow, D.W. and Heidelberger, C. (1978). *Science* **201**, 1141-1142.
6. Ashby, J., Styles, J.A., Anderson, D. and Paton, D. (1978). *Food Cosmet. Toxicol.* **16**, 95-103.
7. Chowaniec, J. and Hicks, R.M. (1979). *Br. J. Cancer* **39**, 355-375.
8. Taylor, J.M., Weinberger, M.A. and Friedman, L. (1980). *Toxicol. Appl. Pharmacol.* **54**, 57-75.
9. Howe, G.R., Burch, J.D., Miller, A.B., Morrison, B.,

    Gordon, P., Welcon, L., Chambers, L.W., Fodor, G. and
    Winsor, G.M. (1972). *Lancet* **2**, 578-581.

10. Newell, G.R., Hoover, R.N. and Kolbye, A.C. (1978). *J. Natl. Cancer Inst.* **61**, 275-276.

11. National Academy of Sciences (USA) (1978). Technical Assessment of Risks and Benefits. Committee for the Study of Saccharin and Food Safety Policy. Report no. 1. Government Printing Office, Washington D.C., USA.

12. Editorial (1980). *Lancet* **1**, 855-856.

13. Sweatman, T.W. and Renwick, A.G. (1979). *Science* **205**, 1019-1020.

14. Mantovani, A., Luini, W., Candiani, G.P., Salmona, M., Spreafico, F. and Garattini, S. (1980). *Toxicol. Lett.* **5**, 287-295.

15. Spreafico, F., Vecchi, A., Mantovani, A., Tagliabue, A., Sironi, M., Luini, W. and Garattini, S. (1981). In "Advances in Immunopharmacology" (eds. J. Hadden, L. Chedid, P. Mullen and F. Spreafico), pp.295-310. Pergamon Press, Oxford.

16. Luini, W., Mantovani, A. and Garattini, S. (1981). *Toxicol. Lett.* **8**, 1-6.

17. Pantarotto, C., Salmona, M. and Garattini, S. (1981). *Toxicol. Lett.* **9**, 367-371.

18. Firestone, D. (1978). *Ecol. Bull.* **27**, 39-52.

19. Reggiani, G. (1980). *J. Toxicol. Environ. Health* **6**, 27-43.

20. Nagayama, J., Kuratsune, M. and Masuda, Y. (1976). *Bull. Environ. Contam. Toxicol.* **15**, 9-13.

21. Bekesi, G. This volume.

22. Rappe, C., Buser, H.R. and Bosshardt, H.P. (1979). *Ann. N.Y. Acad. Sci.* **320**, 1-18.

23. Vos, J.G. (1977). CRC Crit. Rev. Toxicol. **5**, 67-101.

24. Vos, J.G., Faith, R.E. and Luster, M.I. (1980). In "Halogenated Biphenyls, Terphenyls, Naphthalenes, Dibenzo-dioxins and Related Products" (ed. R.D. Kimbrough), pp. 241-266. Elsevier/North Holland Biomedical Press, Amsterdam.

25. Moore, J.A., McConnell, E.E., Dalgard, D.W. and Harris, M.W. (1979). *Ann. N.Y. Acad. Sci.* **320**, 151-163.

26. Vecchi, A., Mantovani, A., Sironi, M., Luini, W., Spreafico, F. and Garattini, S. (1980). *Arch. Toxicol.* Suppl. **4**, 163-165.

27. Mantovani, A., Vecchi, A., Luini, W., Sironi, M., Candiani, G.P., Spreafico, F. and Garattini, S. (1980). *Biomedicine* **32**, 200-204.

28. Vecchi, A., Mantovani, A., Sironi, M., Luini, W., Cairo, M. and Garattini, S. (1980). *Chem. Biol. Interact.* **30**, 337-342.

29   Garattini, S., Vecchi, A., Sironi, M. and Mantovani, A.
     (1982). In "Chlorinated Dioxins and Related Compounds"
     (eds. O. Hutzinger, R.W. Frei, E. Merian and F. Pocchiari),
     pp.403-409. Pergamon Press, Oxford.
30. Poland, A., Greenlee, W.F. and Kende, A.S. (1979). *Ann.*
     N.Y. Acad. Sci. **320**, 214-230.
31. Kociba, R.J. and Schwetz, B.A. (1982). *Drug Metab. Rev.*
     13, 387-406.
32. Kouri, R.E., Rude, T.H., Joglekar, R., Dansettee, P.M.,
     Jerina, D.M., Atlas, S.A., Owens, I.S. and Nebert, D.W.
     (1978). *Cancer Res.* **38**, 2777-2783.
33. Vecchi, A., Sironi, M., Canegrati, M.A. and Garattini, S.
     In "Chlorinated Dioxins and Dibenzofurans in the Total
     Environment" (eds. L.H. Keith, G. Choudary and C. Rappe).
     Ann Arbor Science Publishers, in press.
34. Greenlee, W.F. and Poland, A. (1979). *J. Biol. Chem.*
     254, 9814-9821.
35. Spreafico, F. and Lerner, E.M. (1967). *J. Immunol.* **98**,
     407-416.
36. Pier, A.C. (1978). In "Inadvertent Modification of the
     Immune Response: Effect of Foods, Drugs and Environmental
     Chemicals". Proc. 4th FDA Science Symp., pp.123-127.
     Government Printing Office, Washington DC.
37. Zakany, J., Chihara, G. and Fachet, J. (1980). *Int. J.*
     Cancer **25**, 371-376.
38. Spreafico, F., Malfiore, C., Moras, M.L., Marmonti, L.,
     Filippeschi, S., Barbieri, L., Perocco, P. and Stirpe, F.
     Int. J. Immunopharmacol., in press.

MONOCLONAL ANTIBODY-TOXIN CONJUGATES AS SELECTIVE CYTOTOXIC AGENTS

B.M.J. Foxwell

Imperial Cancer Research Fund,
P.O. Box 123, Lincoln's Inn Fields, London WC2A 3PX, UK

The advent of monoclonal antibodies has opened up several avenues for the application of immunochemistry to clinical medicine. One concept which has received much attention recently is that of the "magic bullet". This idea, similar to that first proposed by Paul Ehrlich nearly a century ago, is to use the high selectivity of antibodies to direct cytotoxic agents to diseased cells. One group of cytotoxic agents which appears well suited for targeting are toxic plant lectins such as abrin and ricin. The likelihood that the entry of one toxin molecule into a cell is sufficient to kill [1] makes these proteins prime candidates for this work.

  Ricin, the toxin from the castor bean, and abrin, the toxin from the jequirty bean, are glycoproteins composed of two polypeptide chains, A and B, linked by a disulphide bond. The cytotoxic effect of these toxins is believed to be the result of a three stage process. Firstly, the toxin binds to galactose-containing cell-surface receptors via a recognition site on the B chain. This is followed by internalization and penetration, at least of the A chain, into the cytosol. Finally, the A chain catalytically inactivates ribosomes by modifying the 60 S subunit, thus abolishing EF-2 catalysed GTPase activity [2] and blocking protein synthesis.

  The aim, in constructing antibody-toxin conjugates, is to replace the low binding specificity of the B chain with the high selectivity of an antibody while retaining fully the membrane penetration and ribosome inactivation qualities of the A chain. Two possible strategies for constructing antibody-toxin conjugates can be envisaged. The simplest option is to couple the intact toxin to the antibody. The alternative is to split the toxin molecule into its constituent subunits and link only the A chain to the antibody.

IMMUNOTOXICOLOGY
ISBN 0-12-282180-7

The following text will show examples of both types of conjugate and illustrate their potential virtues and short-
comings as cytotoxic agents.

Antibody-Intact Toxin Conjugates

A conjugate of monoclonal anti-$Thy_{1.1}$ antibody and abrin was
tested by Thorpe and his coworkers [3,4] for selective cytotoxicity against $Thy_{1.1}$ expressing lymphoma cells in tissue
culture and in animals. The $F(ab')_2$ fragment of the antibody
was used, rather than intact antibody, to prevent non-specific
binding of the conjugate to cells in the mice such as
B-lymphocytes and macrophages which possess receptors for the
Fc portion of the immunoglobulin.

The conjugate was formed using a mixed anhydride derivative
of chlorambucil as the coupling agent [3]. The simple conjugate containing one molecule of antibody and one of toxin
was purified by gel chromatography. No loss of antigen binding capacity of the anti-$Thy_{1.1}$-abrin conjugate was detectable
by indirect immunofluorescence in 100 mM lactose [5].

Figure 1 shows the potent cytotoxic action of the anti-
$Thy_{1.1}$-abrin conjugate on $Thy_{1.1}$ expressing lymphoma cell
lines in tissue culture. Toxicity was assessed from the reduction in protein-synthetic activity of the cells which was
measured by ^{3}H-leucine incorporation into acid-precipitable
material. From dose-response curves, the concentration of
conjugate needed to reduce the uptake of ^{3}H-leucine by AKR-A
and BW5147 cells to 50% of that of non-treated control cul-
tures was 2.5×10^{-11} M and 5×10^{-11} M respectively. A control conjugate, made with a $F(ab')_2$ fragment of normal mouse
IgG2a, was found to be ten times less toxic than the specific
conjugate to AKR-A cells and one hundred times less toxic to
BW5147 cells, showing that the marked toxic action of anti-
$Thy_{1.1}$-abrin upon the lymphoma cells was facilitated by the
antigen-binding of the antibody.

Conjugates with intact abrin and ricin, although highly
effective as cytotoxic agents for target cells in tissue
culture, nevertheless retain substantial non-specific toxicity
to cells which lack the appropriate antigens. This is because
the conjugates can bind via the B chain of their toxin moiety
to galactose-containing receptors which are normally present
on cell surfaces. This is clearly demonstrated by the experiment illustrated in Fig. 2 which showed that in the presence
of excess free galactose the toxicity of abrin and of a
normal IgG-abrin conjugate for a human lymphoma cell line was
abolished whereas that of abrin coupled to anti-lymphocyte
globulin was unimpaired.

The possible *in vivo* potential of these conjugates as anti-

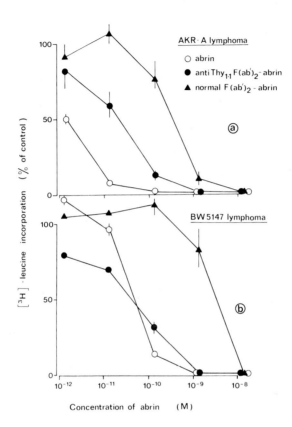

Fig. 1 Cytotoxic effects of anti Thy$_{1.1}$ F(ab')$_2$-abrin conjugate upon Thy$_{1.1}$-expressing lymphoma cells in tissue
culture. Lymphoma cells AKR-A(a) and BW5147(b) were treated
with abrin or the conjugate for 1 h and were then washed;
23 h later 1 μCi of ^{3}H-leucine was added to the cultures.
The ^{3}H-leucine incorporated during a 24 h period is expressed
as a % of that of untreated cultures. Each point in the
figures was calculated from the geometric mean of triplicate
determinations, the standard deviations of which are represented by vertical lines unless smaller than the points as
plotted; abrin (o), anti-Thy$_{1.1}$ F(ab')$_2$-abrin (●), normal
F(ab')$_2$-abrin (▲). (Reproduced from Thorpe and Ross [3].

cancer agents has been tested in a mouse model system.
Immunologically-deprived CBA mice, a strain of mouse which
expresses Thy$_{1.2}$ and not Thy$_{1.1}$, were injected with Thy$_{1.1}$

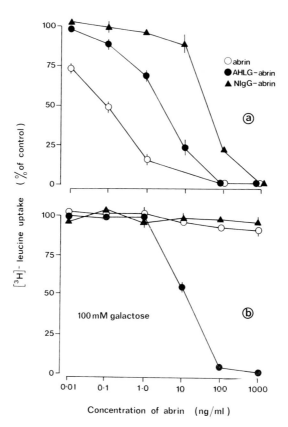

·Fig. 2 Toxic effects of abrin, AHLG-abrin and NlgG-abrin
upon the human lymphoblastoid cell line, Daudi. Daudi lymphoblastoid cells were incubated for 1 h in the presence (b) or
absence (a) of 100 mM galactose, with abrin or conjugates.
The capacity of cells to incorporate ^{3}H-leucine was measured
as for Fig. 1; abrin (o), anti Thy$_{1.1}$F(ab')$_2$-abrin (●), normal
F(ab')$_2$-abrin (▲). (Reproduced from Thorpe et al. (1981)
Clin. Exp. Immunol. 43, 195-200 by permission of Blackwell
Scientific Publications Ltd.)

expressing lymphoma cells. The Thy$_{1.1}$ antigen thus provided
a specific tumour marker which could be used to test the anti-
neoplastic activity of anti-Thy$_{1.1}$-toxin conjugates. If 10^3
cells were administered by intraperitoneal injection followed
by the injection at the same site of 1.5 pmol of anti-Thy$_{1.1}$
F(ab')$_2$-abrin conjugate one day later, 40% of the mice
survive. As the survival of 10 lymphoma cells would

eventually kill, it can be estimated that the conjugate had killed 99% of the lymphoma cells. If 10^5 cells were injected, the survival time of the mice was again prolonged by their treatment with conjugate to an extent corresponding to 99% eradication of lymphoma cells [4]. If the conjugate was administered intravenously instead of intraperitoneally, all anti-tumour activity was abolished, regardless of the number of cells injected.

There are several possible explanations for these results. The different activities between intravenously and intraperitoneally injected conjugate may merely reflect a difference in the final intraperitoneal concentration of conjugate when administered by the two routes. Another possibility is that the intravenously-administered conjugate formed semistable complexes with erythrocytes and plasma glycoproteins in the blood stream, due to the galactose-binding property of the B chain, with the result that diffusion out of the blood was impeded. The non-specific binding of the B chain also contributes to the high *in vivo* toxicity of these conjugates and limits their anti-neoplastic potential.

Conjugates with Toxic A Chain and Similar Inhibitors

A possible method by which the problems of galactose recognition can be circumvented is to use the isolated A chain of the toxin to make the conjugates or to use plant proteins such as gelonin [6] which act like A chains in cell free systems but, possessing no equivalent of the B chain of toxins, are much less toxic to cells.

(a) **Antibody-Gelonin Conjugates** The use of gelonin in the manufacture of conjugates has produced some very promising results. Here, by linking two relatively non-toxic substances, the antibody and gelonin, a highly potent and specific cytotoxic agent was produced. The linkage of the antibody and gelonin was achieved using the hetero-bifunctional reagent N-succinimidyl-3-(2-pyridyldithio)propionate (SPDP) which introduces a disulphide bond between the two proteins. The method was used to mimic the native linkage between the subunits of toxins where it is known that for the A chain to exert its catalytic action, it must be freed by reduction from the B chain [2]. Figure 3 shows the toxicity of monoclonal anti-$Thy_{1.1}$-gelonin conjugate to mouse (AKR-strain) splenic T-cells. At a concentration of 10^{-12} M the conjugate decreased by half the capacity of the cells to synthesize protein. Its potency was equal to that of native abrin, greater than that of ricin and 10^5-fold greater than free gelonin. On cells which lack the $Thy_{1.1}$ antigen, namely

T-cells from CBA mice and B-cells from AKR mice, the conjugate showed less toxicity than free gelonin [7]. When this conjugate was tested *in vivo* in immunologically-deprived CBA mice injected with 10^5 AKR-A lymphoma cells, the conjugate was able to eradicate 99 - 99.9% of injected lymphoma cells.

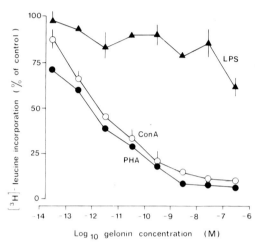

Fig. 3 ^{3}H-leucine incorporation (% of control). Spleen cells from AKR mice were incubated for 1 h with antibody-gelonin conjugate (mol.wt > 300,000) and 1 day later received either B-cell mitogen, bacterial lipopolysaccharide (▲) or one of the T-cell mitogens concanavalin A (o) or phytohaemagglutinin (●). The ^{3}H-leucine incorporation stimulated by the mitogens was measured one day later and is expressed as a % of incorporation in cultures not treated with the conjugates, but stimulated with the corresponding mitogen. The antibody alone at 10^{-6} M was without inhibitory effect. (Reproduced from Thorpe *et al*. [6].)

(b) W3/25-Ricin A Chain Conjugate The W3/25 monoclonal antibody recognizes an antigen expressed by a subpopulation of rat T-lymphocytes [8]. This antibody was linked by a disulphide bond to ricin A chain using the free thiol group on the A chain exposed on splitting ricin into its subunits. Antigen binding activity of the antibody was retained and so was A chain activity. In contrast to the results with the gelonin conjugate above, this conjugate showed no activity against rat T-lymphocytes (Fig. 4a) even at 3 x 10^{-8} M at which concentration the antibody moiety saturated the antigens upon the cells [9]. Immunofluorescence studies with W3/25 ricin A conjugate showed that the conjugate was not capped or

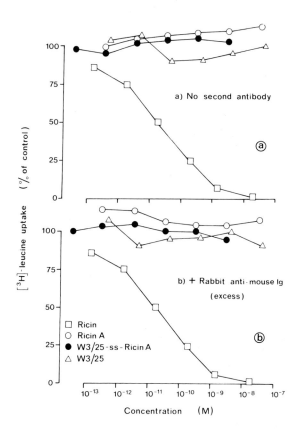

Fig. 4 Ricin A-chain coupled to a monoclonal antibody,
W3/25, is not toxic to rat T-lymphocytes in tissue culture
even when endocytosis of the conjugate is stimulated with
rabbit anti-mouse IgG. Hooded rat spleen cells were treated
for 1 h with ricin, A chain, W3/25-A chain conjugates or
W3/25 antibody and were then washed. The cultures were
incubated for 24 h in the presence (b) or absence (a) of
20 μg/ml of immunopurified rabbit anti-mouse IgG. Phytohaemagglutinin was added to cultures and after 24 h the ^{3}H-
leucine incorporated determined as in Fig. 3; Ricin (□),
ricin A (o), W3/25-S-S-ricin A (●), W3/25 (Δ). (Reproduced
from Thorpe and Ross [3].)

internalized. To investigate whether the inability of
W3/25 to cap was the cause of the conjugate's lack of

toxicity, cross-linking of cell-bound conjugates was induced
with rabbit anti-mouse immunoglobulin antibodies. Under these
conditions capping and internalization did occur but there was
no enhancement of toxicity (Fig. 4b).
    This result highlights the importance of B chain function.
W3/25 linked to intact ricin is a highly potent cytotoxic
agent showing that the B chain in the conjugate could effect
A chain penetration. The B chain could act by binding to
galactose receptors and inducing the internalization of the
conjugate through the toxin entry pathway. The B chain could
also have a function in addition to binding. Studies conducted
by Youle and Neville [10] with an anti-Thy$_{1.1}$-A chain conjugate have shown that the addition of free B chain increases
the toxicity of the antibody-A-chain conjugate. That A chain
conjugates function in a different manner to natural toxins is
further supported by kinetic studies. Ricin shows a dose-
dependent lag time between the addition of toxin to cells and
the onset of inhibition of protein synthesis [2] which, as a
minimum, is 30 minutes. This period is thought to reflect the
time taken for the A chain to enter the cell. The results
obtained with anti-Thy$_{1.1}$-A chain conjugate [10] show no such
lag time.

Conjugates: Their Shortcomings and the Future

The preceding examples of antibody-toxin and antibody-A chain
conjugates have indicated several limitations in both systems.
Conjugates made using intact toxins are very potent but suffer
from a lack of specificity due to the galactose-binding properties of the B chain. The conjugates made with A chains
only or with A chain-like molecules such as gelonin are only
active when attached to antibodies against antigens which
allow translocation of the active species into the cytosol.
One solution to this is to construct conjugates with modified
but intact toxins in which the galactose recognition site has
been blocked and thereby retain the putative penetration
qualities of the B chain. Thorpe and Ross [3] have demonstrated a blockade of the galactose-binding site of abrin
using the SPDP reagent. They reacted abrin with this reagent
and separated the material which had lost binding capacity by
affinity chromatography on a galactose column. The blockade
is probably caused by modification of a lysine residue in, or
close to, the galactose recognition site. The blocked abrin
was 100-fold less toxic to cells in culture than native abrin
and 30-fold less poisonous to animals. The coupling of the
blocked toxin to monoclonal anti-Thy$_{1.1}$ antibody largely
restored the ability of the toxin to kill Thy$_{1.1}$ expressing
T-lymphocytes in culture.

Unfortunately, the blocking of the galactose site may not totally abolish non-specific toxicity *in vivo*. Ricin, abrin and gelonin are all glycoproteins containing mannose and N-acetylglucosamine residues and these residues can be recognized by lectin-like receptors on reticuloendothelial cells. Skilleter *et al.* [11] have shown that Kupffer cells bind ricin using a cell surface mannose receptor and that ricin bound in this way is toxic. Thus antibody-toxin conjugates injected into mice are almost sure to be rapidly cleared from the blood stream with concomitant damage to the reticulo-endothelial system. This may account for the relative success of antibody-diphtheria toxin conjugates as anticancer agents *in vivo* [12], since diphtheria toxin is not a glycosylated protein.

A second problem for consideration is that of the stability of the disulphide linkage used to form conjugates of antibodies and ricin A chain. The disulphide bridge has to be used for the conjugate to be active. However, the *in vivo* studies of Jansen and his colleagues [13] have shown that an anti-DNP-ricin A chain conjugate made with such a bond has a half life of only 30 minutes in the blood. One possible cause of this short half life is the break up of the conjugate by reduction of the disulphide link. The use of intact toxin conjugates with their galactose-recognition site blocked would circumvent this problem by allowing the antibody to be linked to the B chain by a biologically-stable bond while retaining the native disulphide bridge in the toxin.

The problems of making antibody-toxin conjugates for use in animals remain formidable but at present do not seen insuperable. There is, however, one application of conjugates of imminent clinical value which utilizes their great selectivity of cytotoxic action *in vitro*. This is the possibility that bone marrow drawn from patients suffering from leukaemia, lymphoma or certain other malignant diseases could be treated *in vitro* with antibody-toxin conjugates to destroy the infiltrating malignant cells and the cleansed marrow then injected back into the patient after his treatment with high dose chemotherapy and total body irradiation. The experiments of Krolick *et al.* [14] and Thorpe *et al.* [15,16] have validated this approach in experimental animals and there is no obvious reason why it should not also succeed in man. Hopefully, the first clinical application of conjugates may be in the not too distant future.

ACKNOWLEDGEMENTS

I wish to thank Dr Phil Thorpe of the I.C.R.F. for help in writing this manuscript and also Phil and Drs Forrester, Ross

and Edwards, and their colleagues at the Chester Beatty
Research Institute, London, for allowing me to base this
article on a selection of their work.

REFERENCES

1. Eiklid, K., Olsnes, S. and Pihl, A. (1980). *Exp. Cell
    Res.* **126**, 321-326.
2. Olsnes, S. and Pihl, A. (1976). Abrin and ricin and
    their associated agglutinins. In "Receptors and Recog-
    nition" Series B Vol.1: The specificity and action of
    animal, bacterial and plant toxins (Ed. P. Cuatrecasas)
    pp.129-173, Chapman and Hall, London.
3. Thorpe, P.E. and Ross, W.C.J. (1982). *Immunological
    Reviews* **62**, 119-158.
4. Thorpe, P.E., Detre, S.J., Mason, D.W., Cumber, A.J. and
    Ross, W.C.J. (1982). *Adv. in Leukaemia Research* **28(V)**,
    107-111.
5. Ross, W.C.J., Thorpe, P.E., Cumber, A.J., Edwards, P.C.,
    Hinson, C.A. and Davies, A.J.S. (1980). *Eur. J. Biochem.*
    104, 381-390.
6. Barbieri, L. and Stirpe, F. (1982). *Cancer Surveys* **1(4)**,
    489-520.
7. Thorpe, P.E., Brown, A.N.F., Ross, W.C.J., Cumber, A.J.,
    Detre, S.I., Edwards, D.C., Davies, A.J.S. and Stirpe, F.
    (1981). *Eur. J. Biochem.* **116**, 447-454.
8. Mason, D.W., Brideau, R.J., McMaster, W.R., Heeb, M.,
    White, R.A.H. and Williams, A.F. (1980). In "Monoclonal
    Antibodies" (Ed. R. Kennett, T.J. McKearn and K.B. Bechtol)
    pp.251-273, Plenum Publ. Co., New York and London.
9. Mason, D.W. and Williams, A.F. (1980). *Biochem. J.* **187**,
    1-20.
10. Youle, R.J. and Neville, D.M. Hr. (1982). *J. Biol. Chem.*
    257, 1598-1601.
11. Skilleter, D.N., Paine, A.J. and Stirpe, F. (1981).
    Biochem. Biophys. Acta **677**, 495-500.
12. Moolten, F.L., Capparell, N.J., Zajdel, S.H. and Cooper-
    band, S.R. (1975). *J. Nat. Cancer Inst.* **55**, 473-477.
13. Jansen, F.Z., Blythman, H.E., Carriere, D., Casellas, P.,
    Gros, O., Gros, P., Laurent, J.C., Paolucci, F., Pau, B.,
    Poncelet, P., Richer, G., Vidal, H. and Voisin, G.A.
    (1982). *Immunological Reviews* **62**, 185-216.
14. Krolick, K.A., Uhr, J.W. and Vitetta, E.S. (1982).
    Nature **295**, 604-605.
15. Thorpe, P.E., Mason, D.W., Brown, A.N.F., Simmonds, S.J.,
    Ross, W.C.J., Cumber, A.J. and Forrester, J.A. (1982).
    Nature 297, 594-596.
16. Mason, D.W., Thorpe, P.E. and Ross, W.C.J. (1982).
    Cancer Surveys **1(4)**, 389-415.

DRUGS TO MODIFY THE IMMUNE RESPONSE

M.W. Elves

*Cell Biology Division, Glaxo Group Research Ltd,
Greenford Rd, Greenford, Middlesex, U.K.*

INTRODUCTION

The specific immune response occupies the central role in the
defence of the body against invading microorganisms and other
foreign material. It differs from the more primitive inflammatory reaction by virtue of the exquisite specificity for
the antigen and the phenomenon of immunological memory. This
ensures that the subsequent exposures to an antigen result in
a rapid reaction against it. The effectors of the immune response are the antibodies, produced by cells of the lymphoid
system, and the cytotoxic lymphocytes responsible for the
cell-mediated immune response: both are directed specifically
against the challenging antigen. Under normal circumstances
the immunological responses provide an effective mechanism
for rejection of invading pathogens. Under some circumstances the immune mechanisms are defective and the individual then becomes at considerable risk. In other circumstances
the controlling mechanisms of the immune response become altered and result in inappropriate autoaggressive reactions
(autoimmunity). In these latter cases, impairment of the
immune system affords a method of treatment. Such an approach
becomes essential also in the treatment of patients receiving grafts of foreign organs or tissues. This survey will be
confined to a consideration of methods for producing immunodepression.

THE IMMUNE RESPONSES

In order to develop agents capable of inhibiting the immune
system it is important to understand the cellular basis of
the immune responses so that appropriate points in the system which may be targets for drug action can be identified.
The ideal therapeutic requirement, in the transplantation

context, is a drug able to specifically suppress the immune
response to graft-antigens without impairing immunoreactivity
to pathogens. This is a difficult objective to achieve. In
the case of autoimmune diseases the situation is considerably
more complex, as in most cases the antigen(s) is not known
and the nature of the defect in the immune system is ill-
understood.

In the simplest analysis, the immune response can be considered in terms of a reflex arc in which there are three
phases:

a) Afferent arm: during which antigenic recognition occurs
    and the immune response is triggered.

b) Central phase: during which amplification of the cellular
    response by cell proliferation and cellular recruitment
    occurs, and immunological effectors are produced.

c) Efferent arm: during which the immunological effectors
    recognize the antigen and react with it to produce an
    effect.

In practice, the situation is much more complex and involves
a number of cell types in the lymphoid tissues. These can be
only briefly outlined here (Fig. 1), for further details one
of the standard immunological texts should be consulted.

Initial contact with the antigen is made by antigen-reactive
lymphocytes either by direct contact or after its interaction
with antigen-processing cells of the reticulo-endothelial system (RES). There are two principal types of lymphocytes.
The B cells (bone-marrow derived) which ultimately give rise
to the antibody forming plasma cells. They have specific
immunoglobulin (Ig) on their surface which is probably involved in antigen recognition. The T cells (thymus-derived)
are a heterogeneous group and play a part in the regulation
of the immune response by acting as helper cells (T_h), which
are required by B cells before they will react to most antigens, or suppressor cells (T_s) which, as their name implies,
act to reduce or terminate the immune response. A further
group of T cells, the cytotoxic T cells (T_c), are able to
cause tissue damage; these are a product of the immune response. The T_c cells are important in antiviral immunity as
well as in rejection of foreign tissue grafts. The T cell
types can be distinguished by surface antigenic markers.

The immune response is thus a complex process involving
interaction between different lymphocyte populations and RES
elements. The interactions between the different cells involved in the response are determined by receptors on the
cell surfaces which are, so far, poorly defined and also by
a variety of polypeptides or proteins produced by the cells

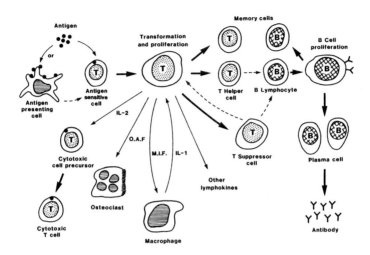

Fig. 1 Cellular interactions during the immune response.
[O.A.F. = osteoclast activating factor; M.I.F. = macrophage inhibitory factor: IL-1 = interleukin 1; IL-2 = interleukin 2].

(lymphokines). The nature and function of these controlling molecules is now becoming better understood. The two best defined are the interleukins (IL) 1 and 2. IL-1 is a product of stimulated RES cells and it causes T lymphocytes to become activated. IL-2 is produced by activated T cells and is necessary for T cell proliferation and differentiation of effector T_c cells from their precursors. Other less well characterized products of activated T cells are lymphokines affecting macrophages (e.g. macrophage activating factor – MAF or MIF), B cells, (B cell-activating factor – BF), osteoclasts (OAF) and a cytotoxic factor (CF). These molecules are all involved in the amplification of immunoinflammatory reactions, initiated as a consequence of recognition of an antigen by a small number of T cells specifically programmed to recognize that antigen.

Cell proliferation is another process by which the immune response is expanded. A consequence of activation of T or B lymphocytes by antigen, lymphokines or other mitogens (e.g. phytohaemagglutinin, poke weed mitogen, etc) is transformation

from the typically small cell into metabolically-active large
blast cells which will divide by mitosis.

The most obvious site for therapeutic intervention is during
the phase of cell proliferation, when the cells will become
susceptible to drugs interfering with DNA synthesis. This
approach is one which has been widely used in the clinic. It
does, however, lack any degree of antigenic specificity and
causes generalized immunosuppression. Interference with antigenic recognition, either during the afferent or efferent
phases of the response, has also been attempted by the use of
specific antibodies against the graft antigens (enhancement).
This approach has enjoyed only limited success and the outcome is unpredictable; graft damage can be caused in some
circumstances. Other targets which suggest themselves are
antagonists of the interleukins and other lymphokines. However, the effects of such agents would not be expected to be
antigenically specific. Another approach, which may offer
some hope of specificity, is the manipulation of T cell subpopulations and, in particular, the suppressor cells. These
may be antigenically specific as will be discussed below.
Finally, attempts have been made, not always successfully,
to reduce the antigenicity of a tissue or organ graft either
by removal of mobile cells such as "passenger leucocytes" or
antigen-presenting cells, which may make a major contribution
to the antigenicity of the graft, or by enzymically treating
the graft. The last situation is futile as either the cells
are killed or, if left alive, will replace the antigens in
due course. Culture of tissues in high O_2 concentrations for
a time before grafting will remove antigen-presenting cells
and render the graft less immunogenic, but this approach is
only possible with few tissues (e.g. pancreatic islets).

It must be admitted that the development of immunosuppressive regimes presently in use have occurred through
serendipity rather than reasoned science. So far, attempts
at specific suppression have not been very successful although,
as will be mentioned below, there are some indications that
this is possible. Current methods used in the clinic, and
some giving encouraging results in the laboratory, will be
reviewed below.

GENERAL IMMUNOSUPPRESSION

A variety of drugs are available which have the capacity to
suppress the immune response, but few have found a place in
the treatment of autoimmune disease or the recipients of
organ grafts. Many of the agents used in the chemotherapy
of cancer have immunosuppressive properties by virtue of
their ability to interfere with cell replication. In the

majority of cases, however, the broad spectrum toxic effects,
and in particular the inhibitory effects upon haemopoietic and
intestinal mucosa cells, mitigate against their use. There
is little evidence of selectivity of action of most of these
drugs and their therapeutic index is unacceptable in anything
other than the cancer context. Some of these compounds have,
however, found a place in the management of organ transplant
recipients and severe autoimmune conditions.

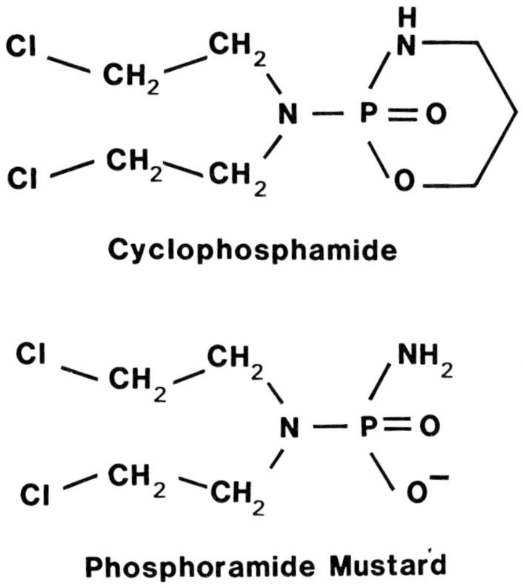

Cyclophosphamide

Phosphoramide Mustard

Fig. 2 Structures of cyclophosphamide and phosphoramide
mustard one of its active metabolites.

Cyclophosphamide

Cyclophosphamide is a drug in the nitrogen mustard group,
which requires metabolism to an active form by the liver
(Fig. 2). This drug is interesting to the immunologist because it appears, when certain treatment regimes are used, to
have an unusual degree of selectivity of action for the lymphoid system, sparing haemopoiesis to a greater than usual
extent; and it also appears to have a major effect upon B
cells rather than T cells. This may reflect the different
proliferative characteristics of these two cell types.
Cyclophosphamide will depress antibody production even when
given up to 48 h after the antigen. It will also inhibit
some cell-mediated immune reactions including allograft rejection and the graft-versus-host reaction (GVH). Paradoxically, however, at high doses in some treatment schedules
cyclophosphamide will cause an enhancement of the delayed
hypersensitivity reaction. Although it is not clear why this

happens, it has been suggested that the drug is selectively inhibiting suppressor cells which would normally dampen down the reaction; alternatively, it may be that production of a "protective" antibody is impaired. A further property of cyclophosphamide is that, if it is used at the same time as antigen administration, it may bring about the development of a state of specific unresponsiveness to that antigen which may be long-lasting. Again, the mechanism underlying this phenomenon is not clear. It has been suggested that it is due to deletion of antigen-reactive lymphocytes, or inhibition of regeneration of surface immunoglobulin receptors on B cells which are needed for antigen recognition and cell triggering.

Cyclophosphamide has not been widely used in the treatment of organ transplant recipients. When it has been used in combination with other agents (anti-lymphocyte serum (ALS) and steroids) results have been satisfactory.

Azathioprine (Aza)

A drug which, at present, forms the principal means of control of anti-graft immune responses, is azathioprine (Imuran; Aza) (Fig. 3). This thiopurine is converted *in vivo* to the

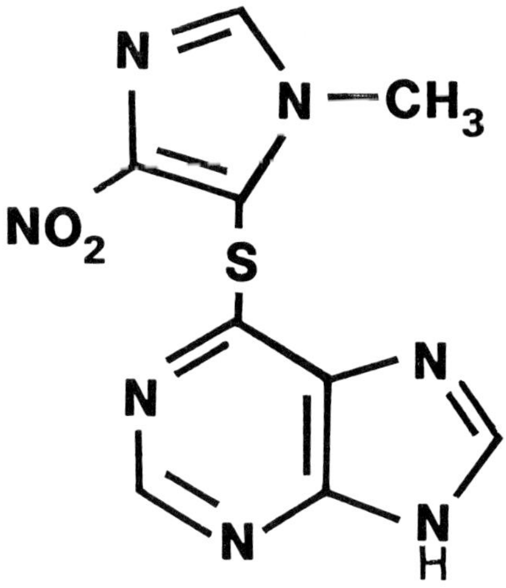

Fig. 3 Structure of Azathioprine.

riboside of 6-mercaptopurine, and this in turn competes with
inosine for the enzyme involved in synthesis of adenylic and
guanylic acids. The result is inhibition, not only of DNA
synthesis and cell proliferation, but also of RNA and protein
biosynthesis.

Both Aza and 6-mercaptopurine will inhibit both antibody
production and cell-mediated immune responses. There is,
however, some evidence to suggest that T cells are more
susceptible to them than B cells, giving rise to greater
effects against T cell-dependent immune responses. For example, production of cytotoxic T cells is impaired. One
consequence of this, which may be relevant in the clinical
context, is that anti-viral immunity is more seriously impaired in Aza treated subjects. Production of lymphokines by
cells reacting to antigens is not affected by Aza.

The immunosuppressive action of these compounds cannot be
explained entirely upon the basis of an inhibitory effect on
cell proliferation. Delay in starting treatment until after
exposure to antigen, when DNA synthesis is at its peak, is
not as effective as treatment before antigen (cf. cyclophosphamide). It is clear that Aza will also inhibit production of precursors of monocytes and macrophages by the
bone marrow, and a lack of these cells may contribute to the
inhibition of delayed type hypersensitivity reactions.

It was first demonstrated in 1962, that in experimental
animals, Aza and 6-mercaptopurine were effective in prolonging survival of kidney grafts, and this paved the way for
their use in human transplant patients. At present, Aza is
the drug of choice by most centres for the prophylactic
treatment of transplant patients to prevent rejection. Invariably, this treatment has to be life-long and, therefore,
it is important that lowest possible doses are used. By
reducing the degree of antigenic disparity between host and
graft for the major histocompatibility system (e.g. HLA in
man; H-2 in mice) the dose of Aza can be kept at a reasonable level, to avoid toxic side-effects or overwhelming
bacterial infection.

Both drugs have been used for the treatment of severe forms
of rheumatoid arthritis but their toxicity limits their use,
in this and other autoimmune conditions, to situations in
which response to other drugs has failed.

Methotrexate (MTX)

There are other drugs affecting DNA synthesis which have
been considered for use as immunosuppressives, but these have
not gained wide acceptance except perhaps for the treatment
of severe autoimmune conditions resistant to other drugs.

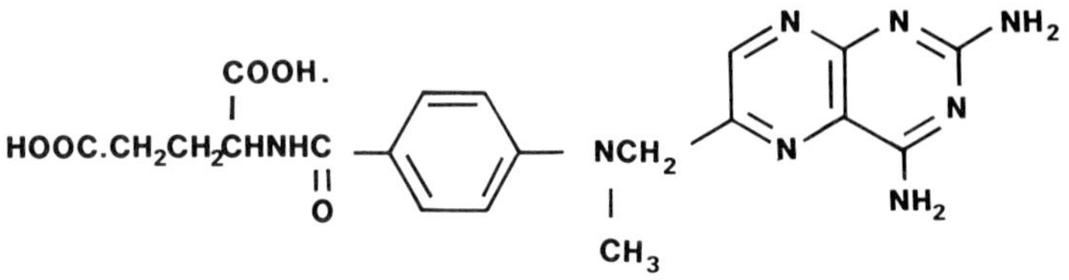

Fig. 4 Structure of methotrexate

The most important of these is methotrexate (amethopterin),
an inhibitor of folic acid metabolism (Fig. 4). MTX has been
found to be of value in the treatment of recipients of bone
marrow transplants in order to prevent or overcome graft-
versus-host disease.

One subject which has not been given sufficient attention
in the use of the above drugs is their pharmacokinetics. Invariably, treatment schedules are empirical, the interaction
of compounds metabolized by the liver with drugs such as
cyclophosphamide is not often considered. Competition for
liver mixed function oxidase enzymes by concurrently used
drugs is likely to have an influence, not only on the therapeutic efficacy of the immunosuppressive, but also upon their
side-effect profiles. The cellular aspects of the immune
response, and half-life values for drugs in common use, in
the design of dosage schedules should also be considered. It
is very likely that improved therapeutic indices for existing
drugs could be obtained with more careful dose scheduling.

Glucocorticoid Steroids

The synthetic steroids derive from the naturally occurring
hormone cortisol which is itself a weak immunosuppressive and
anti-inflammatory agent. Of the synthetic steroids, prednisolone and prednisone are the most widely used for systemic
treatment (Fig. 5). In the patient with an organ transplant
these drugs are often used in combination with Aza, and are
particularly valuable in the control of rejection crises.

The mode of action of the glucocorticoid steroids on the
immunoinflammatory reaction is complex. Being highly lipophilic molecules they readily enter the cell and combine with
a receptor in the cytoplasm to form an active complex. This

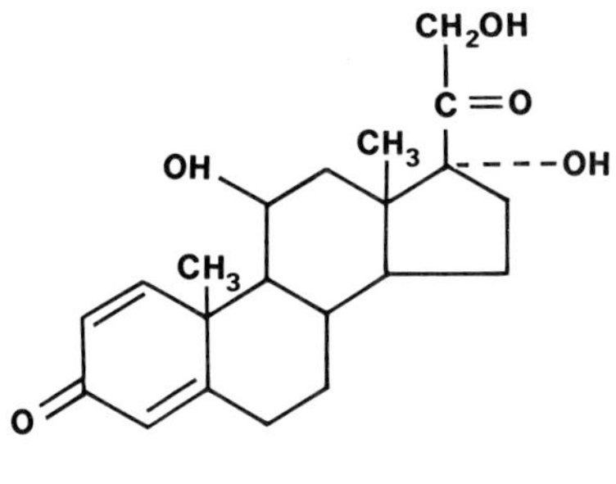

Prednisolone

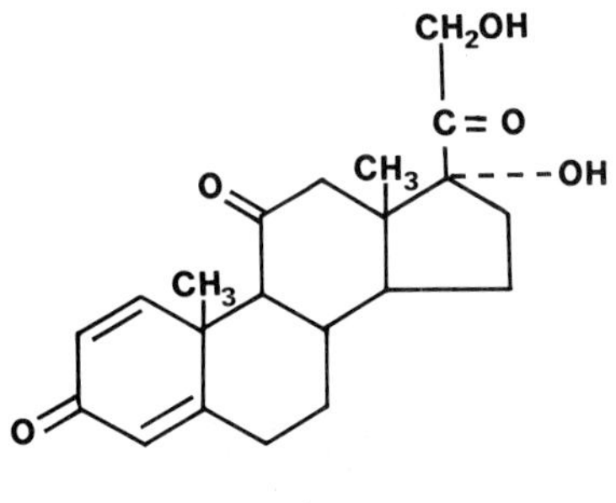

Prednisone

Fig. 5 Structures of prednisolone and prednisone.

is transferred into the nucleus where it combines with nuclear
material and results in the transcription of genes. The product of this process depends upon the cell upon which the
steroid is acting but is usually a protein. Thus in liver
cells, the resulting protein may be induced by enzymes such as
those involved in gluconeogenesis. In the macrophage, two
steroid-induced proteins have been discovered — macrocortin
and lipomodulin — and these are probably the mediators of the
anti-inflammatory effects of these drugs. They cause inhibition of arachidonic acid release and, therefore, reduced
prostaglandin production. Steroids also bring about an
inhibition of neutral protease secretion, etc. These effects
are produced by very low levels of steroid (10^{-9} to 10^{-6} M).
It is not yet clear what the nature of the products of steroid
stimulation of lymphocytes is, nor of its effects. Some
lymphocytes, particularly the immature T cells in the thymus,

are very sensitive to high doses of steroids which cause them
to lyse; hence the thymus atrophy which occurs in steroid
treated animals. The mechanism of this phenomenon is not
known. Other lymphocytes are steroid-resistant. However, a
lymphopenia is a regular finding after steroid treatment.

These synthetic hormones have a variety of other effects
which may be important in immunomodulation. They influence
lymphocyte and macrophage migration patterns, causing re-
distribution of these cells from their normal compartments;
thus, in the case of lymphocytes, interfering with cell interactions and possibly reducing the chance of contact between
lymphocytes and antigen. At higher doses, glucocorticoids
will impair synthesis of DNA, RNA and protein, and this
clearly will affect the amplification stage of the immune
response. On the efferent side of the response it has been
shown, in tissue culture studies, that steroids will revers-
ibly inhibit cytotoxic T cells. The indications are that the
drug is not affecting the binding of the cell to its target
but is affecting the activation of the cytotoxic reaction.
Lymphokine production does not seem to be a steroid sensitive
process, except for IL-2. In this case there is evidence for
inhibition of IL-2 production and this may account for the
effect on T_C cells.

Unfortunately, glucocorticoid steroids have a wide variety
of effects upon other tissues and, as a result, they are far
from specific in their immunosuppressive and anti-inflammatory
properties. Side-effects, which limit their usefulness, include depression of endogenous cortisol production via the
hypothalamus-pituitary-adrenal axis, Cushing-oid changes and
bone necrosis. In most transplant immunosuppressive regimes,
steroids have a place, either at low doses as a chronic
maintenance treatment concomitant with other drugs, or at
higher doses for the control of rejection episodes. They
have also found a place in the treatment of autoimmune diseases, such as rheumatoid arthritis, where they can sometimes
bring about rapid improvement of the condition. In this condition, glucocorticoids may be capable of halting the disease
process as well as ameliorating the symptoms.

Anti-lymphocyte Globulin (ALG)

Anti-lymphocyte (or thymocyte) antibodies have found a place
in some centres for the control of organ graft rejection.
These are heterologous antibodies directed at antigenic
determinants on lymphocytes. Given to rats and mice, ALG is
able to cause a marked prolongation of organ and tissue graft
survival. This will occur even in the situation where the
animal is pre-sensitized to the graft. Immunological memory

is effectively erased. ALG also inhibits antibody production
where help from T cells is required and also GVH reaction.
There is now considerable evidence that the main targets for
ALG are the T lymphocytes. Thus, after treatment, those areas
of the lymphoid tissues occupied by T cells become depleted
whilst B cell areas are, in the main, unaltered. There is
also a depletion of T cells from the peripheral blood of
treated animals. After ALG treatment is stopped the T cells
recover, but for this to occur the thymus is necessary. In
addition to its effect in laboratory rodents, appropriate ALG
has been shown to exert powerful immunosuppressive effects in
man, and has found a place in some immunosuppressive regimes,
particularly as an agent able to arrest rejection episodes.

The most obvious explanation for the immunosuppressive
activity of ALG is that it is killing, or opsonising, circulating T lymphocytes. It thus can attack both the afferent
and efferent arms of the response, and can also ablate
memory cells. Alternatively, it has been suggested that the
antibody "blindfolds" the lymphocytes so that they are unable
to recognize antigens on the target cells. More recently,
however, evidence has begun to emerge which indicates that
ALG might in some way be inducing suppressor cells, which
then hold down the immune response. These may be totally
non-specific or, if graft antigen is present simultaneously,
specific. If this finding is confirmed it would explain why
the effects of ALG last beyond the period of obvious T cell
depletion, and also hold out the hope that, with suitable
treatment regimes employing ALG and graft antigen, specific
immunosuppression may be achieved. Thus, ALG may represent
an agent capable of modifying specific elements of the cellular apparatus of the immune response.

Niridazole

Niridazole is a schistocidal compound which was found to have
a suppressive effect upon cell-mediated immune reactions to
schistosome eggs (Fig. 6). Later, patients receiving the
drug were shown to have reduced skin hypersensitivities to a
variety of antigens. The effect of niridazole upon humoral
immune responses was, however, minimal. Thus, it seemed that
this drug was acting selectively against the cell-mediated
immune response. Experiments with skin grafts in mice and
rats, and heart allografts in rats, indicated useful immunosuppressive properties. Even better graft protection was obtained when niridazole was combined with Aza and prednisone.
Unfortunately, however, when the drug was tested in dogs and
baboons receiving heart and kidney allografts no significant
effect was seen. Studies carried out *in vitro* to elucidate

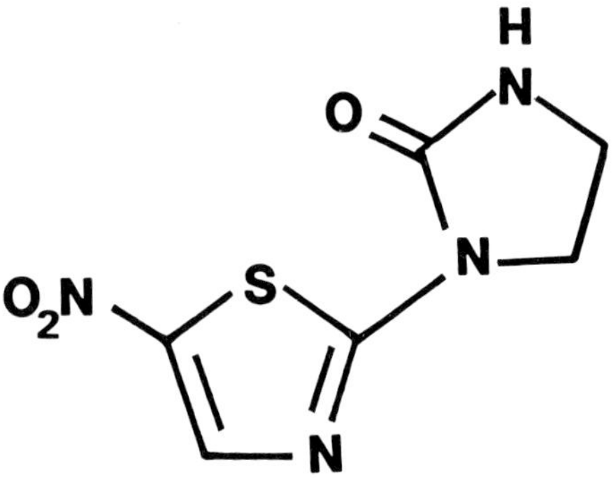

Fig. 6   Structure of niridazole.

the mechanisms of action of niridazole indicated no effect
upon the mixed lymphocyte reaction. However, when serum from
treated humans or rats, or urine from rats, was used in the
culture, inhibitory activity was present. Similarly, the
compound had no effect upon antigen induced lymphokine production. Again, however, serum from treated guinea pigs was
active. In both situations the immunodepressing activity was
found to reside in an unidentified metabolite. This metabolite seems to act at a very early stage in antigen recognition,
as delayed additions to either of these two in vitro systems
results in no activity.
    The major difficulties which stand in the way of this drug
are, firstly, the lack of consistent behaviour in different
species. This is undoubtedly ascribable to species differences in the metabolism of the parent compound to the active
form. The second is the toxicity of niridazole, which again
varies according to species. It is believed that both the
toxicity and the antiparasitic properties of niridazole
reside in the parent molecule. If this is indeed the case,
then there is hope that a useful immunosuppressive niridazole
derivative will be found which lacks its undesirable and
unacceptable side-effects.

Cyclosporin A (CyA)

This fungal metabolite represents the most recent addition
to the immunotherapists armamentarium. This compound is a
cyclic peptide with 11 amino acid residues, and has most
interesting properties (Fig. 7). First and foremost, is its

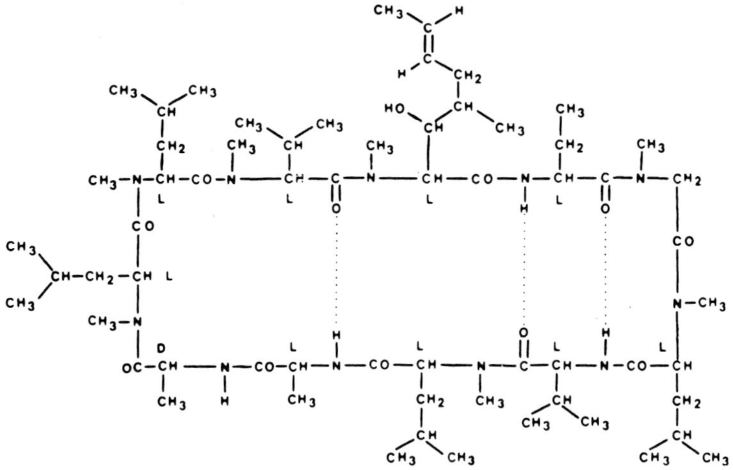

Fig. 7 Structure of cyclosporin A.

virtual lack of myelotoxicity, which is a radical difference
compared with drugs such as Aza and MTX. CyA seems to have
a very specific activity against the T lymphocyte populations
of the immune system, although in man there is an indication
that it may also have anti-B cell effects. There is no evidence that CyA acts as a cytotoxic or antiproliferative agent.
From results of animal experiments, it is clear that this
compound is a very potent immunosuppressive, particularly in
situations involving T lymphocytes. Thus T-cell dependent
antibody production is impaired, whereas antibody production
against T-independent antigens in hardly affected. Delayed
hypersensitivity and other cell-mediated immune responses are
inhibited; and a beneficial effect of CyA has also been shown
in experimental autoimmune disease models such as allergic
encephalomyelitis and adjuvant arthritis. It has been found
to be very effective in producing long-term survival of
tissue and organ grafts in a variety of species, and also in
the prevention of GVH reaction. The drug must, however, be
given at the time of immunization or grafting for maximum
effect. Once a state of immunological unresponsiveness has
been established it will persist for long after cessation of
treatment, and is then quite antigen-specific.

In clinical trials which have so far been carried out,
mainly in renal, liver and cardiac transplantation centres,
results have been very encouraging. CyA has been used both
as sole agent and also in combination with other immunosuppressive drugs (e.g., Aza and steroids). It has also been

used in patients whose grafts were being rejected during Aza
treatment. It has been claimed that patients treated with
CyA have fewer serious rejection episodes which require treatment, and also require significantly less time in hospital.
CyA is also now being used in the context of bone marrow
transplantation for the treatment of leukaemia and aplastic
anaemia in which GVH reactions can be a problem. In some
centres the incidence of GVH reactions in patients given CyA
is significantly lower than in those given MTX.

However, CyA is not without toxic side-effects. The most
serious of these being the development, in some patients and
non-human primates, of lymphomas. Increased incidence of
lymphomas and sarcomas does occur with more conventional
immunosuppressive drugs, but the incidence of tumours connected with CyA treatment was somewhat higher than expected.
There is also a strong link between induction of lymphoma and
the presence of Epstein-Barr (EB) virus in the patients. It
was thought that these lymphomas developed as a result of
unrestrained proliferation of EB-infected B lymphocytes in
the absence of inhibitory T cells. There was an indication,
however, that the incidence of lymphoma was correlated with
the use of high doses of CyA. An important adverse effect of
CyA is its nephrotoxicity. A significant number of treated
patients develop signs of renal damage whilst being treated
with the drug, but this is usually reversible when treatment
is reduced or stopped. However, the problem is made more
serious in renal transplant patients, in whom impaired graft
function may be due to the drug or may indicate rejection.
Stopping treatment with CyA in the former case will improve
the situation; in the latter case it will make rejection
more certain. The development of methods for discerning the
cause of the renal damage in these patients is urgent. Other
toxic side-effects include hepatotoxicity, nausea, tremor,
skin thickening, gum hypertrophy with gingivitis and hirsut-
ism. All of these respond to stopping treatment or reducing
the dose-level.

The cellular basis for the immunosuppressive effects of CyA
is still not clear though a number of clues are emerging,
both from studies in experimental animals and by monitoring
lymphocyte populations in CyA-treated patients. There are
indications that CyA has a differential effect upon T_h and
T_s cells: inhibiting the former whilst sparing the latter.
In patients the $T_h:T_s$ ratio is altered in favour of the T_s
population. There is now evidence that CyA will not affect
activated T cells, but will prevent activation *per se*. This
indicates that it is acting at an early stage of antigen
recognition by the T cell. Production of IL-1, required for
the T_h cell activation, is not impaired. There is, however,

evidence that CyA will block the production by activated
T cells of IL-2. Another possibility is that CyA prevents
the T cells from developing responsiveness to IL-2: there is
evidence that the drug inhibits the expression of IL-2 receptors by stimulated T cells at doses below those which inhibit production of IL-2.

Although the exact mechanism by means of which CyA exerts
its effects upon the immune response remains to be elucidated,
it is clear that this drug opens a new chapter in the history
of immunosuppression. It is the first agent which is clearly
not anti-proliferative and which is selective in its action
upon T cells. There is a very strong possibility that it is
even selective for particular sub-classes of T lymphocytes,
and the soluble mediators that modulate their activity.

ANTIGEN SPECIFIC IMMUNOSUPPRESSION

The ultimate goal for immunosuppression is to produce a state
of immunological unresponsiveness which is specific for
antigen upon grafted tissues (in a transplanting context),
but which leaves the host capable of responding to other unrelated antigenic stimuli (e.g. bacteria). The classical
experiments of Medawar and his colleagues in 1956 achieved
this objective using a laboratory rat model. Allogeneic
cells from one inbred strain of mouse were injected into
immunologically-incompetent neonatal or foetal mice of another
strain. When they reached adulthood these animals accepted
skin grafts derived from animals of the original cell donor
strain. These animals were also chimeric for the donor strain.
In the adult a state of specific tolerance to an antigen is
more difficult to achieve.

Recently, it has been shown that skin grafts between allogeneic mice can be specifically accepted, in the long term,
if the prospective recipient is first injected with a liver
homogenate from the proposed donor strain and then given a
short course of ALG and either *B. pertussis* vaccine or procarbazine, immediately after grafting some 16 days later.
This unresponsiveness can be transferred to sublethally-
irradiated syngeneic hosts indicating that suppressor cells
were probably involved. This group went on to show that the
cells responsible for transferring the unresponsiveness were
T cells. The use of liver extract in this procedure is
again not feasible in the clinical transplantation context.
Brent and his colleagues, however, have also shown quite
clearly that a single injection of about 10^4 white blood
cells could substitute for the liver extract. Again, in this
situation T_S cells were implicated in the unresponsive state.
Why and how these graft antigen specific T_S cells are induced

following this treatment, are unanswered questions. However,
it has also been shown that the pre-grafting exposure to
graft antigen is not necessary in all animals, and ALS with
procarbazine alone is able to induce specific unresponsiveness, but not with the same high frequency. T_S cells have
also been shown to be involved in the maintenance of the
classically neonatally-induced tolerance. What controls their
production, and how T_S cells exert their effect upon other
components of the immune response, are also unanswered questions. Clearly, however, manipulation of this important population of T cells, which are involved in regulation of the
immune response, must represent an attractive target in the
search for new immunomodulating agents.

CONCLUSION

At the beginning of this review the immune response was
represented simply in terms of a reflex arc. Clearly, the
situation is infinitely more complex, and gradually the
intricacies of the immune system are unfolding. The present
approaches to reducing immunoresponsiveness aim mainly at the
central proliferative/amplification step. They are virtually
lacking in any degree of antigenic specificity, although in
experimental animals this is possible as various groups have
shown. So far, however, in man this has not been achieved,
and life-long treatment of the transplant recipient is the
general rule. As we learn more of the details of the immune
response, ways may be found for more subtle modulation of the
various lymphocyte cell types and the soluble mediators they
produce. In Cyclosporin A we may be seeing the beginning of
this new era.

STRUCTURAL DETERMINANTS OF DRUG ALLERGENICITY: IMPLICATIONS IN DRUG DESIGN

R.G. Edwards

*Beecham Pharmaceuticals, Research Division,
Biosciences Research Centre, Yew Tree Bottom Road,
Epsom, Surrey KT18 5XQ, UK*

It is clear that some adverse reactions to drugs in therapeutic use are due to immunologically-mediated reactions and, as such, may be correctly classified as drug allergy. The incidence of such reactions is largely unknown and until diagnostic proficiency improves, no firm figures can be quoted, but it is likely that drug allergy is a relatively infrequent consequence of drug treatment.

Theories on the mechanisms by which simple chemical compounds initiate immune responses are based on the early work of Landsteiner and Jacobs who correlated skin sensitization capacity with ability to form covalent bonds with the amino group of aniline [1]. The chemical grouping introduced in this way onto proteins, is referred to as a hapten. The hapten theory of drug immunogenicity [2] has received general support, and it is not difficult to find examples of chemicals used in the manufacturing industries in which reaction between the chemical and primary amino or sulphydryl groups of proteins provide an adequate explanation of immunogenicity and allergy. The objective of this paper is to try to identify structural features of chemicals and drugs of low molecular weight which predispose to covalent protein binding and thus, by inference, to drug allergy.

Attention has been drawn to anhydrides of carboxylic acids as the result of immunological and allergic reactions in workers handling trimellitic anhydride [3] and phthalic anhydride [4]. These materials would be expected to react with proteins and studies on trimellitic anhydride have confirmed this and identified the haptenic group [3]. Equally reactive products, although inappropriate as drugs, may be encountered as impurities in the final drug product. Acetyl salicylic

IMMUNOTOXICOLOGY
ISBN 0-12-282180-7

anhydride and acetyl salicylsalicylic acid may be present in
commercial forms of aspirin and it has been shown that these
reactive impurities are responsible for immunization of
experimental animals given aspirin preparations containing
them. Purified aspirin proved non-immunogenic [5]. The rare
immunologically-mediated reactions to aspirin might be explained on this basis.

Analysis of sensitization reactions induced by dyestuffs
serves to highlight other structural features leading to
immunological responsiveness. Sensitization to naphtha-
quinone and anthraquinone dyes might be explained on the basis
of the known reactivity of the quinone grouping with amino and
sulphydryl groups present in proteins [6,7]. With azobenzene
dyes initial reduction of the azo link to give an arylamine
could lead to formation of the highly reactive nitrenium ion
via an N-hydroxy arylamine structure (Fig. 1). This could
lead to the introduction of a haptenic grouping and may be
the initiating event resulting in sensitization to these dyes.

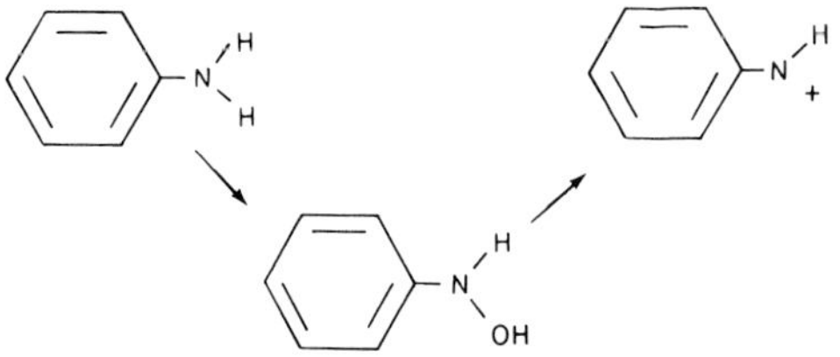

Fig. 1 Route to the formation of the reactive nitrenium ion
from an arylamine.

The Rhus family of plants produce potent sensitizers which
have been identified as substituted catechols. These can be
oxidized by air to produce quinones, the protein reactive
moiety, and this finding underlines the importance of
quinones as sensitizers, as noted above for some dyes. Sensitization resulting from rifampicin, methyldopa and the oestro-
gens, where the catechol structure can be generated by
hydroxylation in vivo, could be explained on this basis. The
plant kingdom also provides an example of an α,β unsaturated
lactone structure in sensitization; the sesquiterpene lactones
of the Compositae, notably allantolactone, are responsible for
sensitization to this family and have been shown to be
protein-reactive via a Michael addition reaction onto the
double bond [8,9]. Prior reduction of the double bond
results in loss of reactivity and of allergenicity [10], providing further evidence for the reactive site. Interestingly,
this knowledge was used to prepare a cross-linked polymer
containing primary and secondary amino groups which could be

used to selectively remove α,β unsaturated lactones from
costus oil, a natural oil used in the cosmetic industry but
which has allergenic properties. The resulting purified oil
had lost this allergenic property whereas components eluted
from the polymer were potent sensitizers. It is possible
that this type of approach could also have application in
drug development.
    The presence of α,β unsaturated ketones in organic molecules
may also result in protein reactivity, again via Michael type
additions to the double bond. For example, Guayulin A and B
are related components isolated from the Mexican rubber plant,
Guayule. Component A (Fig. 2) contains the α,β unsaturated
ketone structure and is a potent contact sensitizer, whereas
component B fails to sensitize [11]. Of similar structure,
esters of cinnamic acid used in sun-screen preparations have
been implicated as allergens and in the drug area, the same
structural features may be responsible for reactions to
ethacrynic acid, griseofulvin, cortisone and virginiamycin.
Factor M, the antibacterial component of this antibiotic,
contains an α,β unsaturated ketone in its structure and is
the allergen.

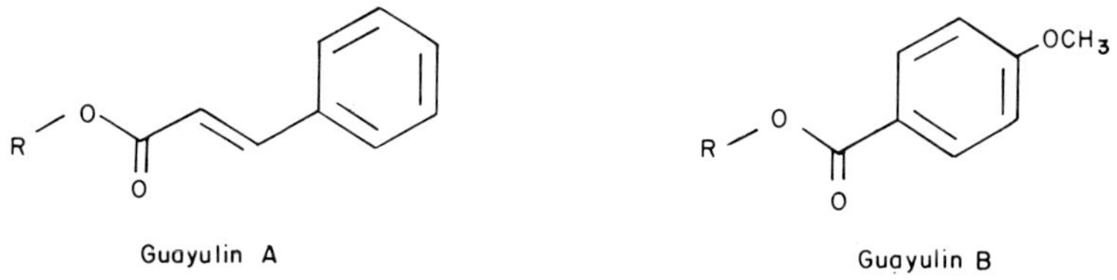

Guayulin A   Guayulin B

Fig. 2 Components isolated from the Mexican rubber plant,
Guayule.

    Another potentially reactive grouping is the aldehyde func-
tion which could react with primary amino groups to form
Schiff bases. An aldehyde function almost certainly accounts
for the immunogenicity and allergenicity of streptomycin.
Glyoxal is a reactive dialdehyde and potent sensitizer and
it has been suggested [12] that this structure could be responsible for allergic reactions to amitriptyline from which
it can be formed by degradation in solution. Substituted
glyoxals are also highly reactive moieties in particular with
protein arginine residues. This is relevant to the question
of the possible allergenicity, albeit rare, of corticosteroids
such as cortisone, hydrocortisone and prednisolone, since on
oxidation in aqueous solution these will spontaneously form
21-dehydrocorticosteroids [13,14] which are substituted
glyoxals with protein reactivity [13,15].
    The penicilloyl group is probably the best documented drug

hapten, formed by reaction of the β-lactam carbonyl group
with primary amino groups, and allergy to the β-lactam antibiotics is the best defined [16].

Clearly, it must also be anticipated that alkylating agents
used in cancer chemotherapy will have a high degree of protein
reactivity. One group is the nitrogen mustards in which the
reactive intermediate is the cyclic aziridinium ion. Certainly,
the simplest member of the group, 2,2'-dichloro-N-methyl-
diethylamine, readily induces contact sensitization in man and
in the guinea pig.

Other potentially reactive groupings are to be found amongst
drug metabolites [17,18]. Some of these, such as aldehydes,
hydroxylated amines and quinones, have already been discussed
but sulphoxides and epoxides are also to be considered. Many
of these metabolites are formed by way of hydroxylation reactions. In particular, aromatic hydroxylations via epoxides
may be a potentially important route as many allergenic drugs
contain aromatic groups.

Knowledge of the structural features which are implicated
in the development of drug allergy may, in some circumstances,
be of value in drug design. This is not the case for the
β-lactam antibiotics, where the β-lactam carbonyl group is
responsible both for the initiation of allergic reactions and
for antibacterial activity. Similarly, the thiazoline ring
of bacitracin A seems to be required for both antibacterial
and allergic properties, as replacement of the thiazoline by
thiazole, as in bacitracin F, is accompanied by loss of both
activities [16]. Other examples include some anti-cancer
drugs and the sulphonamides, where the implicated aromatic
amino group is required for drug action.

It is also possible that structural changes in drugs may
alter allergenic potential both quantitatively and qualitatively and attention has been drawn to this possibility in
relation to prodrugs [19]. Exemplification can be provided
by the diethylaminoethyl ester of benzylpenicillin which
proved to be a contact sensitizer in man, and in animal
models is more sensitizing than the parent molecule benzylpenicillin. Moreover, the antigenic determinant may also
differ, with the C-3 esters of penicillins giving rise to the
penicillanyl determinant, and the parent penicillin primarily
to the penicilloyl determinant [20].

However, other examples show that structural changes of a
relatively minor kind can lead to decrease or abrogation of
allergenicity.

Benzocaine, a local anaesthetic, which is a known contact
sensitizer [21], contains an aromatic amino group which, via
N-hydroxylation reactions, (Fig. 1) could produce haptens.
The amino group is not required for drug action, and

sensitization to the closely related anaesthetics cyclomethy-caine and lignocaine, where the grouping is absent, is extremely rare [21]. Similar manipulations for procainamide and practolol, where again the aromatic amino or acetamido function is not essential for action, should have similar consequences.

Again, streptomycin seems more allergenic and immunogenic than dihydrostreptomycin, presumably due to the lack, in dihydrostreptomycin, of the reactive carbonyl function.

It has been pointed out by many workers interested in drug allergy that few drugs have sufficient intrinsic reactivity with proteins for this reaction to provide a satisfying explanation of their ability to induce antibody formation or sensitization. It is customary thus to argue that the structure that is protein reactive and which introduces new antigenic determinants into proteins, is not the parent drug but a metabolite of it [18]. Reactive epoxides provide such an example, and quite subtle structure modifications can affect their formation or reactivity. Thus substitution of hydrogens in certain critical positions by fluorine or by methyl groups in aromatic systems can often eliminate the formation of epoxides. These types of manipulation have received attention more in relation to considerations of mutagenic or carcinogenic potential but, as the initiating step in both these unwanted effects is probably the interaction of a metabolite with a host macromolecule, changes in allergenic potential might be expected also. Thus, any significant reactivity of this kind might well be identified in a drug during routine safety clearance evaluation and rejected for development without its allergenic potential being realized. However, low molecular weight allergens are not necessarily mutagens or carcinogens, as exemplified most vividly by the penicillins and cephalosporins, and a case can be made for some thought to be given to potential allergenicity in drug design and selection. It is unlikely that this property alone would prevent drug development but the risk-benefit equation would need careful consideration.

REFERENCES

1. Landsteiner, K. and Jacobs, J. (1936). *J. Exp. Med.* **64**, 625-639.
2. Eisen, H.N., Orris, L. and Belman, S. (1952). *J. Exp. Med.* **95**, 473-487.
3. Zeiss, C.R., Patterson, R., Pruzansky, J.J., Miller, M., Rosenberg, M. and Levitz, D. (1977). *J. Allergy Clin. Immunol.* **60**, 96-103.
4. Cronin, E. (1980). In "Contact Dermatitis" pp.635.

Churchill Livingstone, London.

5. Bundgaard, H. and De Weck, A.L. (1975). *Int. Arch. Allergy Appl. Immunol.* **49**, 119-124.

6. Mason, H.S. and Peterson, E.W. (1965). *Biochem. Biophys. Acta.* **111**, 134-146.

7. Liberato, D.J., Byers, V.S., Dennick, R.G. and Catagnoli, Jr., N. (1981). *J. Med. Chem.* **24**, 28-33.

8. Kupchan, S.M., Fessler, D.G., Eakin, M.A. and Giacobbe, T.J. (1970). *Science* **168**, 376-378.

9. Dupuis, G., Mitchell, J.C. and Towers, G.H.N. (1974). *Can. J. Biochem.* **52**, 575-581.

10. Mitchell, J.C., Fritig, B., Singh, B. and Towers, G.H.N. (1970). *J. Invest. Dermatol.* **54**, 233-239.

11. Rodriguez, E., Reynolds, G.W. and Thompson, J.A. (1981). *Science* **211**, 1444-1445.

12. Bundgaard, H. (1977). In "Drug Design and Adverse Reactions" (Eds. H. Bundgaard, P. Juul and K. Kofod), pp.179-180, Munksgaard, Copenhagen.

13. Sunaga, K. and Koide, S.S. (1968). *J. Pharm. Sci.* **57**, 2116-2119.

14. Monder, C. (1968). *Endocrinology* **82**, 318-326.

15. Monder, C. and Walker, M.C. (1970). *Biochem.* **12**, 2489-2497.

16. Dewdney, J.M. (1977). In "The Antigens" Vol. IV. (Ed. M. Sela), pp.73-245. Academic Press, New York.

17. Dewdney, J.M. and Edwards, R.G. (1980). *Chemistry in Britain* **16**, 600-605.

18. Remmer, H. and Schüppel, R. (1972). In "Hypersensitivity to Drugs" (Eds. M. Samter and C.W. Parker), pp.67-89, Pergamon Press, Oxford.

19. Bundgaard, H. (1976). *Acta. Pharm. Suec.* **13**, Suppl. 23.

20. Dewdney, J.M. (1979). In "Drugs and Immune Responsiveness" (Eds. J.L. Turk and D. Parker), pp.164-165, Macmillan, London.

21. Cronin, E. (1980). In "Contact Dermatitis", pp.193-200, Churchill Livingstone, London.

IMMUNOSUPPRESSIVE DRUGS AND CARCINOGENESIS

G. Harris

The Kennedy Institute of Rheumatology,
Division of Experimental Pathology,
Bute Gardens, London W6 7DW, UK

INTRODUCTION

Agents capable of suppressing immune functions have now been
widely used in transplant recipients and in a variety of autoimmune and chronic inflammatory diseases. With more prolonged
survival of such patients it is now possible to accumulate
data concerning the possible carcinogenic risks associated
with immunosuppressive therapy. There is, however, enough
information presently available to justify the conclusion that
exposure to immunosuppressive agents increases the risk of
developing certain types of cancer, particularly of the lymphoid system and skin. A longer period of assessment is needed
with respect to the development of other types of cancer such
as of the stomach and lung.

MECHANISMS OF CANCER PRODUCTION

The cytotoxic modes of action of immunosuppressive agents
have been well-documented. Table 1 lists the presently most
commonly used compounds or agents and their modes of action.
DNA and its dependent processes appear to be the most likely
target for their immunosuppressive effects. However, it is
clear that different agents produce different types of
lesions in the DNA of target cells. Cyclosporin A is an
exception to this and is a novel type of immunosuppressive
agent [1]. Whether it represents a carcinogenic risk is still
to be adequately assessed although higher doses in man may
result in an increased incidence of non-Hodgkin's lymphoma.
In relation to this point we have found (Fig. 1) that Cyclosporin A can prolong the lives of NZB x NZW F_1 hybrid mice
by preventing renal glomerular damage. The mechanism for
this is not yet known and needs further study, but treatment

IMMUNOTOXICOLOGY
ISBN 0-12-282180-7

Table 1 *Commonly used immunosuppressive agents*

Agent	Mode of action
Purine analogues (Azathioprine, 6-mercaptopurine)	Directly incorporated into DNA, RNA; interfere with nucleic acid synthesis by feed-back inhibition of purine synthesis.
Cyclophosphamide	Alkylating agent ⎤ direct reaction with DNA and
Chlorambucil	Alkylating agent ⎦ other cellular macromolecules
Methotrexate	Interferes with single carbon unit transfers by preventing conversion of di- to tetra-hydrofolic acid
Cyclosporin A	Early effect on T-cell response to antigens
Ionizing radiation	DNA damage, membrane damage

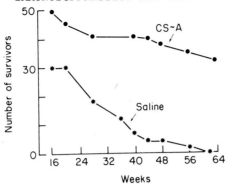

Fig. 1 Mice (NZB x NZW F_1 hybrid) were given Cyclosporin A
(CS-A), 100 mg/kg body weight, dissolved in olive oil, orally
five days a week from 16 weeks of age onwards.

of this hybrid strain has been found to be associated with
an increased incidence of thymic lymphoma as was reported for
penicillamine-D [2]. Ionizing radiation is no longer used in
organ transplantation, but recent reports of the efficacy of
total lymphoid irradiation in rheumatoid arthritis [3] suggests
that it may have some application in this type of condition.
    Table 2 indicates that immunosuppressive drugs are mutagenic,
carcinogenic and clastogenic in many biological systems. A
recent detailed review is available [4]. However the ways in
which they could produce cancer are not understood. It is
therefore pertinent to consider current ideas of tumour
development in this context.

SOMATIC MUTATION/ONCOGENES/SOMATIC RECOMBINATION

Studies of retroviruses and the application of gene transfer
procedures [5] have indicated that oncogenic sequences of
cellular origin exist in normal somatic cells.
    The prototype retroviral onc gene is the Rous sarcoma virus
and its SRC gene. It is now well-established that it is
chimeric; a large portion derived from a replication-competent
avian retrovirus and a small part from the cellular genome of
the chicken [6]. There are now known to be at least 12 such
normal cellular genes which can be mobilized to transforming
activity by a viral gene as the result of transduction. These
cellular genes are highly conserved and widely present in
phylogenetically diverse organisms, thus implying a central
but undefined role for them in normal cell physiology,
possibly differentiation.
    Transfection studies, using isolated DNA, have recently
shown [7] that the transforming activity of the DNA can be
localized to discrete segments present in the donor tumour
cell genome. The DNA of normal cells has been found to

Table 2 *Mutagenicity, clastogenicity and carcinogenicity of some immunosuppressive drugs*

Agent	Mutagenicity			Clastogenicity	Carcinogenicity		
	Pro-karyocytes	Eukarocytes	Mice	Mice	Mouse ⊕	Rat	Man
Azathioprine	+	+	±	+	+	+	+
Cyclophosphamide	+	+	n.d.	+	+	+	+
Chlorambucil	+	+	n.d.	+	+	+	+
Methotrexate	−	−	+	+	−	−	−
Cyclosporin A	−	−	n.d.	−	+*	n.d.	+*

*
possibly a promotional mechanism-production of thymic lymphoma in mice (unpubl. personal observations) non-Hodgkin's lymphoma in man.

n.d. = not determined

⊕ = thymic lymphoma, mammary carcinoma, pulmonary tumours, were most common

contain homologous sequences. Activation of these oncogenes
would appear to involve a process of somatic rearrangement,
or mutations, occurring in target cells during carcinogenesis.
The intervention of virus in this process seems unlikely at
the present time, since there is no evidence of tumour virus
and there is an absence of foreign blocks of DNA sequences
that have become linked to the oncogenes during carcinogenesis.
Six such oncogenes have been defined. This finding of tissue-
associated oncogenes could thus represent a simplifying result
in that different tumours may carry the same activated oncogene.
    There would thus appear to be two groups of oncogenes:

1. Onc genes: defined by their association with retroviruses.
2. Non-viral associated genes.

Homology studies have now shown that there is overlap between
the two groups and suggest that they represent the same genes
activated in different ways; either by recombination with a
retroviral gene or by non-viral somatic mutational events.
There are at least 20 different oncogenes defined on the basis
of sequence studies but it is likely that they derive from a
smaller number of parental genes with distinct enzymic functions. The recent review by Weinberg [8] gives a very clear
and concise account of the current developments in this area.
    An unresolved problem is how physical and chemical agents
which damage DNA can lead to transformed neoplastic cells.
If production of a DNA lesion is the important initiating
event then information about the nature and repair of these
lesions becomes apposite. A variety of rare autosomal re-
cessive conditions in man associated with defects in DNA
repair typically manifest increased susceptibility to develop
skin and lymphoid tumours as well as immune deficiencies [9].
Conversely, immune deficiency states are also associated with
increased susceptibility to develop certain types of cancer,
particularly leukaemias and lymphoreticular malignancies [10].
Table 3 summarizes the data of Kinlen et al. [11] which reviewed the incidence of neoplasia in patients given immunosuppressive treatment for renal transplants or autoimmune
disease. The main types of tumours were non-Hodgkin's
lymphoma or of skin. However, the observational period was
relatively short (4 years) and longer periods are needed
before the risk of developing other types of tumour e.g., in
the lung and stomach can be assessed.
    In view of the types of patients given immunosuppressive
therapy it is therefore important to consider whether those
developing cancer have an increased predisposition. Limited
studies in NZB and NZB/NZW mice [12] indicated that these
SLE-prone strains were highly susceptible to develop thymic

Table 3 [+] *The incidence of neoplasia in patients given immunosuppressive treatment for renal transplants or autoimmune disease*

Patients	Non-Hodgkin's lymphoma		Skin		Other	
	observed	expected	observed	expected	observed	expected
Transplants (renal)	34	0.58	5	1.1	30	17.79
Autoimmune diseases	4[*]	0.34	3	1.94	33	21.44

[+] Summarized from ref.11, with permission

[*] 2 cases of rheumatoid arthritis, 1 case of glomerulonephritis, and 1 case of dermatomyositis

lymphoma as the result of treatment with azathioprine. There
is reported to be an increased incidence of malignant lymphomas
in autoimmune haemolytic disease and Sjögren's syndrome in man,
but the true incidence of malignancy in diseases like systemic
lupus erythematosus and rheumatoid arthritis is not known although there have been occasional sporadic reports indicating
an excess of AML and malignant lymphoma [13]. An important
area for future consideration is therefore the whole question
of carcinogenic risk and predisposition [14].

MECHANISMS OF PRODUCTION OF MALIGNANT LYMPHOMA AND SKIN
CANCER

Initiation-promotion experiments in animals can be readily
interpreted on the basis of a 2-stage model such as that of
Moolgavkar and Knudson [15]. Application of a chemical
(initiator) followed by promotion by an irritant like croton
oil or phorbol ester leads to the development of skin papil-
lomas which then undergo malignant change. The initiators
bind to DNA which thus represents the first event which is
followed by a proliferation-dependent second event needed for
malignant transformation. In more precise terms the initiating event could be the production of a pre-mutagenic DNA
lesion occurring in particular genes in one strand of the
DNA; during replication this will result in an altered base
sequence due to miscoding (specific mutations) in the daughter
strand, which will then be transmitted to future daughter
cells in a heterozygous state. There are, of course, other
processes in DNA, such as error-prone repair and frame shifts,
which can lead to miscoding. It is then postulated that
another mutation or an exchange between homologous chromosomes
leading to homozygosity represents the final stage towards
malignant transformation. In man, several types of cancers
cluster in families, and pedigree data show that an autosomal
dominant cancer gene is sometimes involved. Familial poly-
posus coli and some breast cancers are examples, and 40% of
the rare retinoblastoma type of tumour are estimated to be
due to inheritance of such a dominant gene. This gene may
represent a mutant, occurring in an ancestral germ-line cell,
which acts like an initiating lesion. The second event
could thus be a second mutation at the same site on the homologous chromosome. Other strategies involving exchange between
homologous chromosomes (SCEs) e.g., as in Bloom's syndrome
could also produce the same effect. While this is all somewhat hypothetical it is reasonable to surmise that chemical
and physical carcinogens act by virtue of producing specific
mutations in association with recombinant genetic events, the
latter probably involving viral genomic material. Cancer

production may thus be considered as a multi-stage process
involving alteration of DNA and changes in control of cell
proliferation.

Immunosuppressive agents could thus theoretically act at any
point in this chain of events either as an initiator or by
influencing the rate of proliferation of target, initiated
cells by regulatory means involving growth control or by producing immunological surveillance defects. The development
of primary skin cancer in ultraviolet-irradiated mice [16]
would appear to be a good model for the involvement of immune
surveillance in cancer development.

Cytogenic analysis of B cell lymphomas in mouse and man has
now revealed genetic transpositions to the region of the
immunoglobulin genes which could represent movement of the
oncogene to a region of high promoter activity and greater
transcription function. DNA viral agents, like herpes simplex
or EB virus, may be involved particularly in respect of
lympho-reticular malignancies of B lymphocyte origin in man.
How human viruses could be involved in such a process is not
known but among the possibilities is by interfering with DNA
repair and recombinant process. Some evidence for this is
the finding of chromosomal damage associated with viral infections [17]. Acquired (e.g., viral) as well as inherited
genetic predisposing mechanisms may thus be important in influencing host susceptibility to develop cancer in response
to immunosuppressive and "lympho-modulatory" agents. If this
is so, assessment of these "risk" factors represents a challenge for immunotoxicology.

REFERENCES

1. Brittain, S. and Palacios, R. (1982). *Immunol. Rev.* **65**,
    5-22.
2. Harris, G. and Hutchins, D. (1979). In "Drugs and Immune
    Responsiveness" (Eds. J.L. Turk and D. Parker), pp.41-61.
    The Macmillan Press Ltd., London and Basingstoke.
3. Trentham, D.E., Belli, J.A., Anderson, R.J., Buckley, J.A.,
    Goetzl, E.J., David, J.R. and Austen, K.F. (1981). *New
    Engl. J. Med.* **305**, 976-982.
4. IARC Monographs on the Evaluation of Carcinogenic Risk of
    Chemicals in Humans. (1981). Vol.**26**, W.H.O. Agency for
    Research on Cancer.
5. Cooper, G.M., Okenquist, S. and Silverman, L. (1980).
    Nature **284**, 418-421.
6. Stehelin, D., Varmus, H.E. and Bishop, J.M. (1976).
    Nature **260**, 170-173.
7. Shih, C. and Weinberg, R.A. (1982). *Cell* **29**, 161-169.
8. Weinberg, R.A. (1982). *Cell* **30**, 3-4.

9. Friedberg, E.C., Ehmann, U.K. and Williams, J.I. (1979). *Adv. Rad. Biol.* **8**, 85-174.

10. Good, R.A. (1972). *Proc. Natl. Acad. Sci. (U.S.A.)* **69**, 1026-1032.

11. Kinlen, L.J., Sheil, A.G.R., Peto, J. and Doll, R. (1979). *Brit. Med. J.* **2**, 1461-1466.

12. Casey, T.P. (1968). *Blood* **31**, 396-399.

13. Louie, S. and Schwartz, R.S. (1978). *Semin. Hematol.* **15**, 117-138.

14. Marks, P. (1981). *Surgery* **90**, 132-136.

15. Moolgavkar, S.H. and Knudson, A.G. (1981). *J. Natl. Cancer Inst.* **66**, 1037-1051.

16. Fisher, M.S. and Kripke, M. (1982). *Science* **216**, 1133-1134.

17. Nichols, W.W. (1974). In "The Cell Nucleus" (Ed. H. Busch), Vol. **2**, pp.437-458. Academic Press, New York.

THE USE OF IMMUNOTOXICOLOGICAL DATA
IN THE ENVIRONMENTAL REGULATORY PROCESS

D.E. Gardner, M.J.K. Selgrade and J.A. Graham

U.S. Environmental Protection Agency,
Health Effects Research Laboratory,
Inhalation Toxicology Division,
Toxicology Branch, Research Triangle Park, NC 27711, USA

INTRODUCTION

One of the principal responsibilities of the U.S. Environmental Protection Agency (EPA) is to conduct research necessary to maintain an adequate scientific and technological data
base on which to establish the standards, regulations and
implementation actions required by various Congressional Acts.
We will focus this discussion on two legislative mandates;
the Clean Air Act and the Toxic Substances Control Acts, because most of our research related to immunotoxicity has been
done to provide data for these two Acts.

The Clean Air Act, as amended in 1977, authorizes a national
programme of research directed towards controlling adverse
health effects of airborne chemicals. Research towards this
end falls into two categories, namely, that to support National
Ambient Air Quality Standards (NAAQS) and that to identify,
evaluate and control other hazardous air pollutants.

NAAQS have been set for ozone, nitrogen dioxide, sulphur
dioxide, total suspended particulates, carbon monoxide, and
lead. The goal is to set standards at levels which, in the
judgement of the EPA Administrator, protect the health of
normal and susceptible subpopulations with an adequate margin
of safety. The scientific data bases used in setting these
standards are updated and reviewed every five years. As
scientific information becomes available, uncertainties inherent in NAAQS are reduced, and reliance on judgemental
factors becomes less important.

In addition to the chemicals controlled by NAAQS, there
are a vast number of chemicals in the ambient air, some of
which may be responsible for serious irreversible and/or

incapacitating disease. Over the past several years, increasing attention has been directed towards the identification, evaluation and control of these hazardous air pollutants (HAP) to which no NAAQS is applicable. Hence the EPA has been authorized to regulate mutagens, carcinogens, teratogens and other toxic pollutants. Seven compounds, benzene, asbestos, vinyl chloride, inorganic arsenic, radionuclides, mercury, and beryllium are now listed as hazardous. Of these, only the latter two are listed for non-carcinogenic reasons, and so far no chemical has been regulated on the basis of immunotoxicity.

The objectives of the health effects research being conducted to support these two environmental regulatory programmes are quite different. Updating the relatively large data base to support the maintenance or revision of the NAAQS requires research to 1) better define dose-response relationships; 2) develop more information on sensitive population groups; 3) determine effects of pollutant interactions; 4) confirm and extend important findings of the data base; 5) examine mechanisms of action; 6) increase understanding of the degree of adversity of the observed health effects; and 7) develop exposure estimates for the general as well as the sensitive population. Essentially the data base is being refined. Major objectives of the HAP toxicology programme are to 1) improve and apply identification and screening methods; 2) expand the data base for use in the assessment of potential risk; and 3) better define concentration-response relationship for predicting significant levels of exposure. Thus, under this programme, the data base is essentially being created.

The other legislative mandate, the Toxic Substances Control Act (TSCA) requires that EPA establish chemical testing guidelines for industry to use to assess the toxicity of the chemicals they produce. The research conducted to support this programme differs from that which supports the air programme in that it is done primarily to 1) refine and review existing research guidelines; 2) improve the data base for registration and regulations; and 3) identify methods for testing which can be used in qualified industrial and commercial laboratories. Immunotoxicity testing falls into this last category since at the present time it is not included in the toxicity testing guidelines.

The use of immunological data for regulation of environmental pollutants is obviously in its infancy. In the following discussion we will consider major factors that affect the usefulness of immunological data for regulatory decision making and describe an approach we are presently developing to answer questions related to immunotoxicity of chemicals.

USE OF IMMUNOLOGICAL DATA FOR REGULATORY PURPOSES

Almost any scientifically-sound immunotoxicology study has
some information useful for regulatory decision making. However, there can be a considerable range in the degree of usefulness of such studies. Major factors which influence regulatory relevance are discussed below.

Chemical to be Tested

The chemical to be examined for immunotoxicity must be
environmentally relevant. For those ubiquitous pollutants
regulated by NAAQS, the identity of chemicals of interest is
clear. The only significant exception is for particulate
matter since it is a broad class of chemicals primarily consisting of ammonium sulphate, carbonaceous particles, particles emitted by wood burning, sulphuric acid, alumino-
silicate compounds, ferric oxide, and calcium carbonate.

Other chemicals of interest to EPA under the HAP regulatory
authority are more difficult to identify. In this case the
major problem is the multitude of chemicals, primarily metals
and organics, and the paucity of data bases on environmental
monitoring and health effects. Knowledge of production volumes, industrial waste volume, environmental persistence and
dispersion tendencies, in relationship to the size of populations being exposed, provides guidance on selection of
chemicals. However, information of this sort is often lacking. Also, it is conceivable that a highly toxic chemical
may have low exposure rates, making it difficult to automatically conclude that only high volume chemicals are of
interest. Obtaining health effects data is critical.

A major determinant of regulatory relevance is whether the
chemical form being tested occurs in the environment to a
substantial degree. For instance, the predominant form of
metals in the air is as oxides, not soluble salts, yet most
investigations use the salts. This can make an important
difference as indicated by the following examples: host
defences against bacterial pulmonary infection were more
sensitive to $NiCl_2$ than to $NiSO_4$ and more sensitive to $ZnSO_4$
than $Zn(NH_4)_2(SO_4)_2$ [1,2], primary antibody responses were
significantly reduced by $NiSO_4$ and $NiCl_2$ but not NiO [3];
Pb_2O_3 and NiO caused more alterations in the number of alveolar macrophages in the lung than did $PbCl_2$ and $NiCl_2$ [4,5],
and Waters et al. [6] found that the cytotoxicity of vanadium
was related to the solubility, with the more soluble forms
being more toxic.

The physical state of the chemical is also critical. For
example, several inhalation studies of silica have been performed, but they used smaller particle sizes (< 3 μm, mass

median aerodynamic diameter, MMAD) than typically exist in the
ambient air (about 7 μm, MMAD). As particle size influences
the site of deposition in the respiratory tract and clearance
[7,8], immunotoxicological data developed on a particle size
which is uncommon in the air may have unknown relevance to
EPA. An even more complex issue is that of chemical interactions. Man is exposed to pollutant mixtures, but most toxicological studies are conducted with single chemicals. This
issue requires more experimentation to increase our level of
understanding. Many of the chemicals of interest to EPA are
organics which undergo biotransformation. As there are species
differences in xenobiotic metabolism, it is conceivable that
data developed in a rat might have limited applicability to
man. However, the precise nature of such limits is unknown.

The foregoing indicates how previously conducted research
has strengthened our understanding of the needs for relevance
if data are to be used for regulation purposes. More basic
research in this area will no doubt continue to sharpen our
focus (in terms of relevance) and result in improved experimental protocols in the future.

Exposure Protocol

The route of exposure can be a major determinant of immunotoxic potency. For example, Ni and Cd are more potent when
administered by inhalation than when given intramuscularly
[2]. The time of exposure can also be critical. Following a
prolonged exposure to an H_2SO_4 and carbon mixture and a mixture of SO_2 and carbon, there was immuno-enhancement, followed by no change, followed by immunosuppression as exposure
proceeded [9,10]. Thus, misinterpretations of immunotoxicity
could occur if examinations are only made at one time point
in a study.

As with other toxicological studies, some immunological
research is conducted using only one dose of the chemical.
However, for the most part dose-response data are needed for
regulatory decisions. Several groups are developing risk
assessment and extrapolation (from animal to man) models
which, when developed, will make dose-response data even more
crucial. There is also the issue of potency ranking of chemicals. In the future this might be used to relate the toxicity
of an environmental chemical having no human data base to that
of a chemical having both a human and animal data base.

Interpretability of the Data

Regulators are faced with the problem of interpreting the data
in terms of public health risk. For typical immunotoxicity
data, however, there is no consensus. What is the significant

risk to human health if a chemical causes a 30% statistically
significant decrease in the number of IgM plaque-forming cells
in the spleen of mice? To answer this or similar questions
will require major advancements in our understanding of
immunotoxicity. First is the qualitative extrapolation. Is
a 20% decrease in specific antibody titre of a mouse equivalent to a similar 20% drop in a man, and if so, will man experience an increased incidence or persistence of infection?
Notwithstanding the differences between laboratory animals
and man, there are extensive similarities, making it likely
that if an effect occurs in a number of animal species, the
same type of effect will occur in man. Thus, the greatest
problem is the definition of degree of adversity of a particular experimental observation.

The second problem is the quantitative extrapolation from
animals to man. If an effect occurs at a given dose of chemical in an experimental laboratory animal, what dose will
cause the same effect in man? With such knowledge, one
could determine whether environmental levels were above or
below this human effective dose and take the appropriate regulatory strategy. Quantitative extrapolation has two major
components — dosimetry and species sensitivity [11]. Briefly,
dosimetry involves determining the relationship between inhaled concentration and regional pulmonary tissue delivered
dose for several species, including man. Sensitivity is the
determination of whether the same delivered tissue dose will
produce the same response in different species.

Another major issue in interpreting human risk to immunotoxicological chemicals is host factors which may influence
the outcome of exposure. The developing or senescent immune
system may be more sensitive to chemical exposure than that
of a normal young adult. Other sensitive subpopulations may
exist. Risk factors in immunotoxicity have received relatively minor attention, making it difficult to interpret data
to fashion regulatory strategies to protect the largest numbers of people.

Dissemination of Data

A first major step in developing regulations for air pollutants is a detailed review of the literature. The review is
subject to intense scrutiny. If the papers being reviewed
are not complete and precise, the data contained will have
little use. Papers are reviewed according to criteria which
include nature of publication (peer-reviewed is preferred),
adequacy of experimental design and statistics, and extent of
description of methods and results. Many papers in the peer-
reviewed literature lack details such as number of animals

used, identification of statistical methods, specific identification of chemical levels (including generation and monitoring techniques, calibration of monitors and stability of exposure levels), and specific design elements. For regulatory
use, facts not in evidence in the literature reviews cannot
be considered. Thus, a significant amount of information is
lost because regulatory reviews are, by obvious necessity,
rigorous.

AN APPROACH FOR IMMUNOTOXICITY TESTING

There are now a number of studies [12-16] which indicate that
environmental chemicals depress various aspects of the immune
response as determined by one or more of a myriad of tests
available to assess the functional integrity of specific components. One of the problems which EPA faces in using such
data for regulatory purposes is that few attempts have been
made to correlate changes in immune responses with increased
incidence or severity of disease. Because the Agency needs
to be able to define effects in terms of their degree of adversity, we have taken an approach which is the reverse of
that taken by many other investigators. We are developing a
series of disease susceptibility models and are combining
these with specific immune function tests to determine if any
of the immune responses are depressed in animals exhibiting
increased disease enhancement following exposure to a chemical.

Since more than one host defence mechanism is usually involved in protecting an individual from a given disease, (e.g.,
infectious, neoplastic, allergic, or autoimmune diseases)
susceptibility models usually reflect the combined effects of
a chemical on several immune defence mechanisms and their
interactions. If the mechanisms of pathogenesis and host
response to a particular disease are known, these provide
clues as to the types of specific immune functions which
might be affected in animals exhibiting enhanced symptoms.
Effects of chemicals on these mechanisms can then be tested
using immune function tests and some assessment can be made
as to the degree of immune suppression which is necessary to
exacerbate symptoms. It is theoretically possible to develop
for immunotoxicity testing purposes, a series of disease
susceptibility models, which taken together, may reflect the
health of the entire host defence system.

The practicality of developing an immunotoxicity testing
tier which utilizes disease enhancement as the first step in
the tier has yet to be determined, but it is certain that no
immunotoxicity tier would be valid without providing disease
susceptibility models somewhere in the scheme. We have

developed two such models which utilize infectious agents.
One of these reflects pulmonary defence mechanisms and the
other systemic (primarily cell-mediated) defence mechanisms.

For a number of years, we have used susceptibility of mice
to an aerosol infection with the bacteria *Streptococcus
pyogenes* Group C as an indicator of effects on pulmonary
defence mechanisms [17-19]. Briefly, animals are randomly
selected to be exposed to either clear air or to the test
substance. After the cessation of this exposure, the animals
from both chambers are combined and are exposed to an aerosol
of viable micro-organisms. At the termination of this exposure, some animals from each group are killed. The remainder
of the animals are housed in clean air, and the rate of mortality in the two groups determined during a 15-day holding
period. The control mortality is approximately 10 to 20% and
reflects the natural resistance of the host to the infectious
agent. Other parameters such as number of organisms per lung
at different time periods can also be measured. This particular model has demonstrated toxic effects of numerous gases
and particles (NO_2, O_3, $CdCl_2$, $NiCl_2$, phosgene, toluene, etc)
which can be related to the duration of exposure at different
concentrations [1,17,19, unpublished data].

If host defence mechanisms are functioning normally, there
is rapid inactivation of inhaled bacteria that have been
deposited at the alveolar level [20-21]. However, in
pollutant-exposed animals, the number of microbes in the
lungs increases in number beyond the original number deposited
within four to six hours [22-24]. This acceleration in bacterial growth has been attributed to the pollutant's alteration of the capability of the lungs to destroy bacteria, thus
permitting those with pathogenic potential to multiply and
produce disease.

A number of defence mechanisms operate in the respiratory
system. These include alveolar macrophages, secretory antibody, interferon, cytotoxic T lymphocytes and natural killer
cells, mechanical barriers such as the mucociliary system,
and the various components of the inflammatory system. The
nature of this infectivity streptococcal model allows one to
focus on the possible mechanisms for pollutant enhancement
of disease to the following: 1) production of oedema; 2)
reduction in physical removal by mucociliary mechanisms; and/
or 3) alteration of non-specific cellular defence mechanisms.
A number of studies indicate that the effects of pollutants
on the streptococcal infection are largely a result of adverse effects on the alveolar macrophage [25-28]. Hence,
for any pollutant tested which enhances this infection, the
suspected primary mechanism of action is alveolar macrophage
toxicity.

Another model which we are developing uses susceptibility of mice to murine cytomegalovirus as an indicator of effects on certain systemic defence mechanisms. Human cytomegalovirus is one of the several opportunistic infections which commonly cause disease in immunosuppressed individuals [29-31]. For this reason, it is a good candidate for studies in which increased susceptibility to viral disease is used as an indicator of immunosuppression. Cytomegaloviruses (CMV) are species specific, so human CMV does not infect laboratory animals. However, murine CMV (MCMV) has been extensively developed as an experimental model [32-34]. As in humans, MCMV in mice is usually a benign infection which can be greatly exacerbated by immunosuppression [35-37]. Immune defence mechanisms thought to be important to host defences against MCMV include natural killer (NK) cell activity [38,39], cytotoxic T-cell activity [40], macrophage activity [41], and interferon [42]. It happens that these same defence mechanisms are also prominently mentioned in tumour immunology [43]. MCMV might, therefore, provide a disease susceptibility model which can be more rapidly assessed than increased tumour susceptibility, but yet be predictive of the latter.

Experiments to date have shown that enhancement of acute MCMV by cyclophosphamide and $NiCl_2$ can be correlated with inhibition of natural killer cell activity [44]. With a third pollutant, parathion, mice dosed at the peak of MCMV infection of the liver also exhibited enhanced mortality; however, this occurred too soon after parathion treatment to be indicative of an altered immune response. Such a study indicates that health effects resulting from combined activity between infectious agents and chemicals do not always involve the immune system. While this is not, strictly speaking, an immunotoxicology problem, it is nevertheless important to consider. For instance, most of the theories advanced, which link Reyes syndrome to synergistic activity between toxic chemicals and virus, do not involve immunotoxicity but do involve virus-chemical interactions which affect the liver [45, 46]. It is clear from this example that disease susceptibility models must be accompanied by immune as well as function tests in order to accurately evaluate immunotoxicity.

Obviously the two models we are using do not begin to represent all the host defence mechanisms that could be impaired by chemical exposure. They are merely illustrative of an approach which can be taken to identify substances which are immunotoxic. At the present time, immunotoxicity testing is not required under TSCA, and data from immune function tests and disease susceptibility models have not been used directly in regulating pollutant exposure.

A Case Study of Regulatory Use of Data

Epidemiological studies have been conducted in U.S. and Great Britain which indicate that the incidence of respiratory illness, bronchitis and cough is higher in children living in homes with gas stoves [47-50]. Significantly higher levels of NO_2 in gas versus electric stove homes have been documented [51,52]. In evaluating the evidence, major uncertainties exist regarding what specific agent(s) caused the response and were associated with this effect.

Experimental work with the animal infectivity model has provided sufficient data to demonstrate that NO_2 impairs respiratory defence mechanisms. The findings of these studies indicate that (1) short-term peak exposures may be more important than long-term, low level exposure of equivalent dose (C x T); (2) background concentrations may affect the ability of the host to recover from peak exposures, and (3) that intermittent exposures may not produce an effect that is significantly less than a similar continuous exposure [53-56]. Because of the available data, it was reasonable to suggest that the peaks of NO_2 may be the factor for increased prevalence of respiratory illness for young children living in homes with gas stoves. Thus, the animal data from the infectivity model provided the toxicological plausibility behind the statistically significant associations observed in the epidemiological study, thereby facilitating the use of the entire set of data in decision-making relative to the review of the NAAQS for NO_2.

REFERENCES

1. Gardner, D.E. (1979). In "Aerosols in Science, Medicine and Technology — The Biomedical Influence of Aerosols" (Eds. W. Stober and R. Jaenicke), pp.120-131. Gesell Schaft für Aerosolforschung, Mainz, Germany.
2. Ehrlich, R. (1980). *Environ. Hlth. Perspect.* **35**, 89-100.
3. Graham, J.A., Miller, F.J., Daniels, M.J., Payne, E.A. and Gardner, D.E. (1978). *Environ. Res.* **16**, 77-78.
4. Bingham, E., Pfitzer, E.A., Barkley, W. and Radford, E.P. (1968). *Science* **164**, 1297-1299.
5. Bingham, E., Barkley, M., Zerwes, M., Stemmer, K. and Taylor, P. (1972). *Arch. Environ. Health* **25**, 406-414.
6. Waters, M.D., Gardner, D.E. and Coffin, D.L. (1974). *Toxicol. Appl. Pharmacol.* **28**, 253-263.
7. Brain, J.D. and Valberg, P.A. (1979). *Am. Rev. Respir. Dis.* **120**, 1325-1373.
8. Raabe, O.G. (1982). In "Mechanisms in Respiratory Toxicology" (Eds. H. Witschi and P. Nettesheim),Vol.I, pp.27-76. CRC Press, Boca Raton.

9. Fenters, J.D., Bradof, J.N., Aranyi, C., Ketels, K., Ehrlich, R. and Gardner, D.E. (1979). *Environ. Res.* **19**, 244-257.

10. Zarkower, A. (1972). *Arch. Environ. Health* **25**, 45-50.

11. Miller, F.J., Graham, J.A. and Gardner, D.E. (1982). *Environ. Health Perspect.* (in press).

12. Dean, J.H., Padarathsingh, M.L., Jerrells, T.R., Keys, J. and Nothing, J.W. (1979). *Drug and Chemical Toxicology* **2**, 133-153.

13. Vos, J.G. (1977). *CRC Crit. Rev. Toxicol.* **5**, 67-101.

14. Faith, R.E., Luster, M.I. and Vos, J.G. (1980). In "Reviews in Biochemical Toxicology" (Eds. E. Hodgson, J.R. Bend and R.M. Philpot), Vol.2, pp.173-212. Elsevier, New York.

15. Dean, J.H., Luster, M.I., Boorman, G.A. and Laner, L.D. (1982). *Pharmacol. Rev.* **34**, 137-148.

16. Gardner, D.E. (1982). *Environ. Health Persp.* **43**, 99-107.

17. Gardner, D.E. (1979). In "Assessing Toxic Effects by Environmental Pollutants" (Eds. Lee and Mudd), pp.78-103.

18. Ehrlich, R., Findlay, J.C. and Gardner, D.E. (1979). *J. Toxicol. Environ. Health* **5**, 631-642.

19. Gardner, D.E. and Graham, J.A. (1977). In "Pulmonary Macrophage and Epithelial Cells" (Eds. Sanders, Schneider, Dagle and Ragan). ERDA Symposium Series 43, pp.1-21.

20. Kass, E.H., Greer, G.M. and Goldstein, E. (1966). *Bacteriol. Rev.* **30**, 488-497.

21. Rylander, R. (1968). *Acta Physiol. Scand. Suppl.* **306**, 1-89.

22. Miller, F.J., Illing, J.W. and Gardner, D.E. (1978). *Toxicol. Lett.* **2**, 163-169.

23. Coffin, D.L. and Gardner, D.E. (1972). *Ann. Occup. Hyg.* **15**, 219-234.

24. Gardner, D.E. (1982). In "Air Pollution — Physiological Effects" (Eds. McGrath and Barnes). (in press). Academic Press, New York.

25. Graham, J.A., Gardner, D.E., Waters, M.D. and Coffin, D.L. (1975). *Infect. Immun.* **11**, 1278-1283.

26. Waters, M.D., Gardner, D.E., Aranyi, C. and Coffin, D.L. (1975). *Environ. Res.* **9**, 32-47.

27. Gardner, D.E. (1982). In "Pulmonary Toxicology" (Ed. J. Hook). (in press). Raven Press, New York.

28. Goldstein, E., Tyler, W.S., Heoprich, P.D. and Eagle, C. (1973). *Arch. Environ. Health* **26**, 202-204.

29. Fiala, M., Payne, J.E., Berne, T.V., Moore, T.C., Henle, W., Montgomerie, J.Z., Chatterjee, S.W. and Gaze, L.B. (1975). *J. Infect. Dis.* **132**, 421-433.

30. Neiman, P.E., Reeves, W., Ray, G., Flournoy, N., Lerner, K.G., Sale, G.E. and Thomas, E.D. (1977). *J. Infect. Dis.*

136, 754-767.
31. Pollard, R.B., Rand, K.H., Arvin, A.M. and Merigan, T.C. (1978). *J. Infect. Dis.* **137**, 541-549.
32. Wright, H.T. (1973). In "The Herpes Viruses" (Ed. A.S. Kaplin), pp.353-388. Academic Press, New York.
33. Smith, M.G. (1959). *Progr. Med. Virol.* **2**, 171-202.
34. Osborn, J.E. (1982). In "The Mouse in Biomedical Research II" (Eds. Fox *et al.*). (in press). Academic Press, New York.
35. Agatsuma, Y. (1977). *Sapporo Ishi* **46**, 240-251.
36. Henson, D., Smith, R.D., Gehrke, J. and Neapolitan, C. (1967). *Amer. J. Pathol.* **51**, 1001-1007.
37. Jordan, M.C., Shandley, S.D. and Stevens, J.G. (1977). *J. Gen. Virol.* **37**, 419-423.
38. Quinnan, G.V. and Manischewitz, J.E. (1979). *J. Exp. Med.* **150**, 1549-1554.
39. Bancroft, G.J., Shellam, G.R. and Chalmers, J.E. (1981). *J. Immunol.* **126**, 988-994.
40. Quinnan, G.V., Manischewitz, J.E. and Ennis, F.A. (1980). *J. Gen. Virol.* **47**, 503-508.
41. Selgrade, M.J.K. and Osborn, J.E. (1974). *Infect. Immun.* **10**, 1383-1390.
42. Grundy (Chalmer), J.E., Trapman, J., Allan, J.E., Shellam, G.R. and Melief, C.J.M. (1982). *Infect. and Immun.* **37**, 143-150.
43. Herberman, R.B. and Ortaldo, J.R. (1981). *Science* **214**, 24-30.
44. Selgrade, M.J.K., Daniels, M.J., Hu, P.C., Miller, F.J. and Graham, J.A. (1982). *Infect. Immun.* (in press).
45. Colin, A.R., Pando, V. and Sandberg, A.(1975). In "Reyes Syndrome" (Ed. J.D. Pollack), pp.199-213. Grune and Stratten, Inc., New York.
46. Crocker, J.F., Ozere, R.L., Sabe, S.H., Rigout, S.C., Rozee, K.R. and Hutzinger, O. (1976). *Science* **192**, 1351-1353.
47. Melia, R.J.W., Florey, C. DuV., Altman, D.S. and Swan, A.V. (1977). *Brit. Med. J.* **2**, 149-152.
48. Melia, R.J.W., Florey, C. DuV. and Dhinn, S. (1979). *Int. J. Epid.* **8**, 333-338.
49. Goldstein, B.D., Melia, J.W., Chinn, S., Florey, C. DuV., Clark, D. and John, H.H. (1979). *Int. J. Epidemiol.* **8**, 339-346.
50. Florey, C.V., Melia, R.J.W., Chinn, S., Goldstein, B.D., Brooks, A.G.F., John, H.H. and Webster, X. (1979). *Int. J. Epidemiol.* **8**, 347-354.
51. Wade, W.A., Cote, W.A. and Yocom, J.E. (1975). *J. Air Pollut. Contr. Assoc.* **25**, 893-939.
52. Cote, W.A., Wade, W.A. and Yocom, J.E. (1974). In "Final

Contract No. 28-02-0745, EPA-650-4-74-042".

53. Gardner, D.E. (1980). In "Nitrogen Oxides and their Effects on Health" (Ed. Lee). pp.267-288. Ann Arbor Science, Ann Arbor.

54. Gardner, D.E., Miller, F.J., Blommer, E.J. and Coffin, D.L. (1979). *Environ. Health Perspect.* **30**, 23-29.

55. Gardner, D.E., Coffin, D.L., Pinigin, M.A. and Sidorenko, G.I. (1977). *J. Toxicol. Environ. Health* **3**, 811-820.

56. Coffin, D.L., Gardner, D.E. and Blommer, E.J. (1976). *Environ. Health Perspect.* **13**, 11-15.

IMMUNOTOXICOLOGY — A VIEWPOINT FROM INDUSTRY

G.E. Davies

Imperial Chemical Industries PLC,
Central Toxicology Laboratory,
Alderley Park, Nr Macclesfield, Cheshire SK10 4TJ, UK

As an immunologist working in Industry I am confronted with
two aspects of the problem we are here discussing, namely:
i) will a new compound, of potential commercial interest, be
"immunotoxic" and ii) are apparent immune dysfunctions
observed in human populations the result of exposure to
chemicals? Each aspect demands a separate approach. Determination of potential immunotoxicity requires, in the first
instance, a clear definition of the term "immunotoxicity",
I have elsewhere [1] defined immunotoxicity as: "the undesirable effects of an inappropriate response of the immune
system". I wish to emphasise the word "inappropriate"; many
of the *effects* which, in one set of circumstances we might
classify as "immunotoxic", would, in another set be regarded
as highly desirable. For instance, inhibition of an immune
response might be undesirable in the general population but
highly beneficial in patients with organ grafts. Secondly,
it might be argued that an immunotoxic effect revealed in a
prospective toxicity screen is relevant only in the absence
of other, more generally recognized evidence of toxicity. A
compound causing, for example, kidney necrosis or testicular
atrophy would be classified as "toxic" irrespective of any
effect it might produce on the immune response.

With these two basic provisos in mind I would like to discuss the present status of immunotoxicity from my own personal
viewpoint, and I will present my thoughts under two major
headings: "determination of potential immunotoxicity" and
"*post hoc* investigation".

DETERMINATION OF POTENTIAL IMMUNOTOXICITY

A number of schemes, some of which have been presented in
these proceedings, have been proposed for the prospective

detection of immunotoxicity. Two aspects of these schemes
give me some cause for concern. Firstly, the highly complex
nature of the immune response leads inevitably to discordant
conclusions. Sharma and Zeeman [2] have tabulated the published effects of DDT on the immune response which, according
to the conditions of testing, may have either no effect, or
may increase or decrease antibody formation in animals. This
of course comes as no surprise to any immunologist aware of
the profound influence on the immune response of such considerations as strain, age, sex and species of animals; size
and route of administration of antigen and test chemical;
season of year; time of day etc., but if we are to draw conclusions, affecting the ultimate fate of the test substance,
from such experiments in animals, interpretation of the results becomes a matter of supreme importance. The second
cause for concern is the debatable relevance to man of some
of the animal models. At a recent NATO Advanced Study Institute on Immunotoxicology held in Nova Scotia, eight out of
ten "experts" listed as one of their two chosen techniques,
the estimation of the numbers of plaque-forming cells in the
spleens of mice. Now this method estimates the number of
antibody-forming cells present in the spleen four or five
days after immunization, usually following intravenous administration of antigen, that is before free antibody appears in
the serum. Results are frequently submitted to statistical
analysis (sometimes, indeed, based on the unjustified assumption that the numbers of antibody-forming cells are normally,
rather than log-normally, distributed) and it occasionally
happens that a 50% reduction is stated to be "statistically
significant" — but does this mean anything more than the fact
that one cell division later there will be twice as many active cells present? Certainly it does not mean that there
will eventually be half as much antibody in the treated groups.
The class of affected immunoglobulin must also be considered;
differential effects on IgM, IgG and IgE synthesis are not
uncommon.

The large battery of tests advocated by some authors as
"Tier 2" screens probably add to, rather than diminish, the
difficulties of interpretation and decisions on relevance.
In response to these difficulties a number of so-called
"functional tests" have been proposed. This seems a logical
proposition since our concern about immunotoxicity is, after
all, a concern about disturbed function. Tests involving
bacterial and or virus infections coupled with experimental
models of neoplasia [3] appear to have more to commend themselves than do the more conventional "immunological" types of
tests. We must however be assured of relevance and reproducibility — and by this I do not mean simply the ability to

obtain the same answer by replicating experiments, but that
the same conclusion should be derivable by following different
approaches to the same problem.

It might be expected that some help could be gained from a
comprehensive study in animals of those compounds which have
already shown immunotoxic effects in man. Such evidence in an
unequivocal, independently confirmed form, is difficult to
obtain and I have dealt elsewhere with the apparent discrep-
ancies between studies in animals and effects in man — evidence which is particularly elusive if we seek for specific
immunotoxicity in the absence of other toxic manifestations.
Indeed the reverse is more frequently seen — 2,3,7,8-tetra-
chlorobenzo-p-dioxin (TCDD), for example, was not found to
affect the immune function of children exhibiting other
aspects of TCDD-related toxicity [4]. All these considerations lead me inescapably to the conclusion that we cannot
yet, with confidence, accept any of the proposed schemes for
prospective immunotoxicity testing. This of course is not
intended to undervalue the scientific knowledge gained from
much of the excellent published work. I am submitting the
proposal that we are not yet ready to place our total reliance
on the presently available schemes for large scale screening
of new chemicals. The banal sequel is that more research
is necessary. What then are we to do, since we cannot simply
shut our eyes and hope that the problem will go away? I am
going to suggest a little later on that we should pay more
attention to effects observed in man, but before doing so I
would like to spend a little time on some aspects of undesirable, inappropriate responses of the immune system that
do not appear to be taken into account by much of the current
work on experimental immunotoxicity — namely the idiosyncratic
and "pseudo-immune" responses. The meaning of the term "idiosyncratic" has led in the past to some confusion: I here
adopt the definition of the Concise Oxford Dictionary — "a
physical constitution peculiar to a person". This definition
says nothing about mechanisms but does imply that some people
respond differently from others and this fact is drawn to our
attention more forcibly when idiosyncratic responses are rare.
Such responses will of course include those which are genetically determined but even these are germane to immunotoxicological consideration. Examples of such idiosyncratic responses include the lupus-like phenomena frequently associated
with procaineamide [5], hydralazine [6] and some other drugs
used for the treatment of cardiovascular disorders; autoimmune glomerulonephritis seen after exposure to mercury [7]
or some organic solvents [8] and the major problems associated
with allergy to chemicals about which we have heard a great
deal during the present symposium. Among "pseudo-immune"

responses I would include effects dependent on activation of
the alternative complement pathway, histamine release, etc
[9]. A final category of immunotoxic responses are those revealed when the functions of suppressor cells are interfered
with [10].

It seems to me that in the present state of knowledge immunologists would be well advised to pay more attention to
chemically-induced immune dysfunction in man, either *post hoc,*
by intensive investigation of existing untoward events of a
relevant nature, or by the careful monitoring of immune function during limited release of a new substance to which the
human population may be exposed. It is in connection with
these aspects that I feel animal experiments might prove to
be of most value. Prospective evaluation demands of course,
that very sensitive indicators of dysfunction should be available so as to provide a warning before the actual damage
occurs. It is also apparent that the investigations themselves should not put the population at risk by, for example,
challenge studies. The problem therefore devolves into a
series of investigations which, preferably, can be performed
on samples of blood. Many of the current investigations of
immune function in man rely very heavily, sometimes exclusively, on the response of lymphocytes to mitogens *in vitro.*
Further work is necessary before absolute reliance can be
placed on the relevance of such tests which are notoriously
liable to non-specific effects. Stimulation by antigen (including mixed lymphocyte responses) are probably of more
value, but reproducibility of the tests leaves room for improvement.

In summary, then, my present attitude is to maintain a
watching brief with respect to screening tests in animals for
potential immunotoxicity. If my suggestions for more studies
in man, followed by animal experimentation, are followed, it
may be possible to build up a body of test procedures of proven relevance. At first sight the early history of short
term tests for carcinogenicity would appear to provide a situation analogous to the current state of immunotoxicology, but
the analogy is false. There was a good deal of evidence that
a significant number of chemicals were carcinogenic in man.
I remain to be convinced that equivalent evidence is available for immunotoxicity in man.

REFERENCES

1. Davies, G.E. (1982). In "NATO Advanced Study Institute
    on Immunotoxicology". Nova Scotia, Canada. (in press).
2. Sharma, R.P. and Zeeman, M.G. (1980). *J. Immunopharmacol.*
    2, 285-307.

3. Dean, J.H., Luster, M.J., Boorman, G.A., Leubke, R.W. and
    Lauer, L.D. (1982). *Env. Health Persp.* **43**, 81-88.
4. Seveso. "The Escape of Toxic Substances at the ICMESA
    Establishment on 10th July 1976 and the Consequent Dangers
    to Health and the Environment due to Industrial Activity".
    A translation by the Health & Safety Executive of the
    official report of the Parliamentary Commission of Enquiry
    by permission of the Parliament of the Republic of Italy.
5. Dubois, E.L. (1969). *Medicine (Baltimore)* **48**, 217-228.
6. Perry, H.M. and Schroeder, H.S. (1954). *J. Amer. Med.
    Assoc.* **154**, 670-673.
7. Bucket, J.P., Roels, H., Bernard, A. and Lauwerys, R.
    (1980). *J. Occup. Med.* **22**, 741-750.
8. Beirne, G.J. and Brennan, J.T. (1972). *Arch. Env. Health*
    25, 365-369.
9. "PAR Pseudo-Allergie Reactions" (1980). (Eds. P. Dukor,
    P. Kallos, H.D. Schlumberger and G.B. West). Vols. 1-3,
    Karger, Basel.
10. Loose, L.D. (1982). *Env. Health Persp.* **43**, 89-97.

PERSORPTION OF UNDEGRADABLE MACROMOLECULES: UPTAKE, DISTRIBUTION AND IMMUNOLOGICAL IMPLICATIONS

S. Nicklin and K. Miller

Immunotoxicology Department,
The British Industrial Biological Research Association,
Woodmansterne Road, Carshalton, Surrey, U.K.

Previous work has demonstrated that degraded carrageenan can initiate lesions within the gastro-intestinal tract of a number of experimental animals [1]. On this and other supportive evidence, the FDA ruled that only carrageenans with a molecular weight in excess of 100,000 should be used in foods. However at present there is no firm data available concerning the immunological/toxicological consequences that may occur following the uptake of carrageenans and other macromolecules with molecular weights in excess of 100,000.

A comprehensive view of the biological effects of carrageenan was conducted by DiRossa [2], but since this survey in 1972 several authors have reported that carrageenan when injected systemically markedly affected normal immune responses. These findings extend not only to the effects of carrageenans on macrophages, towards which some grades of carrageenan appear to be selectively cytotoxic [3], but also includes the modification of humoral antibody production [4], allograft rejection [5], and delayed hypersensitivity reactions, [6]. However, no one had considered the effect of oral administration on immune competence until Bash and Vago [7] reported that the oral administration of carrageenan could suppress T-lymphocyte proliferative responses.

In view of the potent biological properties of carrageenan and its wide application in the food and drug industry, a study of the effects of orally-imbibed macromolecules on the immune system was considered particularly relevant. In the present study we have fed three high molecular weight "food grade" carrageenans and Guar gum to rats and investigated firstly carrageenan uptake into the body tissues and secondly

IMMUNOTOXICOLOGY
ISBN 0-12-282180-7

Table 1 *Effect of feeding regimes on biliary immunoglobulin A (IgA) concentration and antigen specificity*

Group	Treatment	IgA concentration (mg/ml)	Anti *E. coli* titre*	Anti gut flora titre**
1	Guar gum	2.50 ± 0.11	2.33 ± 0.20	2.60 ± 0.60
2	Guar gum	2.15 ± 0.07	2.41 ± 0.37	2.80 ± 0.20
3	Carrageenan L100	2.73 ± 0.14	2.00 ± 0.51	3.00 ± 0.49
4	Carrageenan L100	2.63 ± 0.25	2.33 ± 0.42	2.20 ± 0.49
5	Carrageenan CSP	2.45 ± 0.23	2.00 ± 0.36	3.20 ± 0.80
6	Carrageenan CSP	2.80 ± 0.11	3.00 ± 0.44	3.20 ± 0.80
7	Carrageenan J	2.65 ± 0.16	1.83 ± 0.16	2.80 ± 0.37
8	Carrageenan J	2.85 ± 0.18	2.50 ± 0.34	4.00 ± 0.66
9	Control	2.33 ± 0.17	2.16 ± 0.30	2.60 ± 0.41
10	Control	2.23 ± 0.26	3.00 ± 0.25	2.60 ± 0.82

Results are mean values ± S.E. of 6 rats per group.

Groups 2,4,6,8 and 10 were sensitized to sheep erythrocytes.

* Anti *E. coli* antibody titre ($\log_2$ end-point titre).

** Anti-gut flora antibody titre ($\log_2$ end-point titre).

Table 2 *Effect of feeding regimes on serum antibody levels specific for gut microorganisms*

Group	Treatment	Anti *E. coli* titre*	Anti gut flora titre**
1	Guar gum	2.40 ± 0.74	2.00 ± 0.31
2	Guar gum	5.00 ± 0.31	4.20 ± 0.19
3	Carrageenan L100	2.00 ± 0.31	1.80 ± 0.19
4	Carrageenan L100	5.20 ± 0.37	3.80 ± 0.37
5	Carrageenan CSP	2.00 ± 0.00	2.00 ± 0.31
6	Carrageenan CSP	4.60 ± 0.39	4.20 ± 0.85
7	Carrageenan J	1.80 ± 0.37	1.60 ± 0.50
8	Carrageenan J	4.80 ± 0.19	4.00 ± 0.70
9	Control	2.80 ± 0.58	1.80 ± 0.36
10	Control	4.40 ± 0.67	4.40 ± 0.39

Results are mean values ± S.E. for 6 rats per group.

Groups 2,4,6,8 and 10 were sensitized to sheep erythrocytes.

* Anti-*E. coli* antibody titre ($\log_2$ end-point titre).

** Anti-gut flora antibody titre ($\log_2$ end-point titre).

considered the effect of carrageenan and Guar gum on the
following immunological parameters, (I) the immune response
to gut microflora, (II) the immune response to a specific
antigen presented orally and (III) the immune response to
antigen presented systemically.

Experimental Design

Groups of 12 PVG male rats were maintained on normal drinking
water, drinking water containing 0.5% Guar gum or drinking
water containing either 0.5% carrageenan type CSP, 0.5%
carrageenan type J or 0.5% carrageenan type L100 (trade
names, Hercules Co. Ltd.). In each group half of the rats
were sensitized to sheep red blood cells by the intra-
peritoneal injection of sheep erythrocytes on day 55 and day
62 of the feeding study. All groups received an oral
challenge of sheep erythrocytes on days 76 and 83.

Blood samples for serum were taken for analysis on days 62,
69, 76, 83 and 90. In addition a 90-day bile sample was obtained by bile duct cannulation prior to post-mortem
pathology procedures.

Histology

Peyer's patches including a section of gut immediately above
and below each patch were taken from the top, mid and
terminal regions of the gut and processed for light microscopy. Sections were examined for the presence of carrageenan-
containing cells using the Alcian Blue staining technique [8].

Routine light microscopy revealed no pathological lesions
attributable to treatment. However, Alcian Blue positive
cells were observed within the villi, lamina propria and
basement membrane lymphatics of carrageenan-fed rats; these
cells were assumed to be of macrophage origin.

Macrophages were not readily apparent in the routine
haematoxylin and eosin stained sections, however a fluorescence technique was utilized which revealed numerous
macrophage-like cells within the sub-epithelial zone of the
Peyer's patch. These cells were large and contained granules;
enzyme studies revealed that they were positive for both non-
specific esterase and acid phosphatase; immunofluorescence
studies showed these cells to be immunoglobulin negative and
IgA antigen positive. These criteria in association with
electron microscope evidence identified these cells as
macrophages. A similar population of cells was identified
within the villi.

Effects on Immunity

Following the demonstrated uptake of carrageenan into the
body tissues we investigated its effects on local and systemic
immunity.   The immunoglobulin-A content of test and control
90-day bile samples were measured using the Mancini technique
[9].   It was apparent that none of the treatments affected
immunoglobulin-A output into the bile (Table 1).   Ninety-day
serum and bile samples were also assessed for immune reactivity against a range of microorganisms.   Reactivity against
the gut commensal *E. coli* was determined by a standard

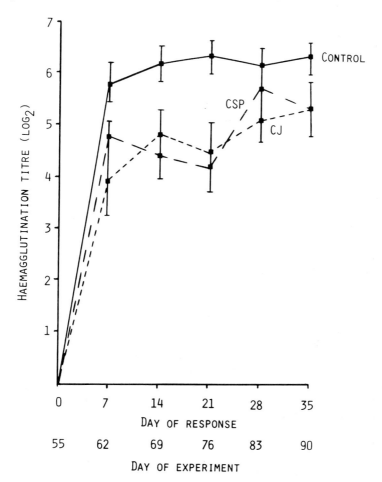

Fig. 1 Effect of feeding carrageenan CJ and carrageenan CSP
on the humoral immune response to sheep red blood cells
(mean ± S.E.).

agglutination procedure. Reactivity against pooled microflora
was assessed using an indirect immunofluorescent procedure.
Anti-*E. coli* antibodies were detected in equivalent amounts
in all test and control bile samples analysed (Table 1).
However when serum samples were assayed for antibody activity
against *E. coli* all of the presensitized animals had higher
levels of anti-*E. coli* antibodies compared with non-
sensitized animals (Table 2). An identical picture emerged
when bile and serum samples were analysed for antibody with
specificity for pooled gut bacteria using the indirect

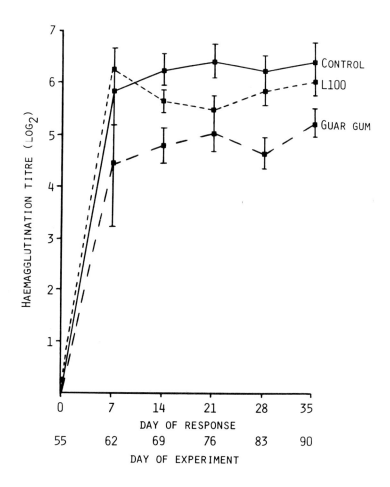

Fig. 2 Effect of feeding carrageenan L100 and Guar gum on
the humoral immune response to sheep red blood cells (mean ±
S.E.).

immunofluorescence assay (Tables 1 and 2). However as equivalent levels of antibody were detected in the appropriate control animals the immunization effect was unrelated to the feeding regime. One possible explanation of these results is that sheep erythrocytes and gut bacteria may possess common epitopes, consequently the immunization procedure boosted the natural immunity against these shared determinants.

We went on to investigate whether food grade carrageenans and/or Guar gum could facilitate immunization to other antigens present in the gut lumen. Test and control animals received a standard sheep red blood cell challenge orally on days 76 and 83 of the feeding study, serum was assessed for anti-sheep blood cell activity on days 83 and 90. In all instances animals failed to produce a haemagglutin response. Similarly 90-day bile samples from these rats contained only background levels of antibody activity.

To investigate any immunosuppressive properties of the test materials, animals were injected with sheep erythrocytes on days 55 and 62 of the feeding study. Serum samples were obtained on days 62, 69, 76, 83 and 90 and assayed for haemagglutinating antibody activity. Guar gum, carrageenan CSP and carrageenan CJ treatment all significantly reduced the haemagglutinin response, carrageenan L100 was less effective (see Figs. 1 and 2).

These data, considered together with the histology results, indicate that the carrageenans at least can penetrate the mucosal barrier of the gut. It appears that macrophages present within the villi and Peyer's patches take up these materials and transport them into the body tissues. Local immune responses are not affected but immune responses against specific systemically-administered antigens do appear suppressed. As some poorly degradable macromolecules are cytotoxic to macrophages it is possible that the observed suppression is due to a deficiency in antigen processing by macrophages rather than a depletion of immunocompetent cells.

ACKNOWLEDGEMENTS

This work forms part of a research project funded by the U.K. Ministry of Agriculture, Fisheries and Food. The results of this research are Crown Copyright.

REFERENCES

1. Sharratt, M., Grasso, P., Carpanini, F. and Gangolli, S.D. (1970). *Lancet* **2**, 932.
2. DiRosa, M. (1972). *J. Pharm. Pharmacol.* **24**, 89-102.
3. Catanzan, P.J., Schwartz, H.J. and Graham, R.C. (1971). *Am. J. Path.* **64**, 387-399.

4. Aschheim, K. and Raffel, S. (1972). *J. Reticuloendothel. Soc.* **11**, 253-261.

5. Rumjanek, V.M. and Brent, L. (1978). *Transplantation* **26**, 113-122.

6. Schwartz, H.J. and Leskowitz, S. (1967). *J. Immun.* **103**, 87-93.

7. Bash, J.A. and Vago, J.R. (1980). *J. Reticuloendothel. Soc.* **28**, 213-229.

8. Gangolli, S.D., Wright, M.G. and Grasso, P. (1973). *Histochemical J.* **5**, 37-48.

9. Mancini, G., Carbonara, A.O. and Heremans, J.F. (1965). *Immunochemistry* **2**, 235-249.

IMMUNOTOXICITY OF ORGANOTIN COMPOUNDS

A.H. Penninks and W. Seinen

*Working-Group Pathology-Toxicology, Department of Pathology
and Department of Pharmacology and Toxicology,
Faculty of Veterinary Sciences,
State University of Utrecht, The Netherlands*

INTRODUCTION

Organotin compounds are used in a variety of applications. They involve such widely divergent fields as: 1) stabilizers for polyvinylchloride (especially dialkyltins); 2) industrial and agricultural biocides (tributyl, triphenyl and tricyclohexyltins are the most important products); 3) wood-preserving and anti-fouling agents (especially tributyltin oxide); 4) catalytic agents in a variety of industrial processes [1-4].

The total production of organotin compounds has grown enormously during the last 20 years. The annual world production of organotins was estimated at 2,000 tons in 1960 whereas the total production nowadays amounts to 25,000 tons a year [4]. This may have profound implications for human and environmental health. Introduction into the environment occurs by their various applications, e.g. the agricultural use, the use in wood preservatives and antifouling paints, and also by leaching from plastic waste disposal. A direct introduction into man may occur by the migration of stabilizers from plastic into food, beverages and drinking water, or from plastic medical devices into body-fluids. Information about degradation and distribution of organotins in the environment is rather scanty or even lacking. On account of their biocidal properties the organotins are potentially hazardous pollutants. However, serious environmental effects of organotins have never been described. A mass poisoning of man occurred in France in 1958 by a preparation (Stalinon) used for treatment of furuncles and other staphylococcal skin infections [5]. The main active components of this preparation were diethyltin diiodide and linoleic acid, but a

IMMUNOTOXICOLOGY
ISBN 0-12-282180-7

certain batch also contained impurities of triethyltin
iodide which is extremely neurotoxic. Two hundred and seven-
teen people are known to have been poisoned, and one hundred
and ten of them died [6]. More recently, in 1975, two outbreaks of dibutyltin dilaurate (DBTD) poisoning involving
cattle, palm doves and mink were recorded in Israel [7]. A
vitamin-mineral supplement containing 1700 ppm DBTD, and
formulated for turkeys were inadvertantly fed to mink of two
farms [7]. They received the supplement at the end of the
whelping season, which resulted in a high mortality in the
mothers with large litters and in the kittens. A second out-
break of DBTD poisoning occurred in cattle by an accidental
addition of a TBTD premix to a calf-rearing concentrate at a
feed-mill. More than 1,000 cattle were poisoned of which
171 died and 287 were slaughtered. Recently we have found
that various di- and tri-substituted organotins induce thymus
atrophy and for some of them, the effects on the immune system have been found to be the most sensitive criteria of
their toxicity [8-12].

Comparative Aspects

In order to compare the immunotoxicity of various organotin
compounds, short term feeding studies were carried out with
weanling rats [10]. These studies revealed that especially
di-n-octyl and di-n-butyltin dichloride induced lymphocyte
depletion of the thymic cortex and the thymus-dependent
lymphoid areas of spleen and peripheral lymph nodes. The
weights of these lymphoid organs decreased in a dose-related
manner and thymus atrophy was already observed at dietary
concentrations of 5 ppm DBTC or DOTC. Of the dialkyltins,
di-n-propyltin and diethyltin dichloride also induced lymphoid atrophy, although to a lesser extent, whereas dimethyltin
dichloride, di-n-dodecyl- and di-n-octadecylin dibromide did
not produce atrophy of lymphoid organs. Of the trialkyltin
compounds tested, only tri-n-butyltin chloride (TBTC) and
tri-n-propyltin chloride caused thymus atrophy comparable to
DBTC and DOTC, at feeding levels which did not induce other
organ changes. Trimethyl- and triethyltin chloride produced
neurological symptoms and increase of brain weight at dietary
concentrations of 5 ppm, which did not reduce thymus weight.
Tri-n-octyltin chloride as well as mono-n-octyltin chloride
and tetra-n-octyltin did not cause any organ changes at
feeding levels up to 150 pp. Of the aryltin compounds, both
di- and triphenyl-tin chloride induced thymus atrophy, but
their thymolytic effect was less pronounced than with DBTC,
TBTC and DOTC. In addition, Ishaaya et al. [13] noted a
reduction of spleen weights and leucocyte counts of mice fed

triphenyltin chloride and acetate, tricyclohexyltin hydroxide or tributyltin oxide, but they did not determine thymus weights, which is the most sensitive criterion of organotin-induced lymphocyte depletion. Probably the extent of organotin-induced thymus atrophy is related to the water-lipid partition of the compounds. The water soluble organotins have no thymolytic properties.

In contrast to rats, DBTC or DOTC did not induce thymus involution in mice, guinea pigs, Japanese quail or chickens upon oral exposure [10]. However, after intravenous administration of DBTC or DOTC, similar thymus effects were found in rats and mice. Thymus atrophy occurred after a single intravenous injection of 1 mg DBTC or DOTC per kg body weight, a dose which did not affect the growth of the animals or the weights and histology of liver and kidney. The difference in the thymus effects of DBTC or DOTC between mice and rats, upon oral treatment, and the similarity of the thymolytic effect upon intravenous administration of these organotin compounds may be explained by differences in uptake from the gastrointestinal tract between rats and mice. Japanese quail and White Leghorn chickens appeared to be very insensitive to the toxic effects of dialkyltin compounds, since feeding levels up to 600 ppm DOTC did not induce any sign of toxicity. In addition, upon intravenous administration, chickens were less sensitive than rats and mice. DBTC or DOTC (10 mg/kg body wt.) reduced thymus weights of two-week-old chickens only marginally, and no thymus effects were noted in older animals.

Reversibility of Thymus Atrophy

In rats fed DBTC or DOTC, thymus atrophy rapidly occurred. After 4 days feeding of 150 ppm DOTC, thymus weight was significantly decreased. However, this effect was completely reversible [10]. A 78% reduction of thymus weight induced by feeding 150 ppm DOTC for four weeks was followed by a fast recovery, when the animals were returned to stock diet. Thymus weights returned to control values within a two-weeks rehabilitation period. This is in accordance with the relatively short half-life of DOTC in the body. In distribution studies with ^{14}C-DOTC in rats, Penninks and Seinen [14] found a half life of 7.8 days.

Selectivity of Thymus Effects

Thymus involution can be mediated by alterations of the hormone system [15,16] e.g. by an increased release of gluco-corticosteroids [17] or by a decreased release of somatotrophic hormone (STH) [18,19]. Therefore the effects

Table 1   *Immune function studies with DBTC and DOTC*

	Effect	Reference
Humoral immunity		
In vivo		
- thymus-dependent antibody synthesis to sheep red blood cells (SRBC)	suppressed	11
- thymus-independent antibody synthesis to *E. coli* lipopolysaccharide (LPS)	not affected	11
In vitro		
- plaque formation against SRBC	suppressed	11
- transformation of lymphocytes by LPS	not affected	12
Cell-mediated immunity		
In vivo		
- delayed type hypersensitivity to tuberculin	suppressed	11
- allograft rejection	delayed	11
- graft-versus-host reaction	suppressed	12
- resistance to Listeria monocytogenes infection	diminished	22
In vitro		
- lymphocyte transformation by phytohaemagglutinin (PHA) and concanavalin A (Con A)	suppressed	12
Phagocytosis by macrophages of carbon particles	not affected	11
Sensitivity to LPS	increased	22

of DOTC were also studied in adrenalectomized [9] and in STH-supplemented rats [14]. It appeared that neither adrenalectomy nor STH supply could abolish the thymus effects of DOTC.

It has also been demonstrated that thymus atrophy is not caused indirectly by inhibition of bone marrow stem cell proliferation [20]. Therefore the organotin-induced thymus atrophy is most probably caused by a direct cytotoxic effect on lymphocytes, which is also supported by their *in vitro* cytotoxicity. However an indirect effect on lymphocyte proliferation in the thymus, mediated by interference with thymus epithelial cells, as suggested by Miller [21], can not be excluded.

Immune Function Studies with DBTC and DOTC

As a consequence of the selective lymphocytotoxicity, DBTC and DOTC impair the immune system. All immune reactions in which T-lymphocytes participate are compromised in DBTC- and DOTC-exposed rats (Table 1).

A dose-related suppression of cell-mediated immunity occurred in such manifestations as tuberculin hypersensitivity, skin graft rejection, graft-versus-host reactivity and lymphocyte transformation by the T-cell mitogens phytohaemagglutinin (PHA) and concanavalin A (Con A). The resistance against Listeria monocytogenes, also a T-cell dependent phenomenon was dose relatedly decreased. The resistance against a Salmonella Dublin strain was decreased by DBTC and DOTC, but this may also be related to an increased susceptibility to Salmonella Dublin endotoxin, since these organotin compounds induce a hypersensitivity for *E. coli* lipopolysaccharide in rats [22].

Inhibition of the humoral immunity is shown by a reduction of plaque-forming cell numbers in the spleen as well as by a reduction of the haemagglutinin and hymolysin titres against sheep red blood cells (SRBC) in the serum of DBTC- and DOTC-exposed rats. In contrast to this inhibition of the antibody response on the thymus-dependent antigen SRBC, neither the response on the thymus-independent antigen *E. coli* LPS, nor the mitogenic response of spleen cells on *E. coli* LPS was suppressed by treatment of rats with DBTC or DOTC. The blood clearance of carbon particles was not impaired by DOTC treatment, nor were the blood monocyte numbers affected by DBTC or DOTC treatment. Therefore it is concluded that these compounds impair T-lymphocytes, and spare B-lymphocytes, which is in agreement with the lymphocyte depletion observed selectively in thymus and thymus-dependent areas of peripheral lymphoid organs of rats exposed to these compounds.

The organotin-induced immunosuppression is probably caused by a selective lymphocytotoxic activity of these compounds. Upon *in vitro* exposure with DBTC and DOTC, the functioning of lymphocytes is markedly impaired [22]. *In vitro* they are

extremely cytotoxic for rat and human thymocytes as well [12].
Rat thymocyte survival decreased in a dose-related and time-
dependent fashion when cultured in the presence of graded
amounts of DBTC or DOTC. A concentration as low as 0.5 µg
DBTC/ml medium still greatly decreased the survival of rat
thymocytes [12]. Although the viability of human thymocytes,
as scored with trypan blue exclusion, was less reduced than
rat lymphocytes, the human cells were definitely damaged by
the organotin compounds. Upon exposure to DBTC and DOTC,
they showed a tendency to aggregate in a dose-related fashion.
The ability of human T-lymphocytes to form E-rosettes with
SRBC was also dose-relatedly decreased and was already
impaired at a level of 0.6 µM DBTC. These results indicate
that these organotins are equally toxic for human as for rat
thymocytes *in vitro*. However, *in vitro* the organotins are
also cytotoxic for other cell types, such as bone marrow
cells, which are not affected upon *in vivo* exposure and in
various tumour cell lines. Therefore the selectivity of the
organotin-induced lymphoid atrophy can not be correlated
directly with the *in vitro* observed cytotoxicity.

Anti-proliferative Effects of Organotins

The selectivity of organotin-induced lymphoid atrophy is
particularly pronounced for DBTC and DOTC. In rats fed 50 or
150 ppm DOTC for four weeks, thymus weights were reduced by
52% and 84% respectively [9].

Histologically, lymphocyte depletion was observed in thymus
and thymus-dependent areas of spleen and lymph nodes, whereas
in other organs no treatment-related histopathological
changes were noted. Although most of the thymus lymphocytes
disappeared upon DBTC or DOTC treatment, signs of cell destruction (karyorrhexis and "starry sky" formation) as seen
after treatment with corticosteroids, antimetabolites,
alkylating agents and other anti-tumour compounds were never
observed. This does not exclude a lymphocytotoxic action,
since population dynamic studies on the thymus [23-25] have
shown that thymocytes die *in situ* without histological evidence of cell destruction. After four weeks feeding 50 or
150 ppm DOTC, the viability of cells isolated from thymus
and spleen was dose-relatedly decreased. However, the effect
on thymocyte number was much more pronounced than the effect
on cell viability. Thymocyte number was already decreased
after two days feeding of DOTC and progressively diminished
to 33% and 6% of the control value at week 4 in rats fed 50
or 150 ppm DOTC, respectively. These data indicate that
DOTC primarily induces an inhibition of cell proliferation
and secondarily causes cell death. Inhibition of cell

Table 2 *^{3}H-Thymidine incorporation of rat thymocytes or bone marrow cells at various time intervals after a single intravenous dose of DBTC.*

Time	Ratio of thymus weight (treated/control)	^{3}H-Thymidine incorporation (dpm x 10^4/10^7 cells)	
		Control	Treated
		Thymocytes	
36	0.97	13.7 ± 2.1	5.0 ± 0.4
48	0.76	14.6 ± 1.2	2.2 ± 0.2
		Bone marrow cells	
36		23.6 ± 7.2	24.5 ± 3.1

Thymocytes or bone marrow cells were isolated at various time intervals after exposure to DBTC (2.5 mg/kh i.v.) and incubated with ^{3}H-TdR for 60 min. ^{3}H-TdR incorporation in dpm x 10^4/10^7 cells is expressed as means values ± S.D. of six male rats.

proliferation is further supported by ^{3}H-thymidine incorporation studies. *In vivo* exposure of rats to DBTC resulted in a diminished capacity of thymocytes to incorporate ^{3}H-thymidine (^{3}H-TdR). Thirty-six hours after a single intravenous injection with 2.5 mg DBTC/kg body weight, the incorporation of ^{3}H-TdR into DNA of thymocytes diminished to 37% of the controls (Table 2). This inhibition of the ^{3}H-TdR incorporation further decreased to 20% of the control value at 48 h after the application of DBTC. Thymus weight as well as the number and viability of thymocytes were not affected up to 36 h after injection of DBTC, and it was only after 48 h that the thymus weight decreased, associated with a diminished cell yield. With regard to the selectivity of DBTC-induced thymus involution, it was apparent that the ^{3}H-TdR-incorporation into bone marrow cells isolated from the *in vivo* exposed animals was not diminished. However, *in vitro*, the ^{3}H-TdR incorporation into both thymocytes and bone marrow cells was dose-relatedly decreased (Table 3). At a concentration of 1 µM DBTC, the ^{3}H-TdR-incorporation with thymocytes was already affected and decreased to 60 and 25% of the control value at 2.5 and 5 µM DBTC respectively. Similar effects were found in bone marrow cells but at higher concentrations. A 50% decrease of the ^{3}H-TdR-incorporation into thymocytes and bone marrow cells was observed at 3.6 and 6.3 µM DBTC respectively.

Table 3 *Effect of various concentrations of DBTC on the*
thymidine incorporation into rat lymphocytes or bone marrow
cells.

Concentration (μM)	^{3}H-Thymidine incorporation (dpm x $10^4/10^7$ cells)	
	Thymocytes	Bone marrow cells
0	15.0 ± 0.78	17.7 ± 0.64
1	14.4 ± 0.36	16.4 ± 0.20
2.5	11.6 ± 0.32	14.5 ± 0.82
5	4.1 ± 0.22	10.6 ± 0.39
10	0.8 ± 0.01	3.2 ± 0.24

After 30 min preincubation with various concentrations of
DBTC, ^{3}H-TdR was added and the incorporation was measured
60 min afterwards. ^{3}H-TdR incorporation in dpm x $10^4/10^7$
cells, of a typical experiment performed in triplicate, is
expressed as mean values ± S.D.

The decreased incorporation of ^{3}H-TdR might be caused by a
limited energy supply, as dialkyltins interfere with the
glucose metabolism of thymocytes *in vitro*. Up to a concentration of 5 μM DBTC, the glycolytic activity of thymocytes
was stimulated to a level also observed after anaerobic
incubation of thymocytes [26]. From the accumulation of
pyruvate and lactate it was also obvious that the increased
amount of glucose consumed was only partly oxidatively
metabolized. These results are in agreement with the inhibition of the α-keto-acid dehydrogenase complex, as was
observed in mitochondrial studies [26,27]. It is difficult
however to explain the selectivity for thymocytes by an
interference with the α-ketoacid-dehydrogenase systems only.
Moreover, up to now, there is no evidence for a diminished
energy production of thymocytes after *in vivo* exposure of
rats to DBTC. However, it cannot be excluded that minor
changes in energy production could account for a re-ordering
of metabolic priorities; for instance, processes essential
for cell survival will be favoured to those related to proliferation and differentiation.

From these results we conclude that organotin-induced
immunotoxicity is caused by its selective anti-proliferative
effect upon thymic lymphocytes. However it is doubtful if
the interference of organotins with cell energetics forms
the molecular basis of its antiproliferative effect.

Summary

Various organotin compounds induce lymphocyte depletion in the lymphoid system especially in the thymus. This report reviews the comparative aspects of the lympholytic activity of various organotins. The immunosuppressive effects of di-n-butyltin dichloride (DBTC) and di-n-octyltin chloride (DOTC) as well as their *in vitro* effects upon rat and human lymphocytes are reviewed. It is stressed that the immunotoxicity is caused by a selective anti-proliferative effect upon lymphocytes.

Acknowledgements

The authors thank Dr E.J. Bulten, Institute for Organic Chemistry, TNO, Utrecht, for the supply of the organotin samples.

References

1. Luyten, J.G.A. (1972). In "Organotin Compounds" (ed. A.K. Sawyer), p.931, Marcel Dekker Inc., New York.
2. Ross, A. (1965). *Ann. N.Y. Acad. Sci.* **125**, 107-123.
3. Van der Kerk, G.J.M. (1975). *Chem. Zeitung.* **99**, 26-32.
4. Van der Kerk, G.J.M. (1978). *Chem. Tech.* **8**, 356-365.
5. Barnes, J.M. and Stoner, H.B. (1959). *Pharmac. Rev.* **11**, 211-231.
6. Alajonanine, T., Derobert, L. and Thieffry, S. (1958). *Rev. Neurol.* **98**, 85-96.
7. Schlosberg, A. and Egyed, M.N. (1979). *Vet. Hum. Toxicol.* **21**, 1-3.
8. Seinen, W. (1978). Immunotoxicity of alkyltin compounds. Ph.D. Thesis, University of Utrecht.
9. Seinen, W. and Willems, M.I. (1976). *Toxicol. Appl. Pharmacol.* **35**, 63-75.
10. Seinen, W., Vos, J.G., Van Spanje, I. Snoek, M., Brands,R. and Hooykaasm H. (1977). *Toxicol. Appl. Pharmacol.* **42**, 197-212.
11. Seinen, W., Vos, J.G., Van Krieken, R., Penninks, A.H., Brands, R. and Hooykaas, H. (1977). *Toxicol. Appl. Pharmacol.* **42**, 213-224.
12. Seinen, W., Vos, J.G., Brands, R. and Hooykaas, H. (1979). *Immunopharmacol.* **1**, 343-355.
13. Ishaaya, I., Engel, J.L. and Casida, J.E. (1976). *Pestic. Biochem. Physiol.* **6**, 270-279.
14. Penninks, A.H. and Seinen, W. Manuscript in preparation.
15. Hudson, R.J., Saben, H.S. and Emslie, D. (1974). *Vet. Bull.* **44**, 119-128.
16. Vos, J.G. (1977). *CRC Crit. Rev. Toxicol.* **5**, 67-101.

17. Selye, H. (1950). In "The Physiology and Pathology of Exposure to Stress" 1st edn. p.286. Acta Inc., Medical Publishers, Montreal.

18. Sorkin, E., Pierpaoli, W., Fabria, N. and Bianchi, E. (1972). In "Growth and Growth Hormone" (eds. A. Pecile and E.E. Müller), p.132, Excerpta Medica, Amsterdam.

19. White, A. (1975). In "The Biological Activity of Thymic Hormones", (ed. D.W. Bekkum), p.17, Kooyker Scientific, Rotterdam.

20. Seinen, W. and Penninks, A.H. (1979). *Ann. N.Y. Acad. Sci.* **320**, 499-517.

21. Miller, C. (1982). *Arch. Tox. Suppl.* **5**, 328-330.

22. Seinen, W. (1982). In "Immunological Consideration in Toxicology" (ed. R.P. Sharma), CRC Press Inc.

23. Metcalf, D. and Brumby, M. (1966). *J. Cell. Physiol.* **76**, 149-168.

24. Weisman, I.L. (1967). *J. Exp. Med.* **126**, 291-304.

25. Cleasson, M.G. (1972). *Acta Pathol. Microbiol. Scand.* **80**, 821-826.

26. Penninks, A.H. and Seinen, W. (1980). *Toxicol. Appl. Pharmacol.* **56**, 221-223.

27. Aldridge, W.N. (1976). In "Organotin Compounds: New Chemistry and Applications" (ed. J.J. Zuckerman) *Advances in chemistry series* **157**, 186-196.

MERCURY-INDUCED LYMPHOCYTE AUTOREACTIVITY

L. Pelletier, R. Pasquier, F. Hirsch, C. Sapin and P. Druet

Group de Recherches sur la Pathologie Rénale et Vasculaire,
Laboratoire de Morphologie et d'Immunopathologies Rénales,
INSERM U.28, CNRS ERA 48, Hôpital Broussais,
96 rue Didot, 75674 Paris Cedex 14, France

INTRODUCTION

A number of drugs and toxic agents are able to induce autoimmune disorders. We have developed an experimental model
of autoimmune disease in Brown-Norway (BN) rats injected with
$HgCl_2$. This toxic agent has been chosen because it has been
known for a long time to be associated with the occurrence of
immune glomerulonephritis in man. $HgCl_2$ induces glomerulonephritis in BN rats [1,2], characterized by the successive
appearance of linear and then of granular IgG deposits along
the glomerular capillary walls. Circulating, anti-glomerular,
basement antibodies and circulating immune complexes are
transiently present in BN rats [3]. We have recently demonstrated that $HgCl_2$ acts as a T cell-dependent B cell polyclonal activator [4]. None of these effects could be obtained in Lewis (LEW) rats [4,5,6]. In the present study,
the popliteal lymph node (PLN) assay [7,8] was used to determine whether spleen cells from $HgCl_2$-treated animals were
able to modify the local graft versus host (GVH) reaction or
to induce a PLN enlargement in syngeneic rats. The effect of
spleen cells from rats susceptible (BN) and resistant (LEW)
to the induction of $HgCl_2$ autoimmune disorders was compared.

MATERIALS AND METHODS

Animals

Male and female, eight to ten weeks old, BN and LEW rats as
well as F_1 (LEW x BN) hybrids were purchased from the
C.S.E.A.L. (Orléans, La Source).

IMMUNOTOXICOLOGY
ISBN 0-12-282180-7

Experimental Procedures

Brown-Norway and LEW rats were injected subcutaneously three times a week with $HgCl_2$ at a dose of 100 µg per 100 g body weight or with control solution [2]. They were killed on days 2, 5, 6, 7, 9, 12 or 14 after the first injection.

Popliteal lymph node (PLN) assay

Spleen and lymph nodes from BN or LEW rats injected with $HgCl_2$ or control solution were removed. The cells were prepared as described elsewhere [4] and were suspended in 199 medium (Institut Pasteur Production France) at a concentration of 3.10^8 spleen cells per ml. Normal BN and LEW rats were subcutaneously injected in the rear footpad with 0.1 ml of these syngeneic cells suspension. Cells from $HgCl_2$-injected BN and LEW rats were injected in the right rear footpad of normal syngeneic rats. Cells from rats injected with control solution were injected in the left footpad of the same normal recipients. The weight of right and left PLN was assessed ten days later. The PLN index (ratio of the lymph node weights) was calculated.

In other experiments, spleen cells from BN rats having received $HgCl_2$ were injected in the right footpad of F_1 (LEW x BN) hybrids while spleen cells from BN rats injected with control solution were injected in the left footpad of the same F_1 hybrid. The PLN index was assessed as described above.

RESULTS

PLN Assay in Syngeneic BN Rats

When spleen cells from BN rats having received $HgCl_2$ or control solution for 2, 5, 6 and 7 days were used, a significant enlargement of the right PLN (draining the footpad injected with spleen cells from BN rats injected with HgCl) was found when compared to the left PLN. This was responsible for a significant increase in the PLN index (Fig. 1a).

In contrast, the difference was no longer significant when spleen cells were obtained from BN rats injected with $HgCl_2$ for 9 to 14 days.

PLN Assay in F_1 (LEW x BN) Hybrids

When spleen cells from BN rats having received $HgCl_2$ or control solution for six to seven days were injected in the footpads of normal F_1 hybrids, a significant increase in PLN index was observed (Fig. 1b).

The difference was no longer significant when spleen cells were obtained from BN rats injected for 2, 5, 9, 12 or 14 days.

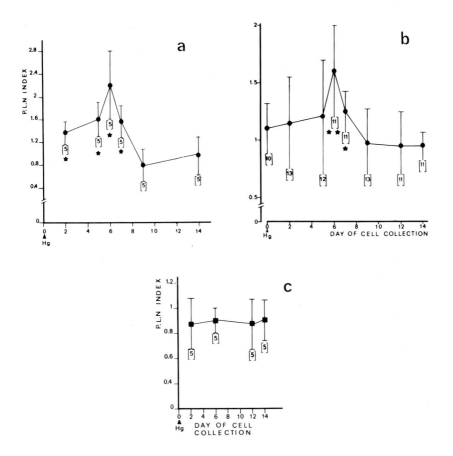

Fig. 1 Popliteal lymph node index (a) in normal BN rats,
(b) in (LEW x BN) F₁ hybrids injected with spleen cells from
BN rats having received HgCl₂ or control solution during two
to 14 days, and (c) in normal LEW rats injected with spleen
cells from LEW rats having received HgCl₂ or control solution
during two to 14 days. $p < 0.01$; $p < 0.001$

PLN Assay in LEW Rats

The PLN index in LEW rats injected with spleen cells from
LEW rats having received HgCl₂ or control solution did not
increase, whatever the days of spleen cell collection (2, 5,
9, 12 or 14 days) (Fig. 1c).

DISCUSSION

It has been previously shown that $HgCl_2$ induces an autoimmune disease [2,3] and a polyclonal activation characterized by lympho-proliferation, autoantibody production and increase in IgE serum level [9] in BN rats. Data now reported demonstrate that spleen cells from BN rats injected with $HgCl_2$ are able to increase the local GVH reaction in F_1 hybrids and to induce an enlargement of the draining PLN in syngeneic BN rats. Similar observations have been recently reported in mice treated with diphenylhydantoin [10]. These findings suggest that several toxic agents are able to modify lymphocyte determinants leading to stimulation of B lymphocytes and to antibody production.

Proliferation of PLN could be induced only when spleen cells were obtained from rats that had received $HgCl_2$ for a limited period of time (up to seven days). This transient effect of $HgCl_2$ is reminiscent of the transient character of the autoimmune manifestations [4] observed in BN rats injected with $HgCl_2$ [1,2] and suggests a common mechanism for both phenomena. Spleen cells from LEW rats injected with $HgCl_2$ were unable to induce lympho-proliferation. Lewis rats do not develop any autoimmune manifestation after $HgCl_2$ injections. Susceptibility of BN rats depends on genes linked to the major histocompatibility complex [3,10]. Differences in susceptibility could be explained by differences in combinations of $HgCl_2$ at the cell surface of lymphocytes. This is important for a better understanding of drug-induced autoimmune disorders.

REFERENCES

1. Sapin, C., Druet, E. and Druet, P. (1977). *Clin. Exp. Immunol.* **28**, 173-179.
2. Druet, P., Druet, E., Potdevin, F. and Sapin, C. (1978). *Ann. Immunol.* (Institut Pasteur) **129 C**, 777-792.
3. Bellon, B., Capron, M., Druet, E., Verroust, P., Vial, M.C., Sapin, C., Girard, J.F., Foidart, J.M., Mahieu, P. and Druet, P. (1981). *Eur. J. Clin. Invest.* **12**, 127-133.
4. Hirsch, F., Couderc, J., Sapin, C., Fournié, G. and Druet, P. (1982). *Eur. J. Immunol.* **12**, 620-625.
5. Druet, E., Sapin, C., Günther, E., Feingold, N. and Druet, P. (1977). *Eur. J. Immunol.* **7**, 348-351.
6. Sapin, C., Mandet, C., Druet, E., Günther, E. and Druet, P. (1982). *Clin. Exp. Immunol.* **48**, 700-714.
7. Ford, W.L., Burr, W. and Simonsen, M. (1970). *Transplantation.* **10**, 258-266.
8. Wander, R. and Hilgard, H. (1981). *Transplantation* **32**, 415-417.

9.   Prouvost-Danon, A., Abadie, A., Sapin, C., Bazin, H. and
     Druet, P. (1981). *J. Immunol.* **126**, 699-702.
10. Gleichman, H. (1981). *Clin. Immunol. and Immunopathol.*
     18, 203-211.

SKIN SENSITIZATION POTENTIAL
OF SATURATED AND UNSATURATED SULTONES

B.F.J. Goodwin*, D.W. Roberts**,
D.L. Williams** and A.W. Johnson*

*Environmental Safety Laboratory, Unilever Research,
Colworth House, Sharnbrook, Bedford MK44 1LQ, U.K.

**Unilever Research, Port Sunlight Laboratory,
Quarry Road East, Bebington, Wirral, Merseyside L63 3JW, U.K.

It is still generally thought that compounds of low molecular weight which cause skin sensitization do so by modifying the structure of native proteins so as to give rise to antigenic determinants against which a cell-mediated immune response develops. This concept was first proposed by Landsteiner [1] nearly forty years ago, and has changed little since then.

There is considerable evidence that in many cases this structural modification involves reaction of the sensitizing compound with protein nucleophilic groupings, such as lysine side chains, to form antigenic determinants covalently linked to the protein. This alkylation reaction can be one of several types, such as Schiff's base formation, a Michael reaction or nucleophilic substitution (Fig. 1).

In this paper we present the result of sensitization tests on a series of saturated and unsaturated sultones, and relate the results to their alkylation chemistry.

The compounds investigated are C_6, C_{14} or C_{16} saturated and unsaturated γ and δ sultones (Table 1).

We have been interested in these compounds for a number of years, since they, or structurally similar compounds, may arise during the manufacture of synthetic detergents. The test compounds were tested by the single adjuvant procedure (SIAT) a modification of the procedure used by Ritz and his colleagues for the study of alkene sultone sensitizers [2].

Sensitization is induced by a single injection of the test material in Freund's adjuvant, and elicited 12 days later by a 6 h occluded patch application on the flank. In recent

IMMUNOTOXICOLOGY
ISBN 0-12-282180-7

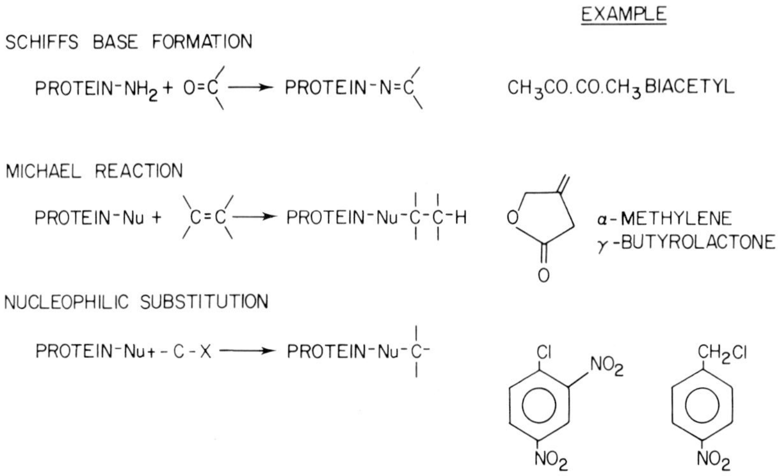

EXAMPLE

SCHIFFS BASE FORMATION

PROTEIN-NH$_2$ + O=C$\Big\langle$ $\longrightarrow$ PROTEIN-N=C$\Big\langle$ CH$_3$CO.CO.CH$_3$ BIACETYL

MICHAEL REACTION

PROTEIN-Nu + $\Big\rangle$C=C$\Big\langle$ $\longrightarrow$ PROTEIN-Nu-C-C-H   α-METHYLENE
γ-BUTYROLACTONE

NUCLEOPHILIC SUBSTITUTION

PROTEIN-Nu+ - C - X $\longrightarrow$ PROTEIN-Nu-C-

Fig. 1 Possible types of alkylation reaction.

Table 1 *Unsaturated and saturated sultones*

STRUCTURE	CARBON NUMBER	SYMBOL
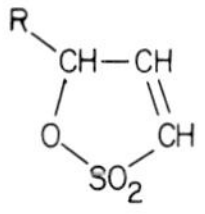 R, CH—CH, O, CH, SO$_2$	C$_6$	C$_6$γ'
	C$_{16}$	C$_{16}$γ'
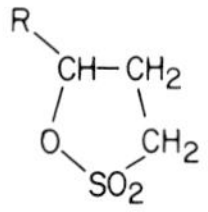 R, CH—CH$_2$, O, CH$_2$, SO$_2$	C$_{14}$	C$_{14}$γ
	C$_{16}$	C$_{16}$γ
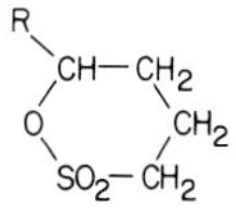 R, CH—CH$_2$, O, CH$_2$, SO$_2$—CH$_2$	C$_6$	C$_6$δ
	C$_{16}$	C$_{16}$δ

Table 2 *Sensitization tests with unsaturated and saturated sultones.*

Sultone	Induction concentration	Challenge concentration	Number of positive reactions/animals treated	
			Challenge 1	Challenge 2
$C_{16}\gamma'$	0.015%	0.01%	8/10	5/10
$C_6\gamma'$	0.5%	0.025%	9/10	7/10
$C_{14}\gamma$	0.015%	0.01%	1/9	0/9
	0.5%	10%	8/10	7/10
$C_{16}\gamma$	0.25%	20%	8/10	7/10
$C_6\delta$	1%	5%	0/10	2/10
$C_{16}\delta$	1%	10%	7/10	8/10

comparison of SIAT with the maximization procedure, SIAT was found to be only slightly less sensitive for the detection of known human contact sensitizers [3].

The results of the sensitization tests are shown in Table 2, from which it can be seen that:

1) All of the sultones tested were sensitizers.
2) The unsaturated sultones were much more potent than their saturated counterparts of similar chain length (compare $C_{16}\gamma'$ with $C_{14}\gamma$ and $C_6\gamma'$ with $C_6\delta$).
3) For both the saturated and unsaturated sultones, the C_6 compounds were much less potent tnan their C_{16} analogues (compare the results for $C_{16}\delta$ and $C_6\delta$ and $C_{16}\gamma'$ and $C_6\gamma'$). In the latter case, although the number of animals reacting was similar, the test concentrations were much higher for $C_6\gamma'$ than for $C_{16}\gamma'$.

A decrease in sensitization potential with decreasing carbon number has previously been observed by Ritz *et al.* [2] for C_{10}-$C_{16}\gamma'$ sultones and by Baer *et al.* [4] for 3-alkyl catechols.

The results of cross challenges are shown in Table 3. The $C_{16}\gamma$ sultone was tested at a later date, and was not available for cross challenge onto the other sultones. From Table 3 it can be seen that:

4) For both saturated and unsaturated sultones, there is no evidence of cross-reactivity between C_6 and C_{16} homologues. This is consistent with the findings of Ritz,

Table 3 *Cross-challenges results with sultones*

Guinea pigs sensitized to	Cross-challenge material	Number of positive cross-challenges/ number of guinea pigs responding
$C_{16}\gamma'$	$C_{14}\gamma$	0/4
$C_6\gamma'$	$C_{16}\gamma'$	0/2
$C_{14}\gamma$	$C_{16}\delta$	2/6
$C_{16}\gamma$	$C_{16}\gamma'$	0/6
	$C_{14}\gamma$	6/8
	$C_{16}\delta$	3/9
	$C_6\delta$	0/6
$C_{16}\delta$	$C_{14}\gamma$	4/4

Connor and Sauter, that over the $C_{10}\gamma'$ to $C_{16}\gamma'$ range, cross-reactivity between pairs diminishes with increasing differences in chain length [2].

5) For similar carbon numbers, γ and δ saturated sultones are mutually cross-reactive. The γ sultones seem to be better than the δ isomers at eliciting sensitization responses (4/4 for $C_{14}\gamma$ used to challenge animals sensitized to $C_{16}\delta$, but only 2/6 and 3/9 for $C_{16}\delta$ used to challenge animals sensitized to $C_{14}\gamma$ and $C_{16}\gamma$ respectively).

6) However, there is no evidence for cross-reactivity between the saturated and the unsaturated sultone types.

With the aim of rationalizing the cross-reactivity relationships among the three sultone types we examined their reactions with n-butylamine (BuNH$_2$), chosen as a simple model for lysine units in proteins. The reaction products obtained are shown in Fig. 2.

The saturated γ and δ sultones give 3-(N-butyl)amino alkane sulphonates and 4-(N-butyl)amino alkane sulphonates respectively. The reaction of unsaturated γ-sultones with n-butylamine is more complicated. The initial reaction is a Michael addition to the double bond, but this is reversible and the Michael addition product cannot be isolated. The driving force for the overall reaction is an intramolecular nucleophilic attack by the nitrogen atom of the Michael adduct, leading to opening of the sultone ring and formation of an aziridinium betaine as the final product. If ethylenediamine is used instead of n-butylamine, an analogous overall reaction

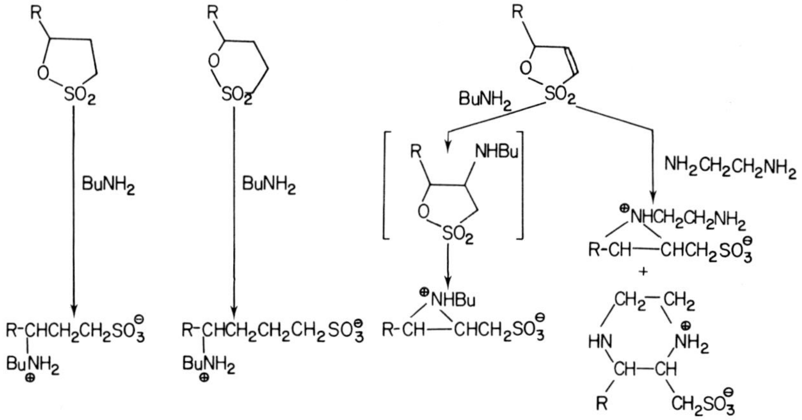

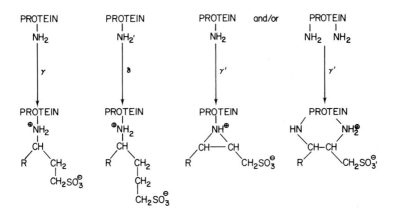

Fig. 2   Reactions of sultones with primary amine.

Fig. 3   Determinant groups corresponding to γ, δ and γ'
sultones.

occurs, but in this case the intramolecular reaction of the
Michael adduct can proceed via attack of the second nitrogen
atom, leading to a pyrazinium betaine. On the basis of this
finding it seems likely that, in reaction with proteins, unsaturated γ sultones can act as cross-linking agents at sites
where two nucleophilic groupings are in close proximity.

On the basis of the observed chemistry with simple nucleophiles, we can now postulate the nature of the determinant
groups produced when the sultones react with skin proteins
(Fig. 3).

It can be seen that the determinant groups corresponding to the saturated γ and δ sultones are very similar to each other, so that cross-reactivity between saturated γ and δ sultones of similar carbon number is not surprising. However, the determinant group corresponding to unsaturated γ sultone is different (particularly if the sultone acts as a cross-linking agent) and this rationalizes the lack of cross-reactivity between the saturated and the unsaturated sultones.

REFERENCES

1. Landsteiner, K. and Jacobs, J. (1936). *J. Exp. Med.* **64**, 625-39.
2. Ritz, H.L., Connor, D.S. and Sauter, E.D. (1975). *Contact Dermatitis* **1**, 349-58.
3. Goodwin, B.F.J., Crevel, R.W.R. and Johnson, A.W. (1981). *Contact Dermatitis* **7**, 248-58.
4. Baer, H., Watkins, R.C., Kurtz, A.P., Byck, J.S. and Dawson, C.R. (1967). *J. Immunol.* **99**, 370-5.

RELATIONSHIPS BETWEEN CHEMICAL STRUCTURE AND SKIN SENSITIZATION POTENTIAL

B.F.J. Goodwin*, A.W. Johnson*,
D.W. Roberts** and D.L. Williams**

*Environmental Safety Laboratory, Unilever Research,
Colworth House, Sharnbrook, Bedford MK44 1LQ, U.K.

**Unilever Research, Port Sunlight Laboratory,
Quarry Road East, Bebington, Wirral, Merseyside L63 3JW, U.K.

INTRODUCTION

We have discussed [1], in qualitative terms, how skin sensitization properties of chemicals are related to their alkylating properties. In this paper we aim to put the relationship on a more quantitative footing by considering the factors which determine the sensitizing potency of a given alkylating agent.

Figure 1 outlines the mechanism of skin sensitization by an alkylating agent. We assume that sensitizing potency of an alkylating agent depends on:

1) The intrinsic antigenicity of the determinant group transferred to carrier protein i.e. the ability of the determinant, when conjugated to carrier, to stimulate the biological processes leading to the sensitized state.
2) The number of determinant groups transferred to carrier proteins, i.e. the degree of carrier alkylation produced, by a given dose of alkylating agent.

At present we cannot quantify intrinsic antigenicity, but we assume that within a series of structurally-related compounds, it can be taken as constant. To quantify the degree of carrier alkylation, we require a mathematical model of the *in vivo* alkylation process.

IMMUNOTOXICOLOGY
ISBN 0-12-282180-7

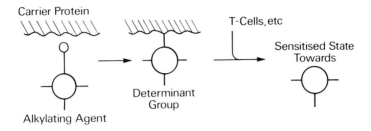

Figure 1
Mechanism of Sensitisation by Alkylating Agents

A MATHEMATICAL MODEL FOR ALKYLATION OF CARRIER PROTEIN

Our mathematical model is described in detail elsewhere [2].
It may be summarized as follows:

1) The carrier protein is in a lipid environment (e.g. a
   cell membrane) which is washed by a polar fluid (e.g.
   lymphatic fluid, blood).
2) The alkylation kinetics are first order.

Based on these assumptions we can set up rate equations for
the alkylation reaction and for the overall disappearance of
test compound from the system (by alkylation and by partition
into the polar fluid). From these equations we can derive an
expression for the extent of *in vivo* carrier alkylation A, in
terms of the *in vivo* alkylation rate constant, the *in vivo*
partition coefficient between the lipid and the polar fluid,
and the dose given. We cannot readily measure *in vivo* rate
constants and partition coefficients, but *in vitro* measurements can give relative values for these parameters. Thus
we obtain an expression for the *relative* extent of carrier
alkylation, A_{rel}:

$$A_{rel} = \left(\frac{kD}{P + P^2} \right)$$

where k is the rate constant for reaction with a standard
nucleophile (we use n-butylamine, as a model for lysine units
in protein), D is the molar dose given and P is the partition
coefficient between a standard polar/non-polar solvent pair
(we use methanol-water/hexane).

A_{rel} is a measure of a "dose" of alkylation. By analogy
with other biological effect-dose relationships [3], we take
log A_{rel} as being an appropriate function to use in comparing
sensitization potential against physico-chemical parameters.
We refer to log A_{rel} as the Relative Alkylation Index,

abbreviated RAI. That is,

$$RAI = \log \left(\frac{kD}{(P + P^2)} \right)$$

Note that RAI is made up entirely of parameters which can be measured *in vitro*.

THE RELATIONSHIP BETWEEN RAI AND SENSITIZATION SCORE

We assume that, for a given determinant group, each animal in a test population has a sensitization threshold for the extent of *in vivo* alkylation, A, below which it will not be sensitized, and a tolerance threshold, above which it will be tolerized so that a sensitization response cannot be elicited. Thus the test population can be represented by two normal distributions (Fig. 2). The number of animals sensitized by a given value of A will be given by the area under the sensitization threshold curve minus the area under the tolerance threshold curve, up to the corresponding log A value.

The theoretical relationship between RAI and sensitization score (i.e. the number of animals found to be sensitized in a sensitization test) can now be obtained by combining the two curves of Fig. 2. The resultant curve is shown in Fig. 3. We divide it into three regions: the sensitization region, where the number of animals sensitized increases with increasing RAI; the saturation region where all animals are sensitized, and the overload region where toleration leads to a decrease in sensitization score as RAI increases.

Figure 2
Representation of a test animal population by sensitisation and tolerance threshold distributions

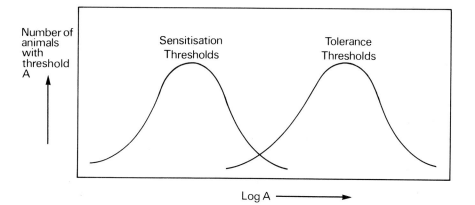

Figure 3
Theoretical relationship between Sensitisation Score and RAI

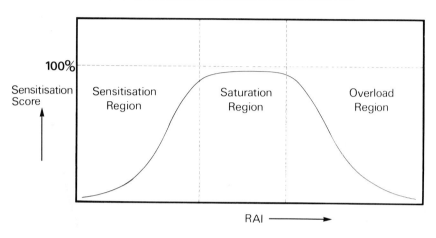

TESTS OF THE THEORY AGAINST EXPERIMENTAL DATA

p-Nitrobenzyl Compounds, $p-NO_2.C_6H_4.CH_2X$

These compounds react with n-butylamine by SN2 displacement
of the benzylic X groups. Physico-chemical and sensitization
test data for a series of these compounds are shown in Table 1.
As expected, the two compounds which do not react (X=H and
X=OH) do not sensitize. When we obtained these data we were
looking for a simple correlation between alkylating reactivity
and sensitization, and the data for the halogen compounds
appeared to give such a correlation, sensitization score increasing as k increases. However, this correlation did not
extend to the tosyl derivative; although its k value puts it
between the chloro- and the bromo-compound in terms of reactivity, its sensitization score was lower than that for the
chloro-compound, and this was confirmed when the test was
repeated. However, the P-value for the tosyl compound is
relatively high, and when we calculated RAI values for the
compounds tested, we found that the tosyl compound was in
line with the other compounds. The graph of sensitization
score against RAI is shown in Fig. 4; it is of the same form
as the sensitization region of the theoretical curve (Fig. 3).

Saturated γ and δ Sultones

We had sensitization test data, some of which was presented
in our previous paper [1] on several of these compounds,
tested at various induction doses by the SIAT method. We

Table 1 *Data for p-nitrobenzyl compounds, $p\text{-}NO_2.C_6H_4.CH_2X$*

X	k*	Sensitization score (SIAT method)	P (methanol-water/hexane)
I	2.3×10^{-1}	9/10	1.7
Br	8.0×10^{-2}	8/10	2.4
Tosyl	2.5×10^{-3}	4/10	8.5
Cl	4.9×10^{-4}	5/10	2.9
F	ca. 5×10^{-9}	1/10	2.7
H	No reaction	0/10	–
OH	No reaction	0/10	–

$D = 7.6 \times 10^{-9}$ mole.   Challenge dose $= 19.2 \times 10^{-9}$ mole.
*Second order rate constant (min^{-1} $mole^{-1}$ litre) for reaction with n-butylamine in dioxan at $23°$.

Figure 4
Sensitisation Score against RAI for p-nitrobenzyl compounds

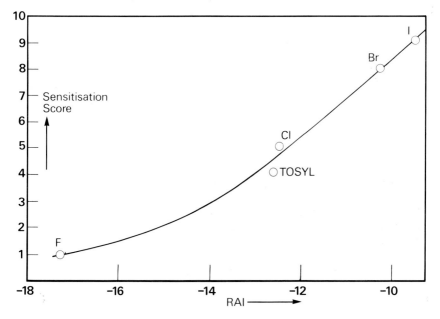

obtained the following P-values for the system methanol-water (87:13, v/v)/hexane:

$$C_{16} \ \gamma \qquad P = 0.65$$

$$C_{14} \ \gamma \qquad P = 1.75$$

$$C_{16} \ \delta \qquad P = 0.61$$

$$C_{6} \ \delta \qquad P = 9.46$$

We used k values of 1 (δ sultones) and 11 (γ sultones), based on relative rate data for reaction with n-butylamine in ethanol at 100°C.

A plot of sensitization score vs. RAI is shown in Fig. 5. It is of the same general form as the theoretical curve shown in Fig. 3.

Unsaturated γ Sultones

These sultones react differently to saturated sultones with nucleophiles, as we discussed in our previous paper [1]. An extensive set of sensitization data for these compounds has been published by Ritz, Connor and Sauter [4]. They tested C_{10}, C_{12}, C_{14} and C_{16} unsaturated γ sultones, using six induction doses (0.071×10^{-9} mole) for each sultone, and obtaining sensitization scores for three challenge doses (200,

Figure 5
Sensitisation Score against RAI for Saturated Sultones

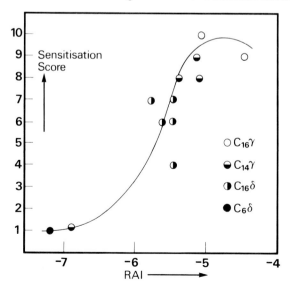

20 and 2 x 10^{-9} mole). Our analysis of the complete set of
data is presented elsewhere [2]; here we will show our findings for the data obtained at the 200 x 10^{-9} mole challenge
dose.

   Since the reactive grouping for all the compounds is the
same, we took a k value of one unit in all cases. We obtained P-values by experiment for the C_{16} sultone and by
interpolation, using our data for the C_{16} and the C_6 sultone,
for the C_{10}, C_{12} and C_{14} homologues. The P-values so obtained
were:

$$C_{10} \text{ sultone} P = 10.78$$

$$C_{12} \text{ sultone} P = 6.49$$

$$C_{14} \text{ sultone} P = 3.24$$

$$C_{16} \text{ sultone} P = 1.33$$

A plot of sensitization score vs. RAI is shown in Fig. 6. It
is of the same form as the theoretical plot (Fig. 3). It may
be seen that in the overload region there is separation into
a different curve for each carbon number. This effect is
rationalized elsewhere [2].

Figure 6
Sensitisation Score against RAI for Unsaturated Sultones

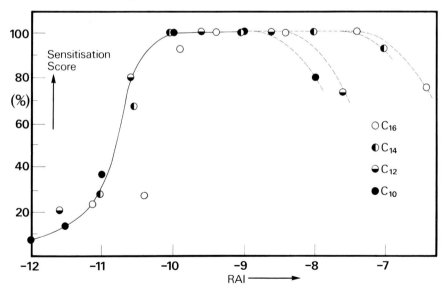

CONCLUSIONS

Our theoretical model is supported by experimental data on three sets of compounds: p-nitrobenzyl compounds, saturated sultones and unsaturated sultones. It can be applied when the compounds under consideration are structurally related to one another, so that intrinsic antigenicity does not vary, and when they all alkylate by the same reaction mechanism (if this is not the case, the proportionality constant between the *in vivo* and *in vitro* rates may vary substantially).

The model applies to sensitization test methods where induction is by intradermal injection. It does not, as it stands at present, apply to tests where induction is by epicutaneous application: for such test methods, skin penetration would have to be taken into account.

Notwithstanding the above limitations, our model enables us to obtain the maximum amount of information we get from the animal-testing we do in the context of product safety.

REFERENCES

1. Goodwin, B.F.J., Roberts, D.W., Johnson, A.W. and Williams, D.L. (1982). This volume.
2. Roberts, D.W. and Williams, D.L. (1983). *J. Theor. Biol.* in press.
3. Bliss, C.J. (1935). *Ann. Appl. Biol.* **22**, 134-67.
4. Ritz, H.L., Connor, D.S. and Sauter, E.D. (1975). *Contact Dermatitis* **1**, 349-58.

PROSPECTIVE TESTING FOR ALLERGENICITY

B. Guerin*, B. Hewitt* and W.D. Brighton[+]

*Laboratoire des Stallergenes, 160 quai de Polangis,
94349 Joinville Le Pont, France

[+]Allergy Advisory Services,
33 Bedhampton Hill, Havant, Hampshire, U.K.

It is perhaps wrong to enquire whether a substance is a
sensitizer or to prepare lists of sensitizers and non-
sensitizers. It is perhaps more appropriate to presume that
most substances have sensitizing activity in some humans and
that the difference between them is one of degree. The
appropriate question therefore is not whether a substance is
sensitizing but how sensitizing it is, and the problem
becomes one of a quantitative assessment with allergens
ranked according to potency.

A pragmatic decision that should perhaps be taken is that
if there is an otherwise good product with a defined small
allergenic risk, is it not better to accept this risk rather
than to search for and test a new material that might have a
much greater risk?

It has been recognized by physicians for many years that
patients suffer clinical symptoms of allergy to many constituents of diet which are quite innocuous in other individuals. Amongst these the food colours have been recognized
as potential sources of trouble but skin prick tests have
proved rather ineffective for diagnosis. Brighton [1]
recently showed that IgE antibodies that reacted with four
different food colours, namely amaranth, green S, sunset
yellow and tartrazine, could be detected in the sera of
patients with food allergy.

We have tested a further thirteen sera taken from patients
suspected of immediate hypersensitivity to tartrazine.
Tartrazine-serum albumin conjugates were prepared using
phosphorus pentachloride, and the quantity of tartrazine
bound determined by differential spectrometry. Both free

IMMUNOTOXICOLOGY
ISBN 0-12-282180-7

Table 1 *Tartrazine-specific IgE measured by RAST*

Serum	RAST titre*
1	4.20
2	1.90
3	2.01
4	0.72
5	1.98
6	0.77
7	0.71
8	1.11
9	0.96
10	1.59
11	10.16
12	7.77
13	2.42

*RAST titre $= \dfrac{\text{cpm test serum}}{\text{cpm negative control serum}}$

Positivity threshold: titre ≥ 2.0

dye and conjugated tartrazine gave maximum absorption at 430 nm. The tartrazine-serum albumin conjugate was then coupled to sepharose 4 B-cyanogen bromide and used as the solid phase in the RAST [2]. Specific serum IgE against tartrazine was detected in five of the sera (Table 1).

What is the significance of these IgE antibodies, however? It is known that IgE is frequently raised by injections of tetanus toxoid, for example, as well as to other substances, but fortunately not every patient with raised IgE levels shows hypersensitivity to the antigen.

A true test for allergenicity in man should be the ability to sensitize an individual with a given substance and then to provoke an allergic reaction in that individual with the same substance. This is not a way in which, for ethical reasons at least, it is practicable to test prospectively new drugs, food additives, or other chemicals, and we must therefore seek other possibilities for a testing protocol.

The obvious alternative in seeking tests for allergenicity,

is to use animals. Some caution is required in interpreting results from animal experiments, however, as it is known that man and animals sometimes recognize different antigenic and allergenic sites on the same molecule.

It is also important to try to understand the kind of structures that are likely to prove allergenic. In testing our experimental model we used tartrazine for which there was already some evidence of allergenicity. Ryan et al. [3,4] have shown that in the rat single oral doses of tartrazine were excreted in the urine, not as free dye but as traces of sulphanilic acid and 4-sulphophenylhydrazine. Tartrazine is prepared from sulphanilic acid and 3 carboxy-1-(4-sulphophenyl)-pyrazol-S-one. Sulphanilic acid was therefore biologically freely available and we included it in our test programme so as to test not only the parent molecule but also one of its principal metabolites, something which we feel to be of fundamental importance. Moreover, when three of the sera that had shown specific IgE to tartrazine were retested by RAST using sulphanilic acid, specific IgE was found to this metabolite (Table 2).

Table 2 *Specific IgE measured by RAST*

	RAST titre to:	
Serum	Tartrazine	Sulphanilic acid
1	4.20	7.48
3	2.01	1.63
11	10.16	6.47
12	7.77	9.12
13	2.42	n.t.*

*n.t. = not tested

In designing our experimental programme we have assumed that the sensitizing potential of a molecule is related to one or more of the following: (a) structure; (b) route of entry; (c) the frequency with which it is encountered. The following test programme was used:

    (i) IgE sensitizing potential (rat)
    (ii) immunizing potential (rabbit)
   (iii) photosensitizing potential (guinea pig)
    (iv) cell-mediated allergic potential (guinea pig).

Table 3 *Sensitizing potential of tartrazine in rats*

Administration	Intraperitoneal plus adjuvant	Intraperitoneal no adjuvant	Oral
Maximum response %	80	50	20
on day:	33	13	13

The IgE sensitizing potential by both the oral and intra-peritoneal route was tested both with and without aluminium hydroxide adjuvant. The number of rats responding to a particular sensitization protocol was determined by passive transfer of serum into normal animals. We found that the IgE response to tartrazine varied according to the route of administration (Table 3). In rats injected with tartrazine together with aluminium hydroxide as adjuvant, 80% of the animals showed detectable levels of reaginic antibody on day 33, whereas when administered by the same route but without adjuvant a maximum of 50% of the animals responded at day 13. By the oral route only 20% of the animals gave detectable levels of antibody at day 13.

The class of the antibody was tested using heated and un-heated serum. On heating the serum to 60°C for one hour no response was observed when it was subsequently used in passive transfer tests even though unheated samples of the same sera illicited a positive response, indicating that the cytophilic antibody responsible for the passive transfer reaction was heat labile IgE.

It should perhaps be emphasized that in all our experiments performed so far with tartrazine the IgE response in the rat has been one of only very low titre antibody. On titrating the sera in passive transfer tests no serum has proved positive beyond a 1:8 dilution

The immunizing potential of tartrazine was tested using Freunds complete adjuvant. Precipitating antibodies shown by counter immunoelectrophoresis were found in the sera of rabbits 35 days after starting the immunization programme.

The photosensitization potential [5] of tartrazine was tested using repeated application to a shaved skin site on a guinea pig over a nine day period followed by ultra violet irradiation after each application. A 14-day rest period followed and then on day 23 a fresh application of tartrazine was made to a naive site which was subsequently irradiated. This site was observed for signs of erythema, skin thickening and unusual dryness at 1, 6, 24 and 48 hours after treatment. No evidence to suggest that tartrazine is photoallergic has so far been obtained.

The cell mediated allergic potential was tested using the Magnusson Kligman Maximization test [6]. Twenty animals were used per test group and results were recorded according to the following classification system:

Percentage of animals showing a reaction	Class	Classification
0 - 8	I	Weak
9 - 28	II	Mild
29 - 64	III	Moderate
65 - 80	IV	Strong
81 - 100	V	Extreme

A modification of the Magnusson Kligman test in which the test product was administered orally was also used.

When using tartrazine and sulphanilic acid we again found some variation in the response according to the route of administration (Table 4), although both tartrazine and sulphanilic acid proved moderately allergenic by this test.

Table 4 *Cell-mediated allergic potential*

| Administration: | Tartrazine | | Sulphanilic acid | |
	Intradermal	Oral	Intradermal	Oral
Sensitizing concentration	1%	1%	2.5%	2.5%
Reaction class	III	III	1/0	III

In conclusion, therefore, we feel that this experimental programme may be used to test the allergenic potential of a molecule. Tartrazine, for which some evidence of allergenicity in man was available, has been shown to have a moderate allergenic potential in both the rat and the guinea pig for both type I and type IV reactions respectively. We feel that these tests could suitably be applied to other small molecular weight compounds including drugs and could be of particular interest for testing known metabolites of such compounds when available.

REFERENCES

1. Brighton, W.D. and Su (1981). *Clinical Allergy* 191-192.
2. Wide, L., Bennich, H. and Johansson, S.G.O. (1967). *Lancet* **2**, 1105.
3. Ryan, A.J., Welling, P.J. and Roxan, J.J. (1969). *Fd. Cosmet. Toxicol.* **7**, 297-299.
4. Ryan, A.J., Welling, P.J. and Wright, S.E. (1969). *Fd. Cosmet. Toxicol.* **7**, 287-295.
5. Herber, L.C., Targovrik, S.E. and Baer, R.L. (1968). *J. Invest. Derm.* **51**, 373-377.
6. Magnusson, B. (1980). *Contact Dermatitis* **6**, 46-50.

THE MODULATION OF MACROPHAGE ACTIVITY BY EXOGENOUS ARACHIDONIC ACID

G.R. Elliott, M.J.P. Adolfs and I.L. Bonta

*Department of Pharmacology, Faculty of Medicine,
Erasmus University of Rotterdam,
P.O. Box 1738, 3000 DR Rotterdam, The Netherlands*

INTRODUCTION

The essential fatty acid (EFA) arachidonic acid (AA) can be metabolized *in vivo* to a plethora of compounds with a variety of different biological activities, the expression of which depends upon the tissue involved and the presence or absence of other mediators. For example, prostaglandin E_2 (PGE_2), synthesized via the cyclo-oxygenase pathway of AA metabolism causes local vasodilatation and vascular permeability when injected intradermally and also provokes hyperalgesia that becomes overt pain upon the subsequent addition of bradykinin [1,2]. These effects, plus the discovery that the non-steroidal anti-inflammatory drugs (NSAID), such as aspirin, inhibit PG formation, resulted in the concept that these metabolites of AA were pro-inflammatory [3]. It is now known that the steroidal anti-inflammatory drugs also block PG synthesis by inhibiting the phospholipase A_2-mediated release of AA from the cellular phospholipid pool, via the synthesis of specific regulatory proteins such as macrocortin and lipo-modulin [4,5]. More recently, products of the lipoxygenase pathway of AA metabolism, for example the hydroxy acids and leukotriene B_4, have been shown to possess chemotactic properties and contribute to cellular infiltration during the inflammatory response [6,7].

Despite this wealth of evidence to suggest that AA metabolites are pro-inflammatory there has accumulated, over the last few years, a considerable amount of data to show that PGs of the "E" series have anti-, as well as pro-inflammatory properties depending on the model used. The most important targets for these anti-inflammatory actions are lymphocytes

IMMUNOTOXICOLOGY
ISBN 0-12-282180-7

and macrophages. PGEs have been shown to suppress B, T and NK-cell activities, and to reduce the severity of the chronic phase of adjuvant-induced arthritis in rats and immune-complex glomerulonephritis in NZB/NZW mice [8-12]. All these effects appear to be mediated by activation of the lymphocyte adenyl cyclase [13]. Similarly, many functions associated with the active macrophages, such as lysosomal enzyme release, phago-cytosis and locomotion are inhibited by the increase in cyclic AMP (cAMP) that occurs upon exposure to PGE [14,15]. Indeed, PGE injected into carrageenin-induced granulomas reduced the severity of the reaction by inhibiting cellular activation via the increase in cell cAMP levels [16,17].

On the basis of the type of results outlined above, it was suggested that the dietary administration of EFAs, aimed at increasing the concentration of PG at the site of an inflam-mation, could be beneficial in the treatment of chronic immune-based inflammatory conditions [18]. Recently reports have appeared demonstrating interactions between AA lipoxy-genase products and prostacyclin, and between PGE_2 and leukotriene C_4 [19-21]. The picture is emerging therefore, at least for the macrophage, of multiple interactions between the different metabolites of AA with both stimulation and inhibition of cell function. It is important that the net effect of all these possible reactions on the activity of a cell *in vitro* is determined before any dietary manipulation is attempted. We report now on the effect of exogenous AA on the synthesis of PG-like material (PGL) and cAMP by resident and starch elicited macrophages.

METHODS

The methods used have been described elsewhere [22]. Briefly, resident, 1-day, and 4-day, starch-elicited, peritoneal macrophages were isolated from the wash of rat peritonae by gradient centrifugation. The isolated macrophages were incu-bated with AA. PGL synthesis was measured by bioassay and cellular cAMP levels were assayed using a protein binding method. PGL activity was standardized with reference to PGE_2 and is given as $M/5 \times 10^6$ cells. Macrophage cAMP con-centrations are expressed as $pmol/5 \times 10^6$ cells.

RESULTS

AA, at the concentrations used, had no effect on the cAMP assay. PGL activity could not be detected in those incu-bations carried out to control for the non-enzymic breakdown of the fatty acid (limit of detection 1.4×10^{-9} M). The concentrations of PGL in the incubation media and the levels of macrophage cAMP after incubating the cells with exogenous

Table 1 *The effect of exogenous arachidonic acid (AA) on the synthesis of cyclic-AMP (cAMP) and prostaglandin-like (PGL) material by resident 1- and 4-day starch-elicited rat peritoneal macrophages.*

AA:	control		3×10^{-6} M		1.5×10^{-6} M		3×10^{-5} M	
Macrophages	cAMP[a]	PGL[b]	cAMP	PGL	cAMP	PGL	cAMP	PGL
Resident	12.6 ± 0.3	$<1.4 \times 10^{-9}$	11.0 ± 0.2	1.1 ± 10^{-8}	9.7 ± 0.1	$3.3 \pm 0.5 \times 10^{-8}$	11.5 ± 0.4	$7.6 \pm 1.4 \times 10^{-8}$
1 day	7.3	$<1.4 \times 10^{-9}$	6.6 ± 0.1	$4.5 \pm 0.6 \times 10^{-9}$	9.1 ± 0.1	$9.5 \pm 0.10 \times 10^{-9}$	10.5 ± 0.3	$2.6 \pm 0.6 \times 10^{-8}$
4 day	10.4 ± 0.3	$<1.4 \times 10^{-9}$	9.4 ± 0.6	$7.8 \pm 2.0 \times 10^{-9}$	12.7 ± 0.3	$1.7 \pm 0.5 \times 10^{-8}$	13.4 ± 0.3	$4.0 \pm 0.4 \times 10^{-8}$

Results are the means ± SEM of triplicate samples (Mann Whitney U-test).

a cAMP concentrations are expressed in pmol/5 x 10^6 cells.

b PGL activity is expressed in M/5 x 10^6 cells.

AA are given in Table 1. Resident macrophage cAMP levels
were not elevated by incubating the cells with 3×10^{-6} to
3×10^{-5} M AA whereas there was a dose-dependent increase in
PGL formation. Basal levels of cAMP in 1-day elicited cells
were lower than those found in resident macrophages but,
unlike the resident cells, AA stimulated cAMP production.
There was also a concentration-dependent increase in PGL
formation when 1-day elicited macrophages were used, although
even at the highest concentration of AA these cells produced
less PGL than the resident ones. Both PGL and cAMP synthesis
by 4-day elicited cells were stimulated by exogenous AA.
The changes observed, however, were intermediate between
those seen when resident and 1-day elicited macrophages were
used. If the percentage change in cAMP is plotted against
PGL synthesis it can be clearly seen that the adenyl cyclase
of 1-day elicited macrophages was much more sensitive to low
concentrations of PGL, produced from a given concentration of
AA, than either the resident or 4-day elicited cells (Fig. 1).

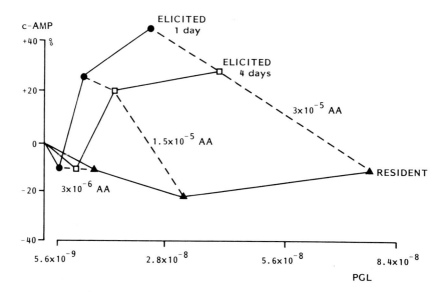

Fig. 1 The percentage change in macrophage cAMP levels in
resident, 1-day and 4-day starch-elicited cells induced by
PGL synthesized from exogenous AA. Solid lines – the
percentage change in macrophage cAMP content related to
medium PGL concentrations. Dashed lines – PGL synthesis by
resident, 1-day and 4-day starch-elicited cells incubated
with exogenous AA. AA and PGL levels are given in molar
concentrations.

Isolation of the macrophages in a buffer containing the cyclo-oxygenase inhibitor aspirin drastically reduced the basal level of cAMP in 1-day elicited cells and prevented the increase normally seen after incubation with AA (data not given).

DISCUSSION

A number of authors have demonstrated that both the basal and stimulated release of AA metabolites from macrophages is lower in elicited cells than in resident ones. This appears to be due to a decrease in activity of phospholipase A_2 and the cyclo-oxygenase pathway [23,24]. The results presented here confirm these reports. It has been reported that the activity of the ectoenzyme, 5'-nucleotidase, is reduced to thioglycollate-elicited cells although the activity of another membrane associated enzyme, leucine aminopeptidase, is increased [25,26]. There is not a general decrease in the activity of membrane-linked enzymes therefore when macrophages are activated and a specific effect upon those necessary for the metabolism of AA is a possibility.

Resident cells had the highest basal levels of cAMP and synthesized most PGL from the exogenous AA. The adenyl cyclase, however, could not be further stimulated by the PGL formed, suggesting that it was optimally activated. The adenyl cyclase of 1-day elicited macrophages was very sensitive to stimulation although it is not possible to say if this was due to an increase in receptor numbers during the activation process or to an increase in the number of unoccupied binding sites due to the low PGL formation. The intermediate character of the 4-day elicited cells could have been due to a decrease in activity of cells present in the peritoneum from day 1 or to an alteration in the cell population with an increase in the percentage of low activity macrophages.

Our results suggest that soon after activation there is an inhibition of both phospholipase A_2 and cyclo-oxygenase activities in the effected macrophages. This results in a drop in PGE formation and, as a consequence, a decrease in the intracellular cAMP concentration. This allows expression of those characteristics associated with the active cell such as lysosomal release, phagocytosis and increased locomotion. The adenyl cyclase of elicited macrophages is very sensitive to stimulation, however, so that even with the reduced activity of the cyclo-oxygenase pathway enough PGL can be synthesized from exogenous AA to enhance cAMP formation. The net beneficial effect of exposing activated macrophages to exogenous AA has recently been demonstrated *in vivo*.

Preliminary results indicate that the free fatty acid can reduce the severity of carrageenans-induced granulomas when injected locally. It appears that although AA can be metabolized to a variety of compounds *in vivo*, some with pro-inflammatory properties, the dominant effect on the granuloma is an anti-inflammatory one.

The sensitivity of the adenyl cyclase-coupled receptor for PGE_2, added exogenously or generated intracellularly from exogenous AA, is greater in elicited cells than in resident ones. It is possible that the regulation of PG synthesis, via the cyclo-oxygenase pathway, together with differences in the sensitivity of the adenyl cyclase-coupled receptor constitutes part of the system for switching the macrophages "on or off". It follows from this concept that any compound that directly, or indirectly, interferes with PG synthesis could also disrupt macrophage, and possibly lymphocyte, function. This would be exacerbated in EFA deficiency conditions [27]. It is suggested that any such drug should be considered for testing for immunological side-effects.

REFERENCES

1. Crunkhorn, P. and Willis, A.L. (1969). *Br. J. Pharmacol.* **36**, 216-217.
2. Ferreira, S.H. (1972). *Nature* (Lond.) **240**, 200-203.
3. Vane, J.R. (1971). *Nature* (Lond.) **231**, 232-235.
4. Flower, R.J. and Blackwell, G.J. (1979). *Nature* **278**, 456-459.
5. Hirata, F., del Carmine, R., Nelson, C.A., Axelrod, J., Schiffmann, E., Warabi, A., De Blas, A.L., Nirenberg, M., Manganiello, V., Vaughan, M., Kumagi, S., Green, I., Decker, J.L. and Steinberg, A.D. (1981). *Proc. Natl. Acad.* (USA) **78**, 3190-3194.
6. Goetzl, E.J. and Gorman, R.R. (1978). *J. Immunol.* **120**, 526-531.
7. Ford-Hutchinson, A.W., Bray, M.A. and Smith, M.J.H. (1979). *J. Pharm. Pharmacol.* **31**, 868-869.
8. Webb, D.R. and Osheroff, P.L. (1976). *Proc. Nat. Acad. Sci* (USA) **73**, 1300-1304.
9. Goodwin, J.S., Bankhurst, A.D. and Messner, R.P. (1977). *J. Exp. Med.* **146**, 1719-1734.
10. Kendall, R.A. and Targan, S. (1980). *J. Immun.* **125**, 2770-2777.
11. Zurier, R.B. and Quagliata, F. (1971). *Nature* (Lond.) **234**, 304-305.
12. Zurier, R.B., Damjanov, I., Miller, P.L. and Blewer, B.L. (1978). *J. Clin. Lab. Immun.* **1**, 95-98.
13. Pelus, L.M. and Strausser, H.R. (1977). *Life Sci.* **20**, 903-914.

14. Zurier, R.B., Dukor, P. and Weismann, G. (1971). *Clin. Res.* **19**, 453 (abstract).
15. Oropeza-Rendon, R.L., Bauer, H.C. and Fischer, H. (1980). *J. Immunopharmac.* **2**, 133-147.
16. Bonta, I.L. and Parnham, M.J. (1979). *Br. J. Pharmac.* **65**, 465-472.
17. Bonta, I.L., Adolfs, M.J.P. and Parnham, M.J. (1981). *Prostaglandins* **22**, 95-103.
18. Bonta, I.L. and Parnham, M.J. (1980). *T.I.P.S.* August 347-349.
19. Moncada, S., Higgs, E.A. and Vane, J.R. (1977). *Lancet* **i**, 18-20.
20. Feuerstein, N., Foegh, M. and Ramwell, P.W. (1981). *Br. J. Pharm.* **72**, 389-391.
21. Schenkelaars, E.J.P.M. and Bonta, I.L. *Eur. J. Pharm.* (in press).
22. Elliott, G.R., Adolfs, M.J.P. and Bonta, I.L. *Agents and Actions* (in press).
23. Humes, I.L., Burger, S., Galavage, M., Kuehl Jr., F.A., Wightman, P.D., Dahlgren, M.E., Davies, P. and Bonney, R.J. (1980). *J. Immunol.* **124**, 2110-2116.
24. Stringfellow, D.A., Fitzpatrick, F.A., Sun, F.F. and McGuire, J.C. (1978). *Prostaglandins* **16**, 901-910.
25. Edelson, P.J. and Cohn, Z.A. (1975). *J. Exp. Med.* **144**, 1581-1595.
26. Wachsmuth, E.D. (1975). *Exp. Cell Res.* **96**, 409-412.
27. Bonta, I.L., Parnham, M.J. and Adolfs, M.J.P. (1977). *Prostaglandins* **14**, 295-307.

ROUND TABLE DISCUSSION

Chairmen: J.L. Turk (Royal College of Surgeons)
D.V. Parke (University of Surrey)

J.L. Turk (Royal College of Surgeons)

First of all I would like to ask the question: "What do we
include under the heading of Immunotoxicology?" There are
two subjects which have been intertwined in this symposium
which we must separate to a certain extent. Firstly, we have
been dealing with compounds that cause direct tissue damage
and secondly, we have considered groups of compounds that
affect immune function.

Among the compounds that cause tissue damage there are
(1) compounds that act directly as haptens, (2) compounds
that have to be degraded or modified *in vivo* to become haptens,
and (3) compounds that result in the production of a response
to an autoantigen, possibly by reacting near to a self antigen.
As an example of this latter instance I would give α-methyldopa
which induces mainly antirhesus antibodies, and that is a
question that we have not dealt with at all. How does autoimmunity develop as a result of drug therapy, and how may we
monitor for it? Having dealt with these three aspects we
should then look at the different types of responses that the
body can make and here we have to deal, of course, with the
anaphylactic response Type I, the haemolytic Type II, serum
sickness and IgE Arthus reactions Type III, and contact
sensitivity Type IV. One of the points that has arisen from
our discussions is that granuloma formation would appear to
be a fifth type of tissue damage, not necessarily related to
delayed hypersensitivity directly, although it has certain
features in common. All these different tissue reactions
have to be monitored.

We then have to discuss compounds that affect immune function and here it is possibly better to look at environmental
pollutants, industrial chemicals at work, industrial chemicals in the home, and therapeutic agents. Another point which
we should consider is the effect on the foetus. We then need
to go into a general discussion of the use of *in vivo* versus

IMMUNOTOXICOLOGY
ISBN 0-12-282180-7

in vitro testing methodology, and end up with a discussion
more at the political rather than the scientific level and
that is, should industry provide its guidelines for testing
rather than leave it to Government bodies to impose guidelines?   I was particularly impressed some years ago when I
was involved with the F.D.A. in the U.S.A., in that they tried
as far as possible to get industry to do the work for them
saving Government money so that there is always an incentive
for Governments to allow industry to provide draft outlines.
This gives industry a chance to get in first, so I think we
should discuss this and perhaps end up with a discussion of
how initiation might occur.   Various countries have different
associations of industrial bodies that are already working in
this field.   I have a number of written questions here, which
are relevant to the topics outlined above.

Let us take first the compounds that cause tissue damage
directly and as I mentioned we have three groups, i.e. the
substances that act directly as haptens, those that have to
be degraded or modified *in vivo* to become haptens, and those
such as α-methyldopa that induce a state of autoimmunity to
a particular antigen.   In this context we are not discussing
compounds such as hydralazine that can produce systemic lupus
erythematosus so much as compounds like α-methyldopa.

To open the discussion may I ask if anyone has experience
of the induction of such a specific autoantibody to a self
antigen by a drug, such as α-methyldopa, which could act as
a hapten?

H.E. Amos (I.C.I.)

I think the α-methyldopa story is a little more complicated,
in that a lot of patients do demonstrate a positive antiglobulin test, but only a few of those go on to produce frank
haemolytic anaemia, which would be the clinical manifestation
of a toxic response.   Therefore the demonstration of even a
specific autoantibody response against a defined hapten is
not necessarily always related to a toxic phenomenon.   I
don't know of any other specific compound like α-methyldopa
which induces a specific adverse immunological effect.   It
may be that we are dealing with a unique compound and mechanism.   Dr Dewdney do you know of other examples?

J.M. Dewdney (Beecham Pharmaceuticals)

No, I do not know of any.

J.L. Turk

There are a number of other compounds that can act to produce

a haemolytic anaemia, for example penicillin. Dr Dewdney
would you care to comment?

J.M. Dewdney

I think the β-lactam antibiotics are *the* prime example of
drugs which can give rise to specific antibodies directed
against the drug as hapten, and can cause all the types of
allergic reactions, with the possible exception of this new
granulomatous reaction we are considering as Type V. Certainly the hapten-specific antibody to the β-lactams can be
responsible for Type I reactions mediated by IgE, haemolytic
anaemia, and other types of reaction and corresponding sensitization. There are very few examples other than the β-lactam
reactions. Further to Dr Amos' comment, we are talking about
a quite common anti-globulin response to α-methyldopa. I
don't know the relevance or the mechanism of this reaction
but it is interesting that amongst the β-lactams you can get
direct globulin (Coomb's test) reactivity to penicillins and
cephalosporins. If you take one of them, cephalothin, and I
doubt if it is alone, you observe a very high incidence of
direct Coomb's test and this is not immunologically based
since it can develop with anti-protein antibodies. This
seems to indicate a non-specific binding of the drug to the
red cell. The basis of the action of α-methyldopa may be of
the same type of mechanism with other structural cells, and
I would suspect this to be true, rather than an immunologically-
mediated effect via a hapten.

J.L. Turk

In this connection could I ask Professor Parke whether a
quinone could react with anything on the cell membrane that
might lead to a change in a rhesus antigen?

D.V. Parke (University of Surrey)

It is possible, yes. That is all one can say without experi-
menting to find out. Certainly there is a precedent for
specific functional groups in a drug molecule to interact
with specific cell membranes and induce immunological responses, for example, the interaction of Sedormid with platelets.

H.E. Amos

I think both α-methyldopa and Sedormid really crystallized
the problems. The phenomena have been characterized, but
mechanisms have not been worked out. Even with Sedormid it
is still not known whether the affinity for the platelet is

by the drug itself, which then binds the antibody and fixes complement, or whether, as Ackroyd suggested, the antigen-antibody complexes are adhering to the platelet as a non-specific phenomenon, and the platelet then becomes damaged as an innocent bystander. Therefore, the specificity of this reaction is in question.

The point is that for both these types of reaction, and I am sure if we thought about it we could think of many more, the mechanisms are not worked out. I would like to ask the question, whose responsibility is it and who would actually work out the detailed mechanisms of these reactions? Even if the mechanisms are known, how would that solve our toxicological problems?

D.V. Parke

The reason I mentioned Sedormid was that I worked on this problem with Ackroyd back in the forties, and we synthesized a series of analogues (many of them radioactively labelled) and one of the features was that the allyl group seemed to be essential for activity. It is now well known that the allyl group can form epoxides and it would be interesting to go back and see if the epoxide of the allyl group is responsible for activity.

To answer your question, Dr Amos, it was the academics who were doing this work, funded by industry, the Medical Research Council, etc., and they were doing it because of their natural inquisitiveness, not for any other reason.

H.E. Amos

Can we rely on that to continue or should industry perhaps be more involved? Should industry perhaps realize its responsibility in this area and perhaps do something about it?

G.T. Brophy (Lilly Research Laboratories)

We've heard several discussions during the meeting, related to testing methods for the evaluation of contact sensitivity. In my own personal experience, some of the problems that we have been encountering have been of the Type II hypersensitivity reaction, haemolytic anaemia, etc. but we have not had any discussion of models that might be predictive. I have not looked at any of those models to address that sort of problem; would the panel or the audience have any comments on this?

J.L. Turk

In fact, you are bringing out the problem that was referred

to by Dr Dewdney, namely, that a penicillin which can be a
very active contact sensitizer can also be bound to a red cell
membrane and be an antigen in haemolytic anaemia.

G.T. Brophy

I think this has happened with some compounds that have similar syndromes but don't necessarily bind, e.g. cephalosporins.
I think this may occur by an "innocent bystander" immune-
complex mechanism, but do we have a short-term model to predict that type of hypersensitivity reaction?

J.M. Dewdney

If you consider a drug which can produce hapten-specific
antibodies, and if it is given in high concentration and
reaches a high blood level, then there is an *a priori* reason
to believe it could, under certain circumstances, cause
haemolytic anaemia through that mechanism. As far as the
other mechanisms are concerned, the "innocent bystander" or
the red cell membrane damage, etc. would you not have expected to pick that up in standard safety clearance procedures, by changes in cell count for example? I've no experience of the latter but that is what I would have anticipated.

G.T. Brophy

In fact we have seen those changes but they have only occurred
after approximately six to eight months of treatment. The
point of my question is really the need to evaluate, on a
short-term immunological basis, to determine whether or not
a compound has potential immunotoxicity. The disadvantages
of long-term drug safety evaluation are clear in terms of
substantial development, time and money.

J.L. Turk

One of the questions that your comment is going to bring up
is that a compound like penicillin can be modified *in vivo*
to a wide range of haptens, some of which will bind to a
particular tissue, and some will bind preferentially to other
tissues, depending on the degree of penetration and the route
by which they are given. This is related to the question of
how compounds can be modified *in vivo* to produce a wide range
of reactants that may react preferentially, and thus you
might get a particular compound causing haemolytic anaemia
and in another situation contact sensitivity.

H.E. Amos

We don't have, of course, good base-line data on the immunological responses to haptens. Very few people actually look
for antibodies to drugs unless that drug is causing some type
of hypersensitivity tissue damage. So we do not know the
base-line, indicating how many compounds administered to man
as small molecular weight haptens actually induce an immunological response. This is because we only investigate the
very few in which activation leads to a hypersensitivity response seen as clinical tissue damage.

   We should be more aware that the compounds we do administer
have a potential for activating the immunological system, and
we ought to think about that in terms of structure-activity
relationships when we know the structure of the compound we
are using. We can obtain information as to how these compounds are metabolised and thus understand, to a certain
extent, just what degree of affinity for macromolecules these
compounds might have. Perhaps if we do start looking at a
very early stage at the immunogenic potential of these small
molecular weight haptens, then we may be able at some later
stage to define how they are going to behave when they get
into man.

J.H. Dean (C.I.I.T.)

I would like to return to Dr Brophy's question.

   I think the question which Dr Brophy raised is an important
issue that's frequently asked in the United States. The problem is very specific in that if you have a compound which
induces autoimmunity, then the problem is how best to look at
a series of other analogues? It has been suggested that one
might use mouse models, especially strains that develop autoimmunity. I do not consider this a problem really; it is
more of a problem of immune regulation as opposed to this
very specific problem of haptenization.

   What model do we have to deal with compounds that facilitate
autoimmunity?

J.L. Turk

I suggest the NZB mouse as an appropriate model.

J.H. Dean

Is that a fair model? The problem is, is it a disease of
regulation as opposed to a disease of haptenization?

F. Spreaficio (Mario Negri)

We have no models, I accept that.

H.E. Amos

We really have to start looking at the immunological potential of chemicals when we actually know their structure. I think this is evident when we consider aspirin. If you assume that aspirin can induce an antibody and you look solely for antibodies against aspirin, you'll find them. Aspirin is supposed to produce intolerance and Richard Farr showed some time ago that if you deacetylate aspirin you can produce an acetyl transfer reaction resulting in the formation of acetylated albumin and subsequent antibody production. Does the acetylated albumin-antibody interaction result in the aspirin intolerance? The point I am trying to make is even if you concentrate solely on antibodies to the specific hapten you really have to take the whole chemistry and metabolism of the structure into account.

R. Hubbard (University of Surrey)

In this symposium we have not had the time nor opportunity to consider photosensitivity as seen with cosmetics and sun-tan lotions. Would the panel or the audience care to comment on this subject?

E.V. Buehler (Procter and Gamble)

Photoallergy, I think, is a special problem. Procter and Gamble have experience of problems in this area with chlorinated salicylanilides and more recently with some perfume materials. These are causing problems under very specific conditions, e.g. with shaving lotions in which the skin is scarified, and in suntan lotions. We are at present developing models to test for photoallergy but it is too early to make any assessment of these. I suspect that such models are going to have limited value in terms of practical safety.

J.L. Turk

We have been discussing mainly organic toxic agents but there are of course many relevant inorganic compounds, one of which Dr Reeves discussed, i.e. beryllium. How do these inorganic compounds act as haptens? Is it just the metal *per se* sticking out from the surface of the protein, or do they modify the tertiary structure of the protein in some way? We know very little about how a metal behaves as a hapten, if it is indeed a hapten. Would you like to comment Dr Reeves?

A.L. Reeves (Wayne State University)

The important aspect of beryllium immunological disorders is the differential reaction to beryllium oxides produced at different firing temperatures. There is excellent evidence that there is a surface characteristic on the solid particle which is responsible for, or at least plays a role in, causing the immune reaction. Otherwise there could be no reason for the different activities of beryllium oxide specimens produced at different firing temperatures. I think that beryllium oxide forms complexes with body proteins leading to beryllium allergy, which might be considered as a form of autoimmune disease.

Aluminium is capable of inducing a similar immune reaction but, in addition, beryllium also causes delayed hypersensitivity of the conventional type.

J.L. Turk

Aluminium doesn't cause an immune response; it can cause a granuloma. I would like to ask how you visualize the protein-beryllium ion interaction? Do you think that the beryllium projects from the surface of the protein or modifies the protein in some way to make it an autoantigen?

A.L. Reeves

I don't think there is any very good evidence one way or the other. This perhaps could be investigated by a microscopic technique.

H.E. Amos

We have looked at the presentation of beryllium to experimental animals and we found that we could adsorb beryllium onto various particles and tissues such as red cells, lymphocytes, etc., but the only tissue which gave a good immunological response to beryllium was when it was presented on a lymphocyte. Beryllium may be modifying a membrane of the lymphocyte, suggesting that the immunological response is in part directed against altered membrane determinants.

J.L. Turk

Could this be related to the major histocompatibility complex?

H.E. Amos

Yes, it could; but we didn't extend the study that far.

A.L. Reeves

I agree with this interpretation which is in agreement with the findings of Skilleter et al. regarding lysosomal membrane rupture. This indicates a specific interaction of an agent with lymphocyte or intracellular membranes.

D.V. Parke

All these metals which are causing immune effects are transitional metals which can form complexes, in which the use of the term "metal" ion is quite wrong. There are groups of metals which can form organometallic complexes and we therefore should be able to predict which metal compounds might be immunogenic. These metal compounds may interact to form complexes with the hydroxyl groups of sugar moieties of glycoproteins and/or with protein amino groups. Thus the metals become an integral part of the membrane and could change the immunogenic character of that membrane from self to foreign. This could be a possible mechanism.

J.L. Turk

How do metal compounds interact with the projecting amino and sulphydryl groups of a protein?

D.V. Parke

I visualize a type of dative covalent binding involving donation of electron pairs to the metal ion forming four and six co-ordination complexes, similar to iron co-ordination in haem complexes. The metal then loses its metallic character and becomes organometallic.

E.D. Wachsmuth (Ciba-Geigy Ltd.)

Could I try just to challenge the concept of a hapten causing immune Type II or III reactions. For example, β-lactam antibiotics, we know, are very effective anti-bacterial compounds *in vivo*. The bacterial products may get into the circulation and be the causal agents of Type II or Type III reactions. We have heard from Dr Hall that physiological changes in response to, e.g. alcohol, may alter gut wall transfer processes. Isn't it feasible that such mechanisms are responsible for the immunological reactions to either antibiotic treatment or due to intake of beryllium.

J.L. Turk

Dr Dewdney, you have had a lot of experience with contaminants in penicillins causing allergies haven't you? I wonder whether these are bacterial products?

J.M. Dewdney

In the case of the penicillins there is no doubt that some of
the allergic reactions are mediated through antibodies. However, there is a major question concerning the most common
adverse reaction to penicillin which has become known as the
ampicillin rash. We have spent many years trying to determine the aetiology of this condition and there is a strong
view that, in fact, it is not immunological at all and may be
mediated by just the sort of mechanism you are describing.
It may relate far more to the release of bacterial products
due to the broad spectrum activity of ampicillin. There are
suggestions to the contrary but I think the point is very
well taken that some of the reactions may not be mediated
immunologically at all.

H.E. Amos

The trouble with the ampicillin rash is that it seems so
specific for ampicillin.

J.M. Dewdney

If it was simply broad spectrum antibiotic activity you would
expect that it would apply to the other broad spectrum antibiotics.

G.E. Davies (I.C.I.)

I have an example I think which supports Professor Wachsmuth's
hypothesis. This was some years ago when there were apparently anaphylactic reactions in calves to levamisole. Our
conclusions were that the first dose of the anthelmintic
released an antigen from the parasite which sensitized the
calf. The second dose of levamisole given later could
release the same antigen into a sensitized animal. Therefore
it was not levamisole that was the hapten or the sensitizing
agent, but it was a result of its pharmacological action.

E.D. Wachsmuth

To take another example, in our experience of toxicity testing a particular cephalosporin we observed haemolytic anaemia,
thrombocytopaenia, immune complexes in the circulation, in
the kidney and in other organs, in dogs. This was clearly
not directly due to the drug since there was no drug hypersensitivity reaction. However, on analysis, the compounds
and their immune complexes were found to contain microbial
products. These microbial products attached to the surface
of the red cells which produced surface complexes.

Alternatively, circulating complexes were absorbed onto the
surface of the red cell producing a similar effect.

J.L. Turk

We should now address ourselves to the question of which tests
might be utilized to predict immunological tissue damage.
We have a whole range of different possible allergic reactions
that can occur, ranging from IgE reactions to serum sickness,
contact reactions, and granulomatous reactions. The question
should be asked, is the demonstration of delayed hypersensitivity enough to predict a granulomatous reaction? Which
models should we use, since this is very relevant. Dr Davies
would you care to respond?

G.E. Davies

I answer this question with some reluctance, because I use
models with some reluctance. A very simple contact test is
to paint the ear of a guinea pig and subsequently challenge,
this test identified at least moderate to strong sensitizers.
I think therefore I would use this test and supplement it
with a Magnusson-Kligman test.

For IgE production I have no model. One would act on the
assumption that an allergen could produce IgE in susceptible
people because it is not always atopic. For example there
is a great deal of recent literature concerning IgE antibodies to trimellitic anhydride. Industrial companies using
trimellitic anhydride in the U.K. were able to identify among
the two or three hundred exposed people, only a few people
who had asthma, none of whom had IgE antibodies to trimellitic anhydride. At the same time I investigated a control
sample which showed the presence of IgE. Therefore there is
no model for IgE production.

Similarly, there is no model for respiratory sensitization
(as Dr Doe has shown) and so we are forced to use inadequate
models, much more inadequate than the models for immunotoxicity for predicting allergy. If we had had such predictive models we may well have made wrong decisions, e.g. penicillin.

H.E. Amos

Professor Turk produced animal data showing a heightened
contact sensitivity response following cyclophosphamide
administration. Would this system be better for selection
of very weak sensitizers, and also for ranking known sensitizers? Assuming that you could rank known sensitizers, of
which you have epidemiological knowledge, then it would be

possible to test and rank a new substance. In this way you
could predict to what extent a particular chemical is likely
to cause an environmental hazard.

E.V. Buehler

I would like to support that view. I suggest that the Buehler
technique is capable of picking up what I would regard as
weak sensitizers. Over the past few years we have taken the
view that by the proper selection of vehicle, and by testing
at high concentration, we do exactly what Dr Amos is suggesting with regard to cyclophosphamide, hence increasing the
sensitivity of the tests. However, because cyclophosphamide
is a known carcinogen this would limit its experimental usage
in the Unites States. Accordingly there is a need for similar
immunomodulators which are not as toxic as cyclophosphamide.
Perhaps there are some available.

G.J.A. Oliver (I.C.I.)

In terms of contact hypersensitivity, the toxicologist is
embarrassed by the models that he can actually use, and I
endorse the viewpoint of Dr Amos regarding known products of
which there is no population experience. In terms of using
agents such as cyclophosphamide to try and increase the test
sensitivity, we have employed similar models using strong,
moderate and weak sensitizers. However we find that these
tests are inadequate for identification of weak sensitizers,
which may be related to Professor Turk's observation that
with certain protein antigens the sensitivity to cyclophos-
phamide-treated animals did in fact vary.

J.L. Turk

It varies according to the strength of the protein as a
sensitizer.
   Dr Dewdney, could you comment on models for contact sensitivity?

J.M. Dewdney

We do not use any contact models in routine safety clearance
except in our products division where we are looking at cosmetics which are applied to the skin. In research we look at
the structure of new drugs being developed because of our
interest in hapten immunology.
   I agree entirely with Dr Davies that there are no models
for IgE production because that in a sense is a patient-
orientated phenomenon. All that one can do is to show whether
the drug is an immunogen in experimental animals. If it is,

then in certain predisposed individuals you probably will get IgE reactions. I certainly do not think that the mouse models of IgE production provide any more information other than that the drug can induce antibodies.

My own view is that if you consider the structure of the drug, and its known major metabolites, then you can make a very good judgement of likely problems. I think that is as much as you can predict, but if I had to introduce a preliminary screen, then I would look at the *in vitro* reactivity of the drug under physiological conditions, e.g. with primary amino and thiol functions. The emphasis, therefore, of this approach is to study the drug reactivity. Now that would, I think, give information on the ability of the parent drug to produce a hapten but gives no information as to the specific binding protein nor their sensitization potential.

P.M. Holmes (Beecham Products)

We have been investigating various methods of contact sensitization over a number of years to identify very weak sensitizers present in cosmetic products. We have used the majority of testing methods available and modified them at various times to suit our own conditions. At present we favour the McGuire method which is a split adjuvant technique and this seems to have the benefits of the Magnussen-Kligman method, but the product is only applied topically. For example, we have been investigating a cosmetic product which went through our normal battery of tests and got on to the market with subsequent problems. With the above type of investigation we are now identifying the offending agent. This is a common problem and it is easy to look back with hindsight and investigate, but it may be that predictability is not completely reliable.

J.H. Dean

Is this routine battery of tests automatically done on all compounds or products during development, or is there a pre-selection of compounds that go through this screen?

P.M. Holmes

There is pre-selection of these compounds. We know the constituents of our products that are likely to cause problems, and Dr Buehler has mentioned perfumes as a further example. We look carefully through new formulae which are often very similar to ones that are already on the market and we investigate the products we think may possibly cause a problem.

E.V. Buehler

We use the guinea pig screen routinely, and look at certain classes of materials more carefully than others, e.g. surfactants and perfumes.

J.W. Hadden (University of South Florida)

What are the regulatory implications of this kind of testing?

D.E. Gardner (E.P.A.)

From an environmental point of view, these tests have not been part of the guidelines at all, so I imagine that someone from industry could respond to that question better than I.

M. Draper (W.H.O.)

Legislation has played a significant role in this conference but maybe we should not place quite so much importance on this subject. I would hope we have learnt sufficiently from our experience with another subject in toxicology introduced ten years ago, namely, mutagenicity. So far attempts to introduce regulatory tests into mutagenicity studies have not been very successful or helpful. We are now trying to decide what to do with the results we are likely to get from mandatory tests carried out in certain parts of the world.

From the point of view of W.H.O., I.L.O. and U.N.E.P. we see our role as trying to get the science right and to give the government regulatory authories a neutral ground where these issues can be presented internationally. We are not in the guideline business and never will be. Our function is to mobilize the experts, get their proper opinions, see what the health implications are, and then see if there is international agreement on guidelines. We have a problem, which amounts to a reduction in the quality of life of some people who may possibly be a special subpopulation for which we could use specific preventative measures. In cosmetics it is in a sense somewhat self-regulatory because if a person buys a particular lipstick and it does not agree with them, they do not buy it again. Similarly we do not regulate the consumption of strawberries or shellfish but there are people who react adversely to these foodstuffs.

From the regulatory point of view, considerable caution is needed; we need a lot more research work, and from our point of view, we want to know what the priorities should be. If we could identify this priority we should then be in a position to facilitate internationally investigations into these priority areas. I return once again to the area of mutagenicity because at the moment some 70 laboratories throughout

the world are trying to solve certain problems concerning
these tests. They are mandatory but we do not know what the
tests mean and hence are endeavouring to produce a better
data base.

It is my view that immunotoxicity is obviously a very important area and has important health implications but I do not
see any necessity to rush to regulation. I think that industry in this situation is probably in the best position to
regulate itself, because of product liability, and this may
be sufficient for the next few years. In the meantime we
must study these immunotoxicological phenomena and we need
more knowledge of how serious is the reduction in the quality
of life for people, not only in our own developed parts of
the world but also in the developing parts of the world.

Dr G. Jones (D.H.S.S.)

There are no specific guidelines for immunotoxicity for new
drugs in the U.K. at the moment, nor is there any prospect in
the near future. The one minor exception is topically-applied
products where there is already a requirement that they are
tested for skin irritation, skin sensitivity and where appropriate, occular irritation. A working party in Brussels
recently considered immunotoxicity and concluded that, in
chronic toxicity studies, lymphoid tissues should be examined
and, if major changes are observed, then the investigation
should be extended. The major reason why we have not issued
any guidelines, nor are we likely to do so in the near future,
is that the science is not solidified enough yet, in that it
is rapidly advancing but there is too much variability and
disagreement as to what tests to use, and how to interpret
the results. Another reason, I think, is that immunotoxic
effects are not really a major problem yet. If in future
they become a major clinical problem then, of course, the
Department will set up a working party.

W.D. Brighton (Allergy Advisory Services)

In the U.K., it is illegal under the terms of the Medicines
Act, for a manufacturer to supply medicines or vaccines without a product licence. Nor may a clinical trial be carried
out by a manufacturer without a clinical trial certificate
or exemption therefrom. In order to achieve either a product
licence, a C.T.C., or a C.T.X., a manufacturer has to provide
experimental data on both the short and long-term toxicity
of the compound. We have now to submit data from both
animals and man but many animal tests may not be relevant to
man. The regulatory authorities have legal power to demand
such information, even though it may not be relevant. Who

is going to decide whether any of these experiments are relevant to man? Secondly, dare a manufacturer not do these tests,
even though they are of very doubtful value, and cost a great
deal of money? The Department already has power to compel a
manufacturer to explain his adverse reactions. We have a
current problem, not a problem which will be solved over the
coming years, we have a problem now.

G. Jones (D.H.S.S.)

The Department has ample power to turn down any licence
application at any time. We do not behave like that, of
course, in an arbitrary way — we give guidelines where needed.

H.E. Amos

There is one aspect of regulation relating more to the hypersensitivity responses, which I think should be borne in mind;
the very rare adverse reaction. For example, halothane,
which causes a reaction in approximately one on 30,000 people.
If the mechanism of this rare reaction is further investigated,
indicating an immunological basis for it, this investigation
comes to the notice of the regulatory authorities. Then the
manufacturer may be required to carry out tests on future
products based on an immunological response of extremely low
incidence. Thus, the direct consequence of investigating a
hypersensitivity reaction of very low incidence, could result
in major regulatory consequences for industry, which could
be commercially very significant.

J. Dean

The United States National Toxicology Programme is not in the
business of regulation nor does it plan to be, but it is in
the business of testing chemicals in lifetime bio-assay for
the potential to produce cancer or any other adverse health
effects. The original intention of the National Toxicology
Programme was to expand the scope of toxicology into newer
areas of target organ systems because many animals had died
in lifetime bio-assays from infectious diseases. On pathological evaluation, some animals had died with thymus atrophy,
had abnormal haematology, or had abnormal bone marrow cellularity, and there was some concern. The issue was, can we
study the kidney, for example, and learn more about individual target organ toxicity so that we could move away from
this rather absurd thing of lifetime testing of animals and
move into more short-term tests that will provide useful information, and be more economical.
    The first question was how do you assess immunity in an

animal, and whether that immunity is normal or abnormal. I
think that this is still an open issue. The decisions taken
were that we would look at several parameters, as few as we
possibly could, and deduce if there is a drug-related effect.
It was decided to include some aspect of host resistance,
either bacterial, viral, or tumour challenge, and seek sensitive ways to look at alteration of immune function and if
there was any correlation with altered host resistance. In
my opinion the best approach is to address the question of
host resistance. The problem here is that there are a variety
of models, many of which have not been well characterized for
immunological end-points. It was necessary to validate the
immune function assays, i.e. for their reproducibility, and
to develop better predictive host-resistance models.

Another aspect was to evaluate previously proposed models.
The National Toxicology Programme saw this as a very broad
area, and so we limited ourselves to the issue of immune
suppression or immune alteration. This was not a simple
matter because it took the contractors almost a year to validate the assays that we had used in our laboratory. Thus we
were able to show the toxicologist that these assays can be
performed with some reproducibility. The question still
remains what is the total relevance of these assays in terms
of the health of man? The Chemical Industry Institute is
dealing with the same issue. If you have a chemical that you
suspect alters the immune response, and benzene is a good
example of a chemical that produces a variety of immune
effects, then how would one predict if that compound is going
to produce an immune response, and how would one assess this?

D.E. Gardner

I would like to add to what Dr Dean said that, after a considerable data base has been established, it is imperative
that the scientist, both in industry, academia and government,
get together and develop these guidelines. I think that industry welcomes the guidelines and these should be used to
give them some indication of what to do and how to do it. In
the USA in many areas, industry has requested from the Federal
Government, specific guidelines on toxicity testing. This
does not mean that they have to follow these guidelines.
However, it is imperative that scientists work together and
develop and agree on these guidelines.

G. Jones

With respect to the drafting and implementation of these
guidelines, may I say that your suggestion is a little naive,
because there has to be close contacts between government and

industry, but in the end, the industry that is being regulated cannot draft the guidelines that are going to regulate them. Obviously industry has to be included and consulted, and the best that could be suggested is that they would take part in a joint working party. I do not think you could really ask industry to produce the first draft and then for Government to respond. It has to be the other way round.

J.L. Turk

However, industry have the best experience of the compounds that they are going to be working with; and they could prepare the problem and present it to Government suggesting tests they propose to use. This may or may not be approved by Government.

G. Jones

Can I say again, that is very naive, because in my experience the pharmaceutical industry would never approach government, to suggest that there is an immunological safety problem at the clinical level with their drug.

D.V. Parke

I would like to point out another facet to this problem in that the foremost companies do submit data, quite voluntarily, on new aspects of toxicity. Large companies do this, partly to safeguard their own products and they are also bound by the U.S. regulations to divulge all information about the new drug or product. This example is followed by all the other major companies until in the end it becomes encompassed in the overall regulations.

H. Amos

Dr Jones is perfectly correct. No industry is going to contact a government agency and indicate that this is a safety problem, which should be investigated and therefore we require guidelines to be produced. It is clear that industry probably do undertake some form of testing, depending on the chemical. No company is going to market a drug if it thinks it is going to cause a problem in a particular organ system. It would just be financial suicide. Industry does carry out immunological testing to safeguard their products. What is questionable, is whether we need guidelines or whether we need a set of regulations imposing tests for industry to do? I would maintain that industry accepts the problem that a compound may have an effect on the immunological system, but I would make a plea, that this is still an early development in toxicology, and industry must have the flexibility to be able to use whatever test system it feels necessary to evaluate their own compounds in this area.

J. Hadden

In analysing the effects of compounds on the immune system, I certainly agree it is difficult to talk about establishing guidelines. In my opinion I would favour resistance model systems and then ask the question if an animal does die of drug exposure, was it an immunological death or an infectious death? With respect to toxic effects on the immune system then, there are no simple approaches to be taken.

J.L. Turk

I think that we have covered the subject fairly comprehensively and may I on your behalf, thank all the speakers and the contributors. Thank you very much.

SUBJECT INDEX

Abietic acid, 117,118
ABPP, as an inducer of interferon,
    340
Abrin, 359,360,362,363,366,367
Acetyl salicylic acid, 385,386
Acetylator status, 29,30
Acetylcholine receptor, 307-315
Adaptive immunity, 13
Adenyl cyclase, activation of,
    464,467,468
Adverse drug reactions
    characteristics of, 102
    classification of, 96,97
    probability scale, 97,103
    scoring system, 97,103
Aflatoxins, 353
Agranulocytosis, drug-induced,
    165,166,168,334
Agricultural biocides, organotins
    in, 427
AID syndrome, 330,337
Air pollutants, 401-409
ALG. *See*: Anti-lymphocyte
    globulin
Alkene sultone sensitizers, 443
Alkylating agents, as skin
    sensitizers, 449
Alkylation
    by nitrobenzyl compounds, 452
    by saturated and unsaturated
        sultones, 443,452-456
    in skin sensitization, 443,449-
        451
Allergenicity
    drug, structural determinants
        of, 385-389
    potential, 125-128
    prospective testing for, 457-
        461
Allergens
    chemical, 108
    cross-linking by, 78-80
    environmental, 111
    quantitative assessment of, 457
    recognition of, 88,93

response to, 77,80,81,92,134
Allergic reactions, 9,27,82,87,92,
    102,103,297-299,301,322
    in beryllium disease, 274-278
    See also: Drug allergy;
        Hypersensitivity
Allergy
    definition of, 107
    drug induced, 247,248
    to food colours, 457
Allograft rejection, 373,419
Althesin, adverse reactions to,
    288,289,300
Aluminium, similarity to beryllium,
    262
Alveolar macrophages,
    as defence mechanisms, 407
    in HCB exposed rats, 226,231-234
    phagocytosis of beryllium by,
        267
Amidopyrine, 166
Aminoglycosides, release of hista-
    mine by, 96
Aminophenazone, 166
Ammonium persulphate, asthma due
    to, 121-123
Ampicillin, reaction to, 112-115
Anaphylactic antibodies, 88,89
    IgG type, 80-83
Anaemia
    aplastic, 167-168
    as evidence of hypersensitivity,
        245
    haemolytic, 101,102,162,164,338
Anaesthetics, as a cause of contact
    dermatitis, 132
    hypersensitivity reactions to,
        283-301
    See also: Halothane
Anaphylactic reactions, 285,297
Anaphylactic shock, in sensitized
    guinea pigs, 153
Anaphylactoid reactions, 71,73,78,
    82-84,91,285,287,296,301
Anaphylatoxin production, 253